Advances in Combination Therapy for Asthma and COPD

ADVANCES IN COMBINATION THERAPY FOR ASTHMA AND COPD

Editor

Jan Lötvall
Krefting Research Centre, University of Gothenburg, Göteborg, Sweden

WILEY-BLACKWELL

A John Wiley & Sons, Ltd., Publication

Library of Congress Cataloguing-in-Publication Data

Advances in combination therapy for asthma and COPD / [edited by] Jan Lötvall, William Busse.
    p.   ;   cm.
  Includes bibliographical references and index.
  ISBN 978-0-470-72702-7 (cloth)
  1. Lungs–Diseases, Obstructive–Chemotherapy.   2. Asthma–Chemotherapy.   3. Polypharmacy.
4. Chemotherapy, Combination.   I. Lötvall, Jan.   II. Busse, W. W. (William W.)
  [DNLM: 1. Asthma–drug therapy.   2. Drug Therapy, Combination.
3. Pulmonary Disease, Chronic Obstructive–drug therapy. WF 553]
  RC776.O3A33   2011
  616.2'3061–dc23
                                                        2011023057

A catalogue record for this book is available from the British Library.

This book is published in the following electronic format: ePDF: 9781119998631; WileyOnline Library: 9781119998624; ePub: 9781119978466; Mobi: 9781119978473

Typeset in 10.5/12.5pt Times by Aptara Inc., New Delhi, India

Printed and bound in Malaysia by Vivar Printing Sdn Bhd

First Impression 2012

Contents

4 LABAs: pharmacology, mechanisms and interaction with anti-inflammatory treatments   53
Gary P. Anderson

5 Long- and ultra-long-acting β_2-agonists   81
Mario Cazzola and Maria Gabriella Matera

6 The safety of long-acting beta-agonists and the development of combination therapies for asthma and COPD   102
Victor E. Ortega and Eugene R. Bleecker

7 Inhaled combination therapy with glucocorticoids and long-acting β₂-agonists in asthma and COPD, current and future perspectives   135

Jan Lötvall

8 Novel anti-inflammatory treatments for asthma and COPD   154

Paul A. Kirkham, Gaetano Caramori, K. Fan Chung and Ian M. Adcock

12   Phosphodiesterase inhibitors in obstructive lung disease   296
Jan Lötvall and Bo Lundbäck

13   Biological therapies in development for COPD   311
J. Morjaria and R. Polosa

14   'Triple therapy' in the management of COPD: inhaled steroid, long-acting anticholinergic and long-acting β_2-agonist   333
Ronald Dahl

Index   343

Contributors

Ian M. Adcock
Airways Disease Section, National Heart and Lung Institute, Imperial College London, London, UK

Gary P. Anderson
Lung Disease Research Group, Departments of Pharmacology and Medicine, University of Melbourne, Parkville, Australia

Peter J Barnes
Section of Airway Disease, National Heart and Lung Institute, Imperial College London, London, UK

Eugene R. Bleecker
Wake Forest University Health Sciences, Center for Human Genomics and Personalized Medicine, Medical Center Boulevard, USA

William W. Busse
Division of Allergy and Immunology, Department of Medicine, University of Wisconsin, Madison, USA

Gaetano Caramori
Centre of Research on Asthma and COPD, University of Ferrara, Ferrara, Italy

Mario Cazzola
Unit of Respiratory Diseases, Department of Internal Medicine, University of Rome 'Tor Vergata', Rome, Italy

K. Fan Chung
Airways Disease Section, National Heart and Lung Institute, Imperial College London, London, UK

Ronald Dahl
Department of Respiratory Diseases, Aarhus University Hospital, Denmark

Sebastian L. Johnston
Department of Respiratory Medicine, National Heart and Lung Institute, MRC and Asthma UK Centre in Allergic Mechanisms of Asthma, Imperial College London, London, UK

Paul A. Kirkham
Airways Disease Section, National Heart and Lung Institute, Imperial College London, London, UK

Jan Lötvall
Krefting Research Centre, University of Gothenburg, Göteborg, Sweden

M. Diane Lougheed
Department of Medicine, Division of Respirology, Queen's University, Ontario, Canada

Bo Lundbäck
Krefting Research Centre, University of Gothenburg, Sweden

Jonathan D.R. Macintyre
Department of Respiratory Medicine,
National Heart and Lung Institute, MRC and
Asthma UK Centre in Allergic Mechanisms
of Asthma, Imperial College London,
London, UK

Maria Gabriella Matera
Unit of Pharmacology, Department of
Experimental Medicine, Second University
of Naples, Naples, Italy

J. Morjaria
Department of Infection, Inflammation and
Repair, University of Southampton,
Southampton, UK

Desmond M. Murphy
McMaster University Medical Center,
Ontario, Canada

Sharmilee M. Nyenhuis
Division of Allergy and Immunology,
Department of Medicine, University of
Wisconsin, Madison, USA

Paul M. O'Byrne
McMaster University Medical Center,
Ontario, Canada

Denis E. O'Donnell
Department of Medicine, Division of
Respirology, Queen's University,
Ontario, Canada

Josuel Ora
Clinical Research Fellow, Respiratory
Investigation Unit, Kingston General
Hospital and Queen's University,
Ontario, Canada

Victor E. Ortega
Wake Forest University Health Sciences,
Center for Human Genomics and
Personalized Medicine, Medical
Center Boulevard, USA

Riccardo Polosa
Ospedale Santa Marta, U.O.C di Medicina
Interna e Medicina d'Urgenza, Catania, Italy

J. Christian Virchow
Department of Pneumology / Intensive Care
Medicine Klinik I / Zentrum für Innere
Medizin Universitätsklinikum, Rostok,
Germany

Preface

The management of both asthma and COPD has improved substantially over the last 25 years, with the introduction of new inhaled therapies, primarily through local treatment with inhaled glucocorticoids and long-acting beta-2-agonists as well as long-acting anti-cholinergic drugs. Despite this improvement, evidence argues that there are extensive unmet needs in both disease groups, and further development of management is needed. In recent years, a substantial number of new medicines are being developed, and many of those are due to become clinically available shortly. For example, new once daily long-acting beta-2-agonists have become available for the treatment of obstructive lung disease. Furthermore, a series of combination products that have the potential to have advantages to current therapies are in different stages of development. The specific mechanisms by which these therapies function, how the components affect disease processes, and how these drugs can interact, are discussed in detail in the different chapters of this book.

In parallel with progress being made in older classes of drugs for asthma and COPD, totally new drugs are being developed as we are learning more and more about mechanisms of these diseases. Thus, a vast number of biological compounds, targeting specific processes within the immune system, are currently being developed for both diseases. These are especially exciting, as they may have the capacity to fundamentally stop specific disease processes.

This book is suitable for any clinician or scientist interested in mechanisms of COPD and/or asthma, and principles by which these diseases can be managed in both the short- and long-term future. It is suitable both as a reference, and as an inspiration for future research and management.

Finally, I wish to thank all the authors of the chapters in the book for having believed in the project, and for having authored their respective sections very professionally. Every author is an undisputed leader in his respective field, and this work would not have been possible without their strong commitment. I also wish to thank the project manager of the book, Mr Jonathan Gregory, who has been very supportive during its development.

Jan Lötvall
Editor

1

Similarities and differences in the pathophysiology of asthma and COPD

J. Christian Virchow

Department of Pneumology, University Medical Clinic, Rostock, Germany

1.1   Introduction

In the early 1960s, when pulmonary function testing was limited to spirometry, a hypothesis was put forward that pulmonary diseases with similar clinical symptoms and spirometry findings such as asthma, chronic bronchitis and emphysema might be different expressions of one disease entity, in which both endogenous (host) and exogenous (environmental) factors would play a role in the pathogenesis.[1] More refined diagnostic tools such as bodyplethysmography or helium-based pulmonary function analysis, which can measure pulmonary hyperinflation, were not available at that time. Pathophysiological as well as immunological characteristics of asthma such as IgE, mast cells and their mediators, leukotrienes, T-cell subsets, cytokines and chemokines had not been discovered. Still, the proposal that asthma, chronic obstructive pulmonary disease (COPD) and chronic bronchitis or emphysema might have a common pathogenic background has been repeated,[2] and even now there is some debate about whether asthma and COPD should be regarded as:

- two different diseases in one lung;
- two diseases with one common pathogenesis; or
- one disease with different clinical phenotypes.

These hypotheses reflect some of the clinical uncertainties that can arise when end-stage COPD and bronchial asthma have to be distinguished based on spirometry and clinical findings alone. This can be especially challenging in patients who smoke on top of an atopic background.

Advances in Combination Therapy for Asthma and COPD, First Edition. Edited by Jan Lötvall.
© 2012 John Wiley & Sons, Ltd. Published 2012 by John Wiley & Sons, Ltd.

Epidemiological, genetic and pathophysiological data collected in the past 50 years, however, allow a relatively clear separation of COPD and asthma into rather distinct entities. These findings, which will be summarized below, make a common pathogenic origin for bronchial asthma and COPD most unlikely.

Among the epidemiological features that can separate asthma from COPD are differences in the age of onset,[3,4] different risk factors[5–10] and comorbidities,[11–16] differences in the genetic background[17–20] and differences in prognosis. While asthma is generally associated with a normal life expectancy, this is significantly reduced in COPD. Furthermore, marked differences in inflammatory cells and mediators[21,22] present in the airways and lungs result in different patterns of inflammation and their intrabronchial and intrapulmonary distribution. As a consequence of these there are distinctly different features in the respective impairment of pulmonary function, different responses to airway irritants in bronchoprovocation tests,[23,24] as well as marked differences in response to treatment and a different prognosis. These will be discussed in more detail below:

The clinical hallmark of asthma is episodic symptoms related to airflow limitation, often in response to external specific (allergen) or non-specific (airway irritants) factors. The characteristic feature of COPD in industrialized countries (which is also its main risk factor) is the long-term exposure to inhaled tobacco smoke or biomass combustion (the latter being more relevant to developing countries).

Asthma and COPD can sometimes be difficult to separate due to similarities in reported symptoms, airflow limitation and response to treatment. While individual patients may occasionally evade a clear separation into either asthma or COPD these patients are more likely an exception than the rule. These are often patients with asthma who have a longstanding smoking history or patients with a smoking history who develop intrinsic asthma. However, they do not support the hypothesis of a common pathogenetic origin or common pathogenetic pathways. The fact that end-stage asthma and COPD can display a number of pathophysiological similarities rather reflects the fact that the lung and its airways have a limited spectrum of responses to endogenous or exogenously induced inflammation irrespective of the origin of the insult. It would be unscientific to understand this limited spectrum of reactions, however, as evidence for a common pathogenesis. In an analogy, while end-stage fibrosing lung disease can appear with similar symptoms and even histopathology, irrespective of the underlying interstitial lung disease and the causative agents, a common pathogenesis is not suspected.

Accordingly, the so-called Dutch hypothesis from 1961 has been refuted in the past decades due to increasing knowledge about the underlying inflammatory processes in asthma and more recently in COPD.

From a clinical perspective, early stages of asthma as well as COPD can be differentiated based on patients' history and clinical, laboratory and pulmonary function findings (Table 1.1).

It should be noted that none of the clinical features on its own clearly distinguishes asthma from COPD. Recent studies indicate that the forced expiratory

Table 1.1   Typical clinical features of COPD.

Feature	Asthma	COPD
Age of onset	Childhood/adolescence	>40 years
Smoking history prior to onset	Rare	Common
Nocturnal symptoms	Common	Rare
Dyspnoea	Variable	On exertion
Allergy	Common	Rare
Course	Variable	Progressive
Airflow obstruction	Variable	Fixed
FEV$_1$ reversibility	Good, >20%	Limited, <20%
Airway hyperresponsiveness	Characteristic feature	Occasionally
Response to corticosteroids	+++	(+)
Sputum production	+	+ to +++

FEV$_1$, forced expiratory volume in 1 second.

volume in 1 second (FEV$_1$)-reversibility to large doses of brochodilators in COPD can change over time,[25] possibly to a degree indistinguishable from bronchial asthma. Nevertheless, in severe COPD pulmonary function abnormalities are usually not responsive to β_2-agonists and/or corticosteroids and the absolute magnitude of response still differs.

Therefore, with increasing

- smoking history
- irreversibility of the airflow obstruction
- age
- dyspnoea on exertion
- $P_a\text{co}_2$
- comorbidities such as coronary heart disease, arteriosclerosis, depression, osteoporosis, etc.

there is a rise in the likelihood that the patient has COPD.

1.2   Pulmonary function abnormalities in asthma and COPD

Pulmonary function abnormalities in asthma and COPD can be very similar. Both are characterized by airflow obstruction but careful analysis can reveal noticeable differences in pulmonary function testing that help to differentiate asthma from COPD (Table 1.2).

Table 1.2 Pulmonary function abnormalities in asthma and COPD.

Abnormality	Asthma	COPD
Site of airflow obstruction	Central airways	Peripheral airways
Reversibility	From +++ to +	From + to ++
Hyperinflation	From + to ++ (dynamic)	From +++ to ++ (largely fixed)
Airflow obstruction increases in response to hyperinflation	+	+++
Airway resistance	Inspiratory and expiratory ++	Expiratory $\gg$ than inspiratory (expiratory airway collapse)
Hypercapnic respiratory failure	Only in severe, acute asthma attacks	Chronic hypercapnic failure possible
Airway hyperresponsiveness	Characteristic – direct and indirect stimuli	Not uniformly present – only direct stimuli
Diffusion capacity	Not impaired	Reduced

Site of airflow obstruction

In asthma the site of the predominant airflow obstruction is usually located in the central airways. During severe attacks or in severe cases peripheral airways are also affected. In asthma, airway wall thickening due to airway remodelling increases with asthma severity and contributes to fixed airflow obstruction.[26]

Airflow obstruction in COPD, however, especially when associated with emphysema, is usually located in the peripheral airways. One of the mechanisms responsible for airflow obstruction in COPD is a dynamic collapse of the small airways during expiration due to an increase in intrathoracic pressure.[27] Central airway obstruction in COPD is also caused by airway collapse due to tracheobronchial instability.

Bronchodilator response

In addition, the responses to bronchodilators in COPD and asthma differ, although this has been partially challenged by recent data.[25] Asthma is usually associated with a good response to bronchodilators, which can cause a complete reversibility to normal values of airflow obstruction. This is limited, however, in severe and/or longstanding cases. In COPD the administration of high doses of bronchodilators has been associated with an unpredictable variability in airflow obstruction.[25] However, this variability less pronounced than in asthma and more closely related to pulmonary hyperinflation. Airway resistance, as measured by bodyplethysmography, is usually evenly distributed between inspiration and expiration in asthma while in COPD airflow resistance is usually more pronounced during expiration, due to hyperinflation and expiratory airway collapse.

Arterial CO_2 tension ($P_a CO_2$)

Patients with asthma, even during episodes of symptomatic airway obstruction, rarely display hypercapnic respiratory failure. Instead, low to hypocapnic $P_a CO_2$ values are

Table 1.3 Asthma or COPD?

	Asthma	COPD
Symptoms	Episodic	Little variability in symptoms
Age of onset	Childhood/adolescence	>40 years of age
First episode	Usually dramatic	Slowly progressive/unnoticed
Prognosis	Good; usually little or no progress	Limited – chronic progressive
Treatment	Good response to glucocorticosteroids	Little response

characteristic for asthma. Elevated P_aCO_2 levels during symptomatic asthma attacks are indicators of impending respiratory arrest. In contrast, in COPD elevated P_aCO_2 levels and chronic hypercapnic respiratory failure are common in more severe cases due to chronic fatigue of the respiratory pump.

Diffusion capacity

Diffusion capacity for carbon monoxide (DLCO) is rarely if ever impaired in asthma. In COPD, however, a reduction in the diffusion capacity is a typical finding and useful to separate COPD from asthma.

Overlap between asthma and COPD

There is little doubt that asthma can present with features of COPD such as poorly reversible airflow obstruction, and COPD can display a marked reversibility in airflow obstruction. Yet, asthma and COPD are unlikely to represent different ends of a spectrum of similar diseases just because of similar pulmonary function abnormalities that are shared with other acute or chronic lung diseases such as cystic fibrosis, post-tuberculosis-syndromes, end-stage sarcoidosis or bronchiolitis. Neither the fact that some patients with asthma can have a progressive course nor the observation that some patients with COPD can have a marked reversibility of their airflow obstruction are suggestive of pathogenic similarities. It appears likely, however, that patients with asthma who smoke can develop features of COPD in addition to their asthma. Their asthma is usually more severe and responds less well to corticosteroids.[28] These patients have not been studied in detail, and a clinical separation into asthmatic and COPD-related contributions to individual cases' symptoms is difficult.

1.3   Risk factors for asthma and COPD

Genetic

A large number of loci and genes with polymorphisms have been identified as possible susceptibility genes for asthma or special features of asthma such as bronchial hyperresponsiveness.[29] Many of these include genes for mediators and/or receptors associated with atopy such as interleukin-4 (IL-4), IL-13 and others.

In contrast, one of the models for COPD that is associated with a single-gene background is the hereditary alpha-1-antiproteinase deficiency. Whether genetic polymorphisms in other genes encoding for antiproteases or proteases are also linked to COPD pathogenesis is currently under investigation.[30]

However, there is little concordance between genetic risk factors for asthma and COPD, again suggesting that a common underlying pathogenesis is unlikely.

Environmental

Atopy has been identified as a major risk factor for asthma,[31, 32] and a large proportion of patients with asthma experience asthmatic symptoms after inhalation and/or ingestion of allergens. The direct effects of allergens on pulmonary function and symptoms can be demonstrated in challenge models such as inhaled or segmental allergen challenge[33] (Figure 1.1). Accordingly, the prevalence for atopy is significantly increased in asthma (with the exception of intrinsic asthma) while there is no evidence for such an association in patients with COPD.[22] Yet, the precise role of IgE-mediated allergic reactions in the pathogenesis of chronic asthma remains unclear. In contrast, there is no challenge model for COPD. The identified risk factor in the vast majority of cases in the Western world is the chronic inhalation of cigarette smoke.[34]

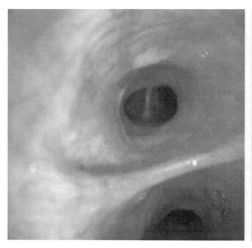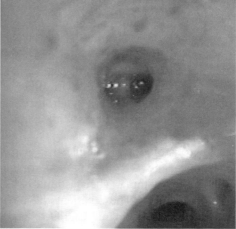

Figure 1.1 Endobronchial changes following segmental allergen challenge. Anterobasal segment of the right lower lobe. Left: Before allergen deposition; right: 5 minutes following allergen challenge. Mucosal oedema, bronchoconstriction and airway secretions can be seen within minutes following endobronchial allergen deposition. This is a feature specific for allergic asthma. Reproduced with permission from Virchow JC Jr, Walker C, Hafner D, Kortsik C, Werner P, Matthys H, and Kroegel C. T cells and cytokines in bronchoalveolar lavage fluid after segmental allergen provocation in atopic asthma, Am. J. Respir. Crit. Care Med. 1995;151:960–968, © American Thoracic Society.

Comorbidities for asthma and COPD

A positive family history for atopy or allergic diseases is a strong risk factor for asthma. Children with a positive family history for asthma who have atopic dermatitis have a high risk of developing asthma themselves. Typically, comorbidities in asthma are also risk factors and they often precede the onset of asthma in individual cases. Allergic rhinitis, atopic dermatitis and sinus disease frequently develop prior to the onset on asthma. A specific subset of patients with asthma, of which about two-thirds are of the intrinsic phenotype, also have an acquired sensitivity to non-steroidal anti-inflammatory drugs (NSAIDs) such as aspirin, indometacin and others.[35] The common mode of action of these drugs is the inhibition of cyclooxygenase I. In these patients ingestion, local application or inhalation of these drugs will result in severe asthma attacks. This acquired syndrome of intolerance against NSAIDs occurs on top of a persistent and progressive asthma. This syndrome, formerly termed aspirin-sensitive-asthma, or AIA, has therefore been labelled as aspirin-exacerbated respiratory disease (EARD).[35] Intolerance to NSAIDs is not associated with COPD.

In contrast, in COPD comorbidities such as coronary heart disease, arteriosclerosis, depression and osteoporosis[36,37] are also consequences of the main risk factor for COPD, namely smoking. There is still debate about whether or not they represent true comorbidities or rather concomitant diseases caused by the same risk factor. True comorbidities of COPD might be differences in risk-taking behaviour and factors associated with social status, both of which have been associated with smoking prevalence. In contrast to asthma there is no association with family history for COPD; the noteworthy exception is that the likelihood for smoking is increased in the offspring of parents who smoke. Whether this is merely a behavioural trait or evidence for a genetic transmission is still debated. Small birthweight (and possibly other susceptibility parameters) have also been associated with COPD.[38] Involvement of the upper airways in COPD has not been studied in detail but appears to be substantially less compared to asthma. The reasons why only a proportion of smoking individuals will eventually develop COPD is still unclear.[39,40] However, the proportion appears to be substantially higher than previously expected. The prevalence of atopy in patients with COPD is not increased.

Atopy as a risk factor for asthma: intrinsic asthma

Allergic asthma has been associated with the atopic phenotype. It is now clear that not all asthma is allergic,[41,42] but many patients, especially of early onset, have elevated IgE concentrations and increased levels of specific IgE. While allergic mechanisms play an important role in acute asthma exacerbations following allergen exposure their role in the pathogenesis of chronic asthma is still unclear. In particular, in intrinsic asthma elevated IgE concentrations cannot be documented, and atopic mechanisms are not involved in the clinical picture of intrinsic asthma, which usually starts in adulthood and includes chronic nasal and sinus polyposis.

1.4   Cellular inflammation in asthma and COPD

Asthma

The pathogenesis of asthma has been associated with a number of inflammatory cells and mediators. The cells that are usually increased in peripheral blood, in sputum and in airway biopsies and that have been associated with asthma severity as well as response to corticosteroid treatment are eosinophils. These cells appear to be causally related to asthmatic inflammation and subsequent symptoms. Therapeutic approaches to reduce eosinophil numbers and/or function have been associated with improvements in asthma of different severity.[43–45]

Other cells present in increased numbers and increased activation status are cells associated with the atopic-allergic phenotype such as mast cells and basophils. Upon interaction of cell-bound allergen-specific IgE and allergen, mast cells and basophils release histamine and other bronchoactive mediators such as leukotrienes. Dendritic cells of the myeloid as well as the plasmacytoid phenotype[46] infiltrate the airways following allergen challenge to orchestrate an immune response. Allergic as well as intrinsic asthma has been associated with an accumulation of activated T-cells of the T-helper cell phenotype, which can release a number of cytokines involved in asthmatic inflammation.[33] In atopic patients there are increased concentrations of cytokines such as IL-4, IL-13 and IL-5. All have been shown to increase eosinophil survival but IL-5 appears to be the most potent cytokine to attract and activate eosinophils. IL-4 and IL-13 are released in response to allergen exposure and are involved in initiating and maintaining an IgE response. Interleukin-5 is crucial for eosinophil activation and survival and can be found in elevated concentrations in allergic as well as in intrinsic asthma.[41] Recent studies suggest that effective blockade of IL-5 in asthma can result in improvement of clinically relevant outcomes such as a reduction in asthma exacerbations.[44, 45] Other mediators of relevance to the eosinophilia in asthma are CCL5 and eotaxin, and the leukotrienes C_4, D_4 and E_4, which are released by a number of cells including mast cells and eosinophils. They are chemotactic for eosinophils and induce a long-lasting contraction of airway smooth muscle. Their pathogenetic role in asthma has been demonstrated by specific leukotriene receptor antagonists that block the CysLT1 receptor and reduce asthma-related symptoms such as airflow obstruction and asthma exacerbations.[47, 48]

COPD

The cellular inflammation in COPD in contrast, is characterized by an increase in macrophages, neutrophils and dendritic cells, especially of the myeloid DC phenotype, which have a reduced expression of chemokine receptors required for the migration to regional lymph nodes.[49]

In addition, there appear to be increased numbers or percentages of CD8$^+$ T-lymphocytes, termed Tc1-type cells. Their precise role has not been established and an exact phenotypic characterization of these cells and their precise function is still lacking. The increase in endobronchial neutrophils seen in a majority of patients with COPD has also been associated with COPD pathogenesis. Neutrophils can release elastase and other proteases that can irreversibly damage pulmonary structures leading to tissue degradation and pulmonary emphysema.

Mediators relatively uniquely expressed in COPD are leukotriene B_4 (LTB_4) and the chemokine CXCL-8 (interleukin-8) while bronchoconstrictory mediators such as histamine or cysteinyl-leukotrienes, which play a role in asthma pathophysiology, are not elevated in COPD.[22] Eosinophils have been recovered mainly during COPD exacerbations but their responsiveness to corticosteroids differs. In stable COPD eosinophil numbers are usually not elevated.

1.5 Distribution and consequences of inflammation in asthma and COPD

Despite some crude similarities between asthma and COPD, the distribution of inflammation and its consequences are markedly different (Table 1.4).[50] In asthma, histopathological examination of endobronchial biopsies reveals epithelial shedding, to which a number of mechanisms contribute. Collagen and myofibroblast deposition below the epithelium, which results in basement membrane thickening, has been described as a feature specific to asthmatic airways.[51] In addition a marked hypertrophy of the smooth muscle layer of the airways can be observed in asthma, which has been related to the degree of airflow obstruction in asthma.[52] Recently, neoangiogenesis in asthmatic airways has been described.[53] Destruction of lung parenchyma and the development of emphysema is not a typical feature of asthma. In contrast to COPD, where mortality has been associated with COPD exacerbations,[54] mortality in asthma has not been linked to the number of exacerbations but rather to the severity of asthma attacks.

The airway epithelium in COPD is characterized by squamous cell metaplasia of the bronchial epithelium and a bronchiolar fibrosis,[55] and the development of emphysema. Smooth muscle constriction or hypertrophy is not a feature of COPD. The inflammation in COPD is arranged in lymphocyte-containing follicles suggesting an adaptive immune response in the airways.[56,57]

Table 1.4 Epithelial injury in asthma and COPD.

Asthma	COPD
Epithelial fragility/shedding	Squamous cell metaplasia
Collagen deposition/basement membrane thickening	Bronchiolar fibrosis
Hypertrophy/hyperplasia of the airway smooth muscle layer	
Glandular hypertrophy	
Angiogenesis	

Table 1.5   Distribution of airway inflammation in asthma and COPD.

Asthma	COPD
Central airways	Small airways
Involvement of peripheral airways in severe asthma	Destruction of lung parenchyma, emphysema

Both asthma and COPD are characterized by submucosal gland hypertrophy, which can contribute to mucus production and airflow obstruction. The precise contribution of submucosal glands to the pathophysiology of asthma and COPD might be considerable but has been insufficiently studied.

1.6   Patterns of epithelial injury in asthma and COPD

Most of the changes described above in asthma can be observed predominantly in the more central airways, from where they can spread to more peripheral airways as observed in more severe asthma. However, COPD is located predominantly in the small airways, where destruction of lung parenchyma leading to pulmonary emphysema occurs (Table 1.5).[55]

1.7   Airway hyperresponsiveness

Airway hyperresponsiveness (AHR) to direct (e.g. histamine, methacholine) as well as indirect (adenosine, cold air, exercise) stimuli is a characteristic pathophysiological feature of asthma. Its pathogenesis in asthma is most likely multifactorial. Several features of asthma pathophysiology contribute to this hyperresponsiveness. These include structural changes to the airways, such as airway remodelling, which result in fixed airflow obstruction, but also inflammatory changes. Recently, the role of neurotrophins and their effects on neurogenic remodelling of the airways has been added to the mechanisms contributing to AHR.[58] While inflammatory contributions to AHR can be reversible following treatment a complete loss of airway hyperresponsiveness in asthma is an uncommon event suggesting that the pathogenesis of AHR cannot be explained by inflammation alone. Airway hyperresponsiveness in asthma does not show a plateau effect to increasing doses of the respective stimulus. Thus, with increasing dose of stimulus the asthmatic airway will constrict further, which is characteristic neither for normal airways nor for airways in COPD.

In contrast to asthma, airway hyperresponsiveness in COPD is typically limited to direct stimuli such as histamine suggesting that the airway response in COPD is largely determined by airway calibre rather than an inflammatory bronchoconstriction.

1.8   Beta-receptor blockers

Asthmatic airways have a peculiar sensitivity to beta-receptor blockers. Exposure of patients with asthma even to low doses or even topical application can result in deterioration of asthma control and severe and long-lasting bronchospasm. The precise mechanisms responsible for this unique pathophysiological feature of asthma are incompletely understood but may be associated with postsynaptic regulation of neurotransmitter release in the airways. While bronchial asthma is a contraindication for beta-blockers their use in COPD is not associated with any deterioration of pulmonary function, again suggesting fundamental differences in asthma and COPD.

Furthermore, the chronic, unbalanced use of β_2-agonists in asthma has been associated with a tachyphylaxis to the bronchoprotective effects of β_2-agonists and possibly a loss in asthma control and an increase in asthma deaths.[59] This has not been observed for COPD, where the bronchodilator response to β_2-agonists is in general lower than in asthma but where chronic use of β_2-agonists has not been associated with a loss of effect or a loss of control of COPD.

1.9   Differential diagnosis of asthma and COPD

The differential diagnosis of asthma and COPD include a large number of diseases such as:

- gastro-oesophageal reflux disease;
- vocal-cord dysfunction syndrome;
- hyperventilation syndrome;
- pulmonary oedema;
- congestive heart failure;
- carcinoid syndrome;
- tumours that obstruct central airways;
- pneumothorax;
- tracheomalacia;
- bronchiolitis obliterans;
- recurrent pulmonary emboli;
- pulmonary vasculitis;
- collagen vascular diseases;
- Swyer-James syndrome, etc.

All of these can, however, also occur together with asthma or COPD, which can further complicate diagnostic accuracy.

However, the fact that end-stage lung disease in severe asthma or COPD can at times be clinically indistinguishable is determined by the possible pattern of response of the affected organ. Whether so-called neutrophilic asthma (in which neutrophils are the predominant inflammatory cell in the airways) represents a 'burned out' variant of chronic (severe) asthma where the asthma-specific cellular inflammation is replaced by a non-specific, neutrophil-dominated pathology is unclear and requires further studies. Similarly, the precise role of neutrophils in the 'neutrophil-dominated' pathology of COPD is uncertain. While neutrophils can contribute to parenchymal destruction with elastin-degrading enzymes their contribution to a COPD-specific inflammation is still unclear.

1.10   Overlap syndrome

It has been emphasized for a long time that there are a number of patients who are not reflected in clinical studies and who present with features of both COPD and asthma. This condition has been referred to as 'overlap syndrome', and it has been proposed that it can be recognized by the coexistence of increased variability of airflow in a patient with incompletely reversible airway obstruction.[60] These patients may have either mild allergic asthma with a smoking history, or a longstanding asthma with progressive decline in pulmonary function, or have developed adult-onset, intrinsic asthma coexistent with a prior smoking history. Although inflammatory (neutrophils) and physiological features (smoking history, decline in pulmonary function, increasing age, recurrent exacerbations) in these patients can resemble classical COPD a prior history of asthma clearly contributes to their pathogenesis. Due to the fact that these patients are generally excluded from clinical trials, mainly based on their incomplete response to bronchodilators, the generalisibility from such trials to the general asthma (and COPD) population is limited.[60] Whether the pathogenetic features of asthma and COPD actually converge[60] in this population or whether different pathologies result in similar outcomes remains a controversial issue and will require future research. Increased attention to the course of bronchial asthma in relation to other chronic obstructive airway disease, especially in older people, is needed to improve care and subsequently prognosis with improved health outcomes.[61]

1.11   Conclusion

Despite the fact that asthma and COPD can at times present with similar symptoms and similar changes in pulmonary function there is little evidence suggesting a common pathogenesis. In some, usually those asthma patients who smoke or who have been smoking, the individual contribution of asthma and smoking to the signs and symptoms of the disease can be difficult to separate. Especially in older patients with longstanding asthma and loss of reversibility, separation from COPD can be difficult. This patient group has usually been omitted from clinical studies. Despite the fact that a considerable number of patients are affected by this condition it is not well represented in guidelines and the general physician's perception. One of the main differences between asthma and COPD today remains that asthma can be treated while COPD can be prevented. However, at present there is little evidence that asthma can be prevented, while the response of COPD to currently available therapy is limited. This calls for future research to address the long-term consequences of either disease in order to develop specific therapies with improved health outcomes for asthma as well as COPD.

References

1. Sluiter HJ, Koeter GH, de Monchy JG, Postma DS, de Vries K, Orie NG. The Dutch hypothesis (chronic non-specific lung disease) revisited. Eur Respir J 1991;4:479–89.
2. Orie NG. The Dutch hypothesis. Chest 2000;117:299S.
3. Abramson M, Matheson M, Wharton C, Sim M, Walters EH. Prevalence of respiratory symptoms related to chronic obstructive pulmonary disease and asthma among middle aged and older adults. Respirology 2002;7:325–31.
4. Turner SW, Young S, Goldblatt J, Landau LI, Le Souef PN. Childhood asthma and increased airway responsiveness: a relationship that begins in infancy. Am J Respir Crit Care Med 2009;179:98–104.
5. Louhelainen N, Rytila P, Obase Y, et al. The value of sputum 8-isoprostane in detecting oxidative stress in mild asthma. J Asthma 2008;45:149–54.
6. Pelkonen M. Smoking: relationship to chronic bronchitis, chronic obstructive pulmonary disease and mortality. Curr Opin Pulm Med 2008;14:105–9.
7. Pelkonen M, Notkola IL, Nissinen A, Tukiainen H, Koskela H. Thirty-year cumulative incidence of chronic bronchitis and COPD in relation to 30-year pulmonary function and 40-year mortality: a follow-up in middle-aged rural men. Chest 2006;130:1129–37.
8. Hukkanen J, Pelkonen O, Hakkola J, Raunio H. Expression and regulation of xenobiotic-metabolizing cytochrome P450 (CYP) enzymes in human lung. Crit Rev Toxicol 2002;32: 391–411.
9. Karki NT, Pokela R, Nuutinen L, Pelkonen O. Aryl hydrocarbon hydroxylase in lymphocytes and lung tissue from lung cancer patients and controls. Int J Cancer 1987;39:565–70.
10. Burgess JA, Lowe AJ, Matheson MC, Varigos G, Abramson MJ, Dharmage SC. Does eczema lead to asthma? J Asthma 2009;46:429–36.
11. Yawn BP, Kaplan A. Co-morbidities in people with COPD: a result of multiple diseases, or multiple manifestations of smoking and reactive inflammation? Prim Care Respir J 2008;17:199–205.
12. Sutherland ER. Obesity and asthma. Immunol Allergy Clin North Am 2008;28:589–602, ix.
13. Peroni DG, Piacentini GL, Ceravolo R, Boner AL. Difficult asthma: possible association with rhinosinusitis. Pediatr Allergy Immunol 2007;18(Suppl. 18):25–7.
14. Thomas M. Allergic rhinitis: evidence for impact on asthma. BMC Pulm Med 2006;6(Suppl. 1): S4.
15. Gern JE. Viral respiratory infection and the link to asthma. Pediatr Infect Dis J 2004;23:S78–86.
16. von HL. Role of persistent infection in the control and severity of asthma: focus on Chlamydia pneumoniae. Eur Respir J 2002;19:546–56.
17. Boyce JA, Broide D, Matsumoto K, Bochner BS. Advances in mechanisms of asthma, allergy, and immunology in 2008. J Allergy Clin Immunol 2009;123:569–74.
18. Moffatt MF. Genes in asthma: new genes and new ways. Curr Opin Allergy Clin Immunol 2008;8:411–17.
19. Bosse Y. Genetics of chronic obstructive pulmonary disease: a succinct review, future avenues and prospective clinical applications. Pharmacogenomics 2009;10:655–67.
20. Molfino NA. Current thinking on genetics of chronic obstructive pulmonary disease. Curr Opin Pulm Med 2007;13:107–13.

21. Barnes PJ. The cytokine network in asthma and chronic obstructive pulmonary disease. J Clin Invest 2008;118:3546–56.
22. Barnes PJ. Immunology of asthma and chronic obstructive pulmonary disease. Nat Rev Immunol 2008;8:183–92.
23. Sterk PJ. Airway hyperresponsiveness: using bronchial challenge tests in research and management of asthma. J Aerosol Med 2002;15:123–9.
24. Postma DS, Kerstjens HA. Characteristics of airway hyperresponsiveness in asthma and chronic obstructive pulmonary disease. Am J Respir Crit Care Med 1998;158:S187–92.
25. Tashkin DP, Celli B, Decramer M, et al. Bronchodilator responsiveness in patients with COPD. Eur Respir J 2008;31:742–50.
26. Awadh N, Muller NL, Park CS, Abboud RT, FitzGerald JM. Airway wall thickness in patients with near fatal asthma and control groups: assessment with high resolution computed tomographic scanning. Thorax 1998;53:248–53.
27. Kurosawa H, Kohzuki M. Images in clinical medicine. Dynamic airway narrowing. N Engl J Med 2004;350:1036.
28. James AL, Palmer LJ, Kicic E, et al. Decline in lung function in the Busselton Health Study: the effects of asthma and cigarette smoking. Am J Respir Crit Care Med 2005;171:109–14.
29. Wills-Karp M, Ewart SL. Time to draw breath: asthma-susceptibility genes are identified. Nat Rev Genet 2004;5:376–87.
30. Hersh CP, DeMeo DL, Silverman EK. National Emphysema Treatment Trial state of the art: genetics of emphysema. Proc Am Thorac Soc 2008;5:486–93.
31. Platts-Mills TA, Wheatley LM. The role of allergy and atopy in asthma. Curr Opin Pulm Med 1996;2:29–34.
32. Gaffin JM, Phipatanakul W. The role of indoor allergens in the development of asthma. Curr Opin Allergy Clin Immunol 2009;9:128–35.
33. Virchow JC Jr, Walker C, Hafner D, et al. T cells and cytokines in bronchoalveolar lavage fluid after segmental allergen provocation in atopic asthma. Am J Respir Crit Care Med 1995;151:960–8.
34. Tashkin DP, Murray RP. Smoking cessation in chronic obstructive pulmonary disease. Respir Med 2009;103:963–74.
35. Stevenson DD, Zuraw BL. Pathogenesis of aspirin-exacerbated respiratory disease. Clin Rev Allergy Immunol 2003;24:169–88.
36. Luppi F, Franco F, Beghe B, Fabbri LM. Treatment of chronic obstructive pulmonary disease and its comorbidities. Proc Am Thorac Soc 2008;5:848–56.
37. Chatila WM, Thomashow BM, Minai OA, Criner GJ, Make BJ. Comorbidities in chronic obstructive pulmonary disease. Proc Am Thorac Soc 2008;5:549–55.
38. Stern DA, Morgan WJ, Wright AL, Guerra S, Martinez FD. Poor airway function in early infancy and lung function by age 22 years: a non-selective longitudinal cohort study. Lancet 2007;370:758–64.
39. Shapiro SD. Evolving concepts in the pathogenesis of chronic obstructive pulmonary disease. Clin Chest Med 2000;21:621–32.
40. Waterer GW, Temple SE. Do we really want to know why only some smokers get COPD? Chest 2004;125:1599–600.
41. Walker C, Bode E, Boer L, Hansel TT, Blaser K, Virchow JC Jr. Allergic and nonallergic asthmatics have distinct patterns of T-cell activation and cytokine production in peripheral blood and bronchoalveolar lavage. Am Rev Respir Dis 1992;146:109–15.
42. Virchow JC Jr, Kroegel C, Walker C, Matthys H. Cellular and immunological markers of allergic and intrinsic bronchial asthma. Lung 1994;172:313–34.

43. Horn BR, Robin ED, Theodore J, Van Kessel A. Total eosinophil counts in the management of bronchial asthma. N Engl J Med 1975;292:1152–5.
44. Nair P, Pizzichini MM, Kjarsgaard M, et al. Mepolizumab for prednisone-dependent asthma with sputum eosinophilia. N Engl J Med 2009;360:985–93.
45. Haldar P, Brightling CE, Hargadon B, et al. Mepolizumab and exacerbations of refractory eosinophilic asthma. N Engl J Med 2009;360:973–84.
46. Bratke K, Lommatzsch M, Julius P, et al. Dendritic cell subsets in human bronchoalveolar lavage fluid after segmental allergen challenge. Thorax 2007;62:168–75.
47. Arnold V, Balkow S, Staats R, Matthys H, Luttmann W, Virchow JC Jr. [Increase in perforin-positive peripheral blood lymphocytes in extrinsic and intrinsic asthma.] Pneumologie 2000; 54:468–73.
48. Bjermer L, Bisgaard H, Bousquet J, et al. Montelukast and fluticasone compared with salmeterol and fluticasone in protecting against asthma exacerbation in adults: one year, double blind, randomised, comparative trial. Brit Med J 2003;327:891.
49. Bratke K, Klug M, Bier A, et al. Function-associated surface molecules on airway dendritic cells in cigarette smokers. Am J Respir Cell Mol Biol 2008;38:655–60.
50. Jeffery PK. Structural and inflammatory changes in COPD: a comparison with asthma. Thorax 1998;53:129–36.
51. Davies DE, Wicks J, Powell RM, Puddicombe SM, Holgate ST. Airway remodeling in asthma: new insights. J Allergy Clin Immunol 2003;111:215–25; quiz 26.
52. Pepe C, Foley S, Shannon J, et al. Differences in airway remodeling between subjects with severe and moderate asthma. J Allergy Clin Immunol 2005;116:544–9.
53. Paredi P, Barnes PJ. The airway vasculature: recent advances and clinical implications. Thorax 2009;64:444–50.
54. Soler-Cataluna JJ, Martinez-Garcia MA, Roman Sanchez P, Salcedo E, Navarro M, Ochando R. Severe acute exacerbations and mortality in patients with chronic obstructive pulmonary disease. Thorax 2005;60:925–31.
55. Hogg JC. Pathophysiology of airflow limitation in chronic obstructive pulmonary disease. Lancet 2004;364:709–21.
56. Hogg JC, Timens W. The pathology of chronic obstructive pulmonary disease. Annu Rev Pathol 2009;4:435–59.
57. Hogg JC, Chu F, Utokaparch S, et al. The nature of small-airway obstruction in chronic obstructive pulmonary disease. N Engl J Med 2004;350:2645–53.
58. Lommatzsch M, Virchow JC. The neural underpinnings of asthma. J Allergy Clin Immunol 2007;119:254–5; author reply 5.
59. Hasford J, Virchow JC. Excess mortality in patients with asthma on long-acting beta2-agonists. Eur Respir J 2006;28:900–2.
60. Gibson PG, Simpson JL. The overlap syndrome of asthma and COPD: what are its features and how important is it? Thorax 2009;64:728–35.
61. Gibson PG, McDonald VM, Marks GB. Asthma in older adults. Lancet 2010;376:803–13.

2

Glucocorticoids: pharmacology and mechanisms

Peter J. Barnes

National Heart and Lung Institute, Imperial College, London, UK

2.1   Introduction

Glucocorticoids (glucocorticosteroids or corticosteroids) are widely used to treat a variety of inflammatory and immune diseases. The most common use of glucocorticoids today is in the treatment of asthma and other allergic diseases, and inhaled glucocorticoids are now established as first-line treatment in adults and children with persistent asthma. Despite intense efforts by the pharmaceutical industry it has proved extraordinarily difficult to find any new treatment that comes close to the therapeutic benefit of glucocorticoids in asthma.[1] This chapter focuses on the cellular and molecular mechanisms of glucocorticoids that are relevant to asthma and also discusses why they do not appear to work in some patients with asthma or in patients with chronic obstructive pulmonary disease (COPD). There have been major advances in understanding the molecular mechanisms whereby glucocorticoids suppress inflammation, based on recent developments in understanding the fundamental mechanisms of gene transcription.[2,3] These advances have important clinical implications, as they will lead to a better understanding of the inflammatory mechanisms of many diseases and may lead to the development of new anti-inflammatory treatments in the future. The new understanding of these molecular mechanisms also helps to explain how glucocorticoids are able to switch off multiple inflammatory pathways, and it also provides insights into why glucocorticoids apparently fail to work in patients with steroid-resistant asthma and in patients with COPD.

2.2   Chemical structures

The adrenal cortex secretes cortisol (hydrocortisone) and, by modification of its structure, it was possible to develop derivatives, such as prednisolone and dexamethasone, with enhanced glucocorticoid effects but with reduced mineralocorticoid activity.

Advances in Combination Therapy for Asthma and COPD, First Edition. Edited by Jan Lötvall.

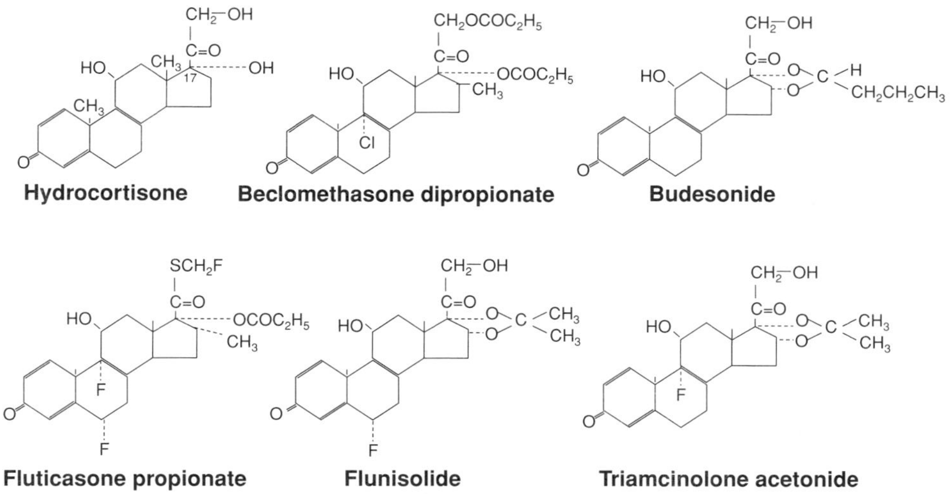

Figure 2.1 Chemical structures of inhaled corticosteroids.

These derivatives with potent glucocorticoid actions were effective in asthma when given systemically but had no anti-asthmatic activity when given by inhalation. Further substitution in the 17α ester position resulted in steroids with high topical activity, such as beclometasone dipropionate (BDP), triamcinolone, flunisolide, budesonide and fluticasone propionate, which are potent in the skin (dermal blanching test) and were later found to have significant anti-asthma effects when given by inhalation (Figure 2.1).

2.3   The molecular basis of inflammation

Understanding the molecular mechanisms involved in asthmatic inflammation is necessary in order to understand how glucocorticoids so efficiently suppress airways inflammation in asthma. Patients with asthma and allergic rhinitis have a specific pattern of inflammation in the airways that is characterized by degranulated mast cells, infiltration of eosinophils and increased number of activated T-helper 2 (Th2 cells).[4] Suppression of this inflammation by glucocorticoids controls and prevents these symptoms in the vast majority of patients. Multiple mediators are produced in allergic diseases, and the approximately 100 known inflammatory mediators that are increased include lipid mediators, inflammatory peptides, chemokines, cytokines and growth factors.[5] There is increasing evidence that structural cells of the airways, such as epithelial cells, airway smooth muscle cells, endothelial cells and fibroblasts, are a major source of inflammatory mediators in asthma. Epithelial cells may play a particularly important role, as they may be activated by environmental signals and they may release multiple inflammatory proteins, including cytokines, chemokines, lipid mediators and growth factors.

Inflammation is mediated by the increased expression of multiple inflammatory proteins, including cytokines, chemokines, adhesion molecules, and inflammatory enzymes and receptors. Most of these inflammatory proteins are regulated by increased gene transcription, which is controlled by proinflammatory transcription factors, such as nuclear factor-κB (NF-κB) and activator protein-1 (AP-1), that are activated in asthmatic cells.[6] For example, NF-κB is markedly activated in epithelial cells of asthmatic patients, and this transcription factor regulates many of the inflammatory genes that are abnormally expressed in asthma. NF-κB may be activated by rhinovirus infection and allergen exposure, both of which exacerbate asthmatic inflammation.

Chromatin remodelling

Chromatin consists of DNA and basic proteins called histones, which provide the structural backbone of the chromosome. It has long been recognized that histones play a critical role in regulating the expression of genes and determine which genes are transcriptionally active and which ones are suppressed (silenced). The chromatin structure is highly organized as almost two metres of DNA have to be packed into each cell nucleus. Chromatin is made up of nucleosomes, which are particles consisting of 146 base pairs of DNA wound almost twice around an octamer of two molecules each of the core histone proteins H2A, H2B, H3 and H4.[7] Expression and repression of genes is associated with remodelling of this chromatin structure by enzymatic modification of the core histone proteins, particularly by acetylation. Each core histone has a long N-terminal tail that is rich in lysine residues, which may become acetylated, thus changing the electrical charge of the core histone. In the resting cell DNA is wound tightly around core histones, excluding the binding of the enzyme RNA polymerase II, which activates gene transcription and the formation of messenger RNA. This conformation of the chromatin structure is described as closed and is associated with suppression of gene expression. Gene transcription only occurs when the chromatin structure is opened up, with unwinding of DNA so that RNA polymerase II and basal transcription complexes can now bind to DNA to initiate transcription.

Histone acetyltransferases and coactivators

When proinflammatory transcription factors, such as NF-κB and AP-1, are activated they bind to specific recognition sequences in DNA and subsequently interact with large coactivator molecules, such as cyclic adenosine monophosphate response element binding protein (CREB)-binding protein (CBP). These coactivator molecules act as the molecular switches that control gene transcription and all have intrinsic histone acetyltransferase (HAT) activity.[7] This results in acetylation of core histones, thereby reducing their charge, which allows the chromatin structure to transform from the resting closed conformation to an activated open form. This results in unwinding of DNA, binding of TATA box binding protein (TBP), TBP-associated factors and RNA polymerase II, which then initiates gene transcription. This molecular mechanism is common to all genes, including those involved in differentiation, proliferation and activation of cells. Of course this process is reversible and deacetylation of acetylated histones is associated with gene silencing. This is mediated by histone deacetylases (HDACs), which act as corepressors, together with other corepressor proteins that are subsequently recruited.

These fundamental mechanisms have now been applied to understanding the regulation of inflammatory genes in diseases such as asthma and COPD.[8,9] In a human epithelial cell line activation of NF-κB, by exposing the cell to inflammatory signals such as interleukin-1β (IL-1β), tumour necrosis factor-α (TNF-α) or endotoxin, results in acetylation of specific lysine residues on histone H4 (the other histones do not appear to be so markedly or rapidly acetylated), and this is correlated with increased expression of genes encoding inflammatory proteins, such as granulocyte-macrophage colony stimulating factor (GM-CSF).[10]

Histone deacetylases and corepressors

The acetylation of histone that is associated with increased expression of inflammatory genes is counteracted by the activity of HDACs, of which 11 that deacetylate histones are now characterized.[11,12] There is now evidence that the different HDACs target different patterns of acetylation.[13] In biopsies from patients with asthma there is an increase in HAT and a reduction in HDAC activity, thereby favouring increased inflammatory gene expression.[14] With this background it is now possible to understand better why glucocorticoids are so effective in suppressing this complex inflammatory process that involves the increased expression of multiple inflammatory proteins. HDACs act as corepressors in consort with other corepressor proteins, such as nuclear receptor corepressor (NCoR) and silencing mediator of the retinoid and thyroid hormone receptor (SMRT), forming a corepressor complex that silences gene expression.[15]

2.4   Cellular effects of glucocorticoids

Glucocorticoids are the only therapy that effectively suppresses the inflammation in asthmatic airways, and this underlies the clinical improvement in asthma symptoms and prevention of exacerbations. At a cellular level glucocorticoids reduce the numbers of inflammatory cells in the airways, including eosinophils, T-lymphocytes, mast cells and dendritic cells (Figure 2.2). These remarkable effects of glucocorticoids are produced through inhibiting the recruitment of inflammatory cells into the airway by suppressing the production of chemotactic mediators and adhesion molecules and by inhibiting the survival in the airways of inflammatory cells, such as eosinophils, T-lymphocytes and mast cells. Epithelial cells may be a major cellular target for inhaled glucocorticoids. Thus glucocorticoids have a broad spectrum of anti-inflammatory effects in asthma, with inhibition of multiple inflammatory mediators and inflammatory and structural cells. It is probably the broad anti-inflammatory profile of glucocorticoids that accounts for their marked clinical effectiveness in asthma. Attempts to find alternative treatments that are more specific, such as inhibitors of single mediators, have usually been

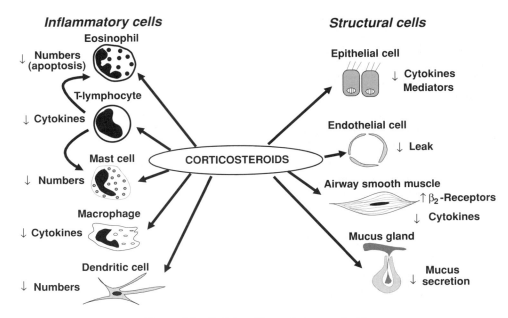

Figure 2.2   Cellular effects of glucocorticoids.

unsuccessful, emphasizing the importance of simultaneously inhibiting many inflammatory targets. Any explanation of the anti-inflammatory effects of glucocorticoids needs to account for this broad spectrum of anti-inflammatory effects.

2.5   Glucocorticoid receptors

Glucocorticoids diffuse readily across cell membranes and bind to glucocorticoid receptors (GR) in the cytoplasm. Cytoplasmic GR are normally bound to proteins, known as molecular chaperones, such as heat shock protein-90 (HSP90) and FK-binding protein, that protect the receptor and prevent its nuclear localization by covering the sites on the receptor that are needed for transport across the nuclear membrane into the nucleus.[16] There is a single gene encoding human GR but several variants are now recognized, as a result of transcript alternative splicing, and alternative translation initiation.[17] The receptor GRα binds glucocorticoids whereas GRβ is an alternatively spliced form that binds to DNA but cannot be activated by glucocorticoids. GRβ has a very low level of expression compared to GRα. The GRβ isoform has been implicated in steroid-resistance in asthma, although whether GRβ can have any functional significance has been questioned in view of the very low levels of expression compared to GRα.[18]

Glucocorticoid receptors may also be modified by phosphorylation and other modifications, which may alter the response to glucocorticoids by affecting ligand binding, translocation to the nucleus, *trans*-activating efficacy, protein–protein interactions or recruitment of cofactors.[19] For example, there are a number of serine/threonines in the N-terminal domain where glucocorticoid receptors may be phosphorylated by various kinases.

Once glucocorticoids have bound to GR, changes in the receptor structure result in dissociation of molecular chaperone proteins, thereby exposing nuclear localization signals. This results in rapid transport of the activated glucocorticoid receptor-glucocorticoid complex into the nucleus, where it binds to DNA at specific sequences in the promoter region of glucocorticoid-responsive genes known as glucocorticoid response elements (GRE). Two glucocorticoid receptor molecules bind together as a homodimer and bind to GRE, leading to changes in gene transcription. Interaction of GR with GRE classically leads to an increase in gene transcription (*trans*-activation), but negative GRE sites have also been described where binding of GR leads to gene suppression (*cis*-repression)[20] (Figure 2.3). There are few well-documented examples of negative GREs, but some are relevant to glucocorticoid side effects, including genes that regulate the hypothalamic-pituitary axis (proopiomelanocortin and corticotrophin-releasing factor), bone metabolism (osteocalcin) and skin structure (keratins).

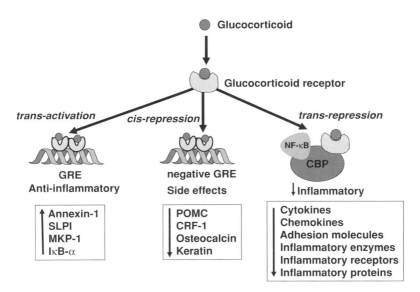

Figure 2.3 Glucocorticoids may regulate gene expression in several ways. Glucocorticoids enter the cell to bind to glucocorticoid receptors (GR) in the cytoplasm, which translocate to the nucleus. GR homodimers bind to glucocorticoid-response elements (GRE) in the promoter region of steroid-sensitive genes, which may encode anti-inflammatory proteins. Less commonly, GR homodimers interact with negative GREs to suppress genes, particularly those linked to side effects of glucocorticoids. Nuclear GR also interact with coactivator molecules, such as CREB-binding protein (CBP), which is activated by proinflammatory transcription factors, such as nuclear factor-κB (NF-κB), thus switching off the inflammatory genes that are activated by these transcription factors. SLPI, secretory leukoprotease inhibitor; MKP-1, mitogen-activated kinase phosphatase-1; IκB-α, inhibitor of NF-κB; GILZ, glucocorticoid-induced leucine zipper protein; POMC, proopiomelanocortin; CRF, corticotrophin releasing factor.

2.6   Glucocorticoid activation of gene transcription

Glucocorticoids produce their effect on responsive cells by activating glucocorticoid receptors to directly or indirectly regulate the transcription of target genes. Relatively few genes per cell are *directly* regulated by glucocorticoids, but many are indirectly regulated through an interaction with other transcription factors and coactivators. Glucocorticoid receptor homodimers bind to GRE sites in the promoter region of glucocorticoid-responsive genes. Interaction of the activated glucocorticoid receptor dimer with GRE usually increases transcription. Glucocorticoid receptors may increase transcription by interacting with coactivator molecules, such as CBP, thus activating histone acetylation and gene transcription. For example, relatively high concentrations of glucocorticoids increase the secretion of the antiprotease secretory leukoprotease inhibitor (SLPI) from epithelial cells.[10]

The activation of genes by glucocorticoids is associated with a selective acetylation of lysine residues 5 and 16 on histone H4, resulting in increased gene transcription[10] (Figure 2.4). Activated GR may bind to coactivator molecules, such as CBP, as well as

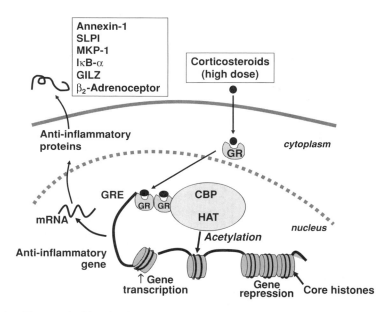

Figure 2.4   Glucocorticoid activation of anti-inflammatory gene expression. Glucocorticoids bind to cytoplasmic glucocorticoid receptors (GR), which translocate to the nucleus where they bind to glucocorticoid response elements (GRE) in the promoter region of steroid-sensitive genes and also directly or indirectly to coactivator molecules such as CREB-binding protein (CBP). The latter have intrinsic histone acetyltransferase (HAT) activity, causing acetylation of lysines on histone H4, which leads to activation of genes encoding anti-inflammatory proteins, such as secretory leukoprotease inhibitor (SLPI), mitogen-activated kinase phosphatase-1 (MKP-1), inhibitor of NF-κB (IκB-α) and glucocorticoid-induced leucine zipper protein (GILZ).

steroid-receptor coactivator-1 (SRC-1) and glucocorticoid receptor interacting protein-1 (GRIP-1 or SRC-2), all of which possess HAT activity.[21]

Anti-inflammatory gene activation

Several of the genes that are switched on by glucocorticoids have anti-inflammatory effects, including annexin-1 (lipocortin-1), secretory leukoprotease inhibitor (SLPI), interleukin-10 and inhibitor of NF-κB (IκB-α). However, therapeutic doses of inhaled glucocorticoids have not been shown to increase annexin-1 concentrations in bronchoalveolar lavage fluid,[22] and an increase in IκB-α has not been shown in most cell types, including epithelial cells.[23] Glucocorticoids also switch on the synthesis of two proteins that affect inflammatory signal transduction pathways: glucocorticoid-induced leucine zipper protein (GILZ), which inhibits both NF-κB and AP-1,[24] and mitogen-activated protein kinase phosphatase-1 (MKP-1), which inhibits p38 MAP kinase and Jun kinase.[25] However, it seems unlikely that the widespread anti-inflammatory actions of glucocorticoids could be entirely explained by increased transcription of small numbers of anti-inflammatory genes, particularly as high concentrations of glucocorticoids are usually required for this effect, whereas in clinical practice glucocorticoids are able to suppress inflammation at low concentrations.

Side effect genes

Relatively little is known about the molecular mechanisms of glucocorticoid side effects, such as osteoporosis, growth retardation in children, skin fragility and metabolic effects. These actions of glucocorticoids are related to their endocrine effects. The systemic side effects of glucocorticoids may be due to gene activation. Some insight into this has been provided by mutant glucocorticoid receptors, which do not dimerize and therefore cannot bind to GRE to switch on genes. In transgenic mice expressing these mutant glucocorticoid receptors glucocorticoids show no loss in their anti-inflammatory effects and are able to suppress NF-κB-activated genes in the normal way.[26] As indicated above several of the genes associated with side effects, including those involving the hypothalamo-pituitary-adrenal axis, bone metabolism and skin structure, appear to be regulated by interaction of glucocorticoid receptors with negative GRE sites.[20]

2.7 Suppression of inflammatory genes

In controlling inflammation, the major effect of glucocorticoids is to inhibit the synthesis of multiple inflammatory proteins through suppression of the genes that encode them (Table 2.1). Although this was originally believed to be through interaction of GR with negative GRE sites, these have been demonstrated on only a few genes, which do not include genes encoding inflammatory proteins.[20]

Table 2.1 Effect of glucocorticoids on gene transcription.

Increased transcription (*trans*-activation)	Decreased transcription (*trans*-repression)
Annexin-1 (lipocortin-1, phospholipase A₂ inhibitor)	**Cytokines**
β₂-Adrenoceptors	IL-1, IL-2, IL-3, IL-4, IL-5, IL-6, IL-9, IL-11, IL-12, IL-13, IL-16, IL-17, IL-18
Secretory leukoprotease inhibitor	TNF-α, GM-CSF, SCF
Clara cell protein (CC10, phospholipase A₂ inhibitor)	
Interleukin-1 receptor antagonist	**Chemokines**
Interleukin-1R2 (decoy receptor)	IL-8, RANTES, MIP-1α, MCP-1, MCP-3, MCP-4, eotaxins
IκB-α (inhibitor of NF-κB)	
GILZ (glucocorticoid-induced leucine zipper protein)	**Adhesion molecules**
	ICAM-1, VCAM-1, E-selectin
MKP-1 (mitogen-activated protein kinase phosphatase-1)	**Inflammatory enzymes**
Interleukin-10 (indirectly)	Inducible nitric oxide synthase (iNOS)
	Inducible cyclooxygenase (COX-2)
	Cytoplasmic phospholipase A₂ (cPLA₂)
	Inflammatory receptors
	Tachykinin NK₁-receptors, NK₂-receptors
	Bradykinin B₂-receptors
	Peptides
	Endothelin-1

Abbreviations: GM-CSF, granulocyte-macrophage colony stimulating factor; ICAM, intercellular adhesion molecule; IL, interleukin; MCP, monocyte chemoattractant protein; MIP, macrophage inflammatory protein; RANTES, released by normal activated T-cells expressed and secreted; SCF, stem cell factor; TNF, tumour necrosis factor; VCAM, vascular-endothelial cell adhesion molecule.

Interaction with transcription factors

Activated glucocorticoid receptors have been shown to interact functionally with other activated transcription factors. Most of the inflammatory genes that are activated in asthma do not have GRE sites in their promoter regions, yet are potently repressed by glucocorticoids. There is persuasive evidence that glucocorticoids inhibit the effects of proinflammatory transcription factors, such as AP-1 and NF-κB, that regulate the expression of genes encoding many inflammatory proteins, such as cytokines, inflammatory enzymes, adhesion molecules and inflammatory receptors.[6] Activated GR can interact directly with other activated transcription factors by protein–protein binding, but this may be a particular feature of cells in which these genes are artificially overexpressed, rather than a property of normal cells. Treatment of asthmatic patients with high doses of inhaled glucocorticoids that suppress airway inflammation is not associated with any reduction in NF-κB binding to DNA, yet is able to switch off inflammatory genes, such as GM-CSF, that are regulated by NF-κB.[27] This suggests that glucocorticoids are more likely to be acting downstream of the binding of proinflammatory transcription factors to DNA and attention has now focused on their effects on chromatin structure and histone acetylation.

Effects on histone acetylation

Activated glucocorticoid receptors may bind to CBP or other coactivators directly to inhibit their HAT activity,[10] thus reversing the unwinding of DNA around core histones and thereby repressing inflammatory genes. More importantly, particularly at low concentrations that are likely to be relevant therapeutically in asthma treatment, activated GR recruit HDAC2 to the activated transcriptional complex, resulting in deacetylation of histones, and thus a decrease in inflammatory gene transcription[10] (Figure 2.5). Using a chromatin immunoprecipitation assay we have demonstrated that glucocorticoids recruit HDAC2 to the acetylated histone H4 associated with the GM-CSF promoter.[10] When using interference RNA to selectively suppress HDAC2 in an epithelial cell line, we have shown that there is an increase in the expression of

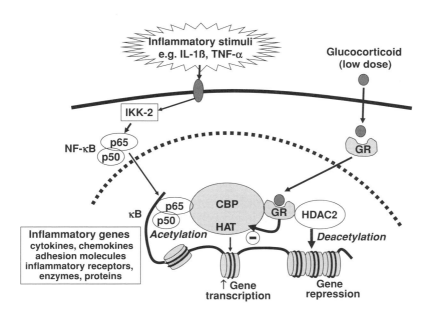

Figure 2.5 Glucocorticoid suppression of activated inflammatory genes. Inflammatory genes are activated by inflammatory stimuli, such as interleukin-1β (IL-1β) or tumour necrosis factor-α (TNF-α), resulting in activation of IKK2 (inhibitor of I-κB kinase-2), which activates the transcription factor nuclear factor-κB (NF-κB). A dimer of p50 and p65 NF-κB proteins translocates to the nucleus and binds to specific κB recognition sites and also to coactivators, such as CREB-binding protein (CBP), which have intrinsic histone acetyltransferase (HAT) activity. This results in acetylation of core histone H4, resulting in increased expression of genes encoding multiple inflammatory proteins. Glucocorticoid receptors (GR) after activation by glucocorticoids translocate to the nucleus and bind to coactivators to inhibit HAT activity directly and recruit histone deacetylase-2 (HDAC2), which reverses histone acetylation leading to suppression of these activated inflammatory genes.

GM-CSF and reduced sensitivity to glucocorticoids.[28] By contrast, knock-down of HDAC1 and HDAC3 had no such effect on steroid responsiveness. An important issue that is not yet resolved is why glucocorticoids selectively switch off inflammatory genes, while having no effect on genes that regulate proliferation, metabolism and survival. It is likely that glucocorticoid receptors only bind to coactivators that are activated by proinflammatory transcription factors, such as NF-κB and AP-1, although we do not yet understand how this specific recognition occurs.

Other histone modifications

It has now become apparent that core histones may be modified not only by acetylation, but also by methylation, phosphorylation and ubiquitination, and that these modifications may also regulate gene transcription.[29] Methylation of histones, particularly histone H3, by histone methyltransferases, usually results in gene suppression. The anti-inflammatory effects of glucocorticoids are reduced by a methyltransferase inhibitor, 5-aza-2′-deoxycytidine, suggesting that this may be an additional mechanism whereby glucocorticoids suppress genes.[30] Indeed, there may be an interaction between acetylation, methylation and phosphorylation of histones, so that the sequence of chromatin modifications (the so-called 'histone code') may give specificity to expression of particular genes.[31]

Glucocorticoid receptor acetylation

It has been increasingly recognized that many regulatory proteins, particularly transcription factors and nuclear receptors, are also regulated by acetylation controlled by HATs and HDACs.[32] Acetylation plays a key role in the regulation of androgen and oestrogen receptors, and this has now been shown to be the case for GR.[33] GR is acetylated within the nucleus at specific lysine residues close to the hinge region and only binds to its DNA binding site in its acetylated form. However, in order to inhibit NF-κB-activated genes it is necessary to deacetylate the receptor, and this is achieved by HDAC2 (Figure 2.6).

Non-transcriptional effects

Although most of the actions of glucocorticoids are mediated by changes in transcription through chromatin remodelling, it is increasingly recognized that glucocorticoids may also affect protein synthesis by reducing the stability of mRNA so that less protein is synthesized. It is increasingly recognized that several inflammatory proteins are regulated post-transcriptionally at the level of mRNA stability.[34] This may be an important anti-inflammatory mechanism as it allows glucocorticoids to switch off the ongoing production of inflammatory proteins after the inflammatory gene has been activated. The stability of some inflammatory genes is determined by regulation of AU-rich elements (ARE) in the 3′-untranslated regions of the gene, which

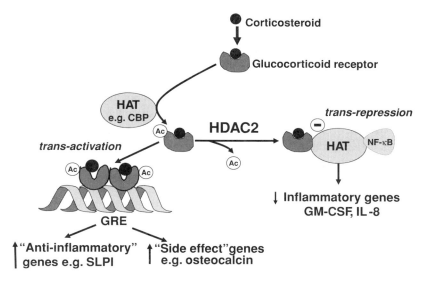

Figure 2.6 Acetylation of glucocorticoid receptors (GR). Binding of a corticosteroid to GR results in its acetylation by histone acetyltransferases (HAT), such as CREB-binding protein (CBP), and a dimer of acetylated GR then binds to glucocorticoid response elements (GRE) to activate or suppress genes (such as side effect genes). Deacetylation of GR by histone deacetylase-2 (HDAC2) is necessary for GR to interact with CBP and inhibit nuclear factor-κB (NF-κB) to switch off inflammatory genes. GM-CSF, granulocyte-macrophage colony stimulating factor; IL-8, interleukin-8; SLPI, secretory leukoprotease inhibitor.

interact with several ARE-binding proteins such as HuR and tristetraprolin that may stabilize mRNA.[35] Some inflammatory genes, such as the genes encoding GM-CSF and cyclooxygenase-2 (COX-2), produce mRNA that is particularly susceptible to the action of ribonucleases that break down mRNA, thus switching off protein synthesis. Glucocorticoids may have inhibitory effects on the proteins that stabilize mRNA, leading to more rapid breakdown and thus a reduction in inflammatory protein expression.[36, 37] Glucocorticoids do not appear to have any effect on human antigen R (HuR) or tristetraprolin expression, however.[38]

Effects on signal transduction pathways

Glucocorticoids have complex effects on signal transduction pathways through trans-repression of critical enzymes involved in inflammatory cascades, or through increased transcription of endogenous inhibitors of these pathways.[39]

Mitogen-activated protein (MAP) kinases play an important role in inflammatory gene expression through the regulation of proinflammatory transcription factors. There is increasing evidence that glucocorticoids may exert an inhibitory effect on these pathways. Glucocorticoids may inhibit AP-1 and NF-κB via an inhibitory effect on c-Jun N-terminal kinases (JNK), which activate these transcription factors.[40] They reduce the stability of mRNA for some inflammatory genes, such as COX2, through an inhibitory action on another MAP kinase, p38 MAP kinase.[35] p38 MAP kinase regulates multiple inflammatory genes, including TNF-α, IL-1β, IL-6, GM-CSF and IL-8, which have ARE sites in their 3'-untranslated regions, by stabilizing their mRNA so that synthesis of the inflammatory protein is increased.[35] The inhibitory effect of glucocorticoids is mediated via the rapid induction of a potent endogenous inhibitor of p38 MAP kinase, MKP-1, which is one of the genes switched on by glucocorticoids[41] (Figure 2.7). Glucocorticoids not only induce the MKP-1 gene, but also reduce its degradation. MKP-1 inhibits all MAP kinase pathways and therefore inhibits JNK and to a lesser extent extracellularly regulated kinase (ERK), in addition to p38 MAP kinase.[41] This indicates that glucocorticoids have the capacity to inhibit all MAP kinase

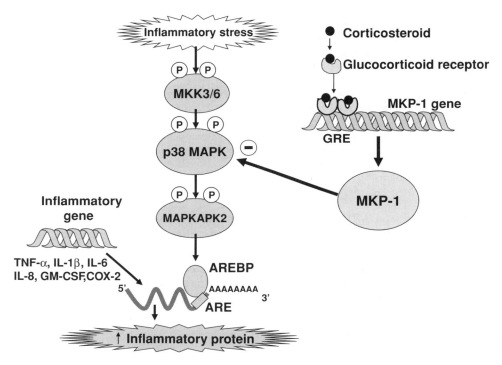

Figure 2.7   Inhibition of p38 mitogen-activated protein kinase (MAPK) by glucocorticoids. p38 MAP kinase is activated by inflammatory stresses through activation of MAP kinase kinase-3 (MKK-3) and MKK-6. p38 phosphorylates (P) MAP kinase-activated protein kinase (MAPKAPK)-2, which plays a role in stabilizing messenger RNA (mRNA) encoding several inflammatory proteins, such as tumour necrosis factor-α (TNF-α), interleukin-1β (IL-1β), IL-6, IL-8, granulocyte-macrophage colony stimulating factor (GM-CSF) and cyclo-oxygenase-2 (COX-2). This mRNA is characterized by AU-rich elements (ARE) in the 3'-untranslated region, which make the mRNA unstable and rapidly degraded. ARE-binding proteins (AREBP) stabilize these proteins and may be activated (probably indirectly) by MAPKAPK-2. Glucocorticoids induce the expression of MAP kinase phosphatase (MKP)-1, which inhibits p38 and thus prevents the stabilization of multiple inflammatory proteins. GRE, glucocorticoid response element.

pathways, but the selectivity of MKP-1 for different MAP kinases appears to vary from cell to cell.[42]

2.8 Steroid resistance

Although glucocorticoids are highly effective in the control of asthma and other chronic inflammatory or immune diseases, a small proportion of patients with asthma fail to respond even to high doses of oral glucocorticoids,[43,44] and patients with COPD are largely unresponsive to glucocorticoids. Resistance to the therapeutic effects of glucocorticoids is also recognized in non-pulmonary inflammatory and immune diseases, including rheumatoid arthritis and inflammatory bowel disease. Steroid-resistant patients present considerable management problems as there are few alternative anti-inflammatory treatments available. The new insights into the mechanisms whereby glucocorticoids suppress chronic inflammation have shed light on the molecular basis for steroid resistance in asthma and COPD.

Steroid-resistant asthma

There may be several molecular mechanisms for resistance to the effects of glucocorticoids, and these may differ between patients.[43,44] It is likely that there is a spectrum of steroid responsiveness, with the very rare resistance at one end, but also a relative resistance seen in patients who require high doses of inhaled and oral steroids (steroid-dependent asthma).

p38 MAP kinase

Biopsy studies have demonstrated the typical eosinophilic inflammation in the bronchial mucosa in these patients, with increased expression of Th2 cytokines. There is also resistance to the anti-inflammatory effects of glucocorticoids in circulating mononuclear cells.[45] Certain cytokines (particularly IL-2, IL-4 and IL-13, which show increased expression in bronchial biopsies of patients with steroid-resistant asthma) may induce a reduction in affinity of glucocorticoid receptors in inflammatory cells such as T-lymphocytes, resulting in local resistance to the anti-inflammatory actions of glucocorticoids. The combination of IL-2 and IL-4 induces steroid resistance *in vitro* through activation of p38 MAP kinase, which phosphorylates glucocorticoid receptors and reduces glucocorticoid binding affinity within the nucleus.[46] The therapeutic implication is that p38 MAP kinase inhibitors now in clinical development might reverse this form of steroid resistance.

Glucocorticoid receptor-β

Another proposed mechanism for steroid resistance in asthma is increased expression of GRβ, which may theoretically act as an inhibitor by competing with GRα for binding to GRE sites or by interacting with coactivator molecules.[18,47] However, there is no increased expression of GRβ in the mononuclear cells of patients with steroid-dependent asthma who have a reduced responsiveness to glucocorticoids *in vitro*. Furthermore, GRα greatly predominates over GRβ, making it unlikely that it could have any functional inhibitory effect,[48] and GRβ protein is undetectable in blood monocytes of asthmatic patients.[49] Furthermore, there is no evidence for induction of GRβ in response to IL-2/IL-4 exposure, which induces steroid-resistance in mononuclear cells, convincingly demonstrating that GRβ cannot account for steroid resistance in asthma.[49]

Interaction with transcription factors

Another proposed mechanism is a failure of GR to inhibit the activation of inflammatory genes by transcription factors, such as NF-κB and AP-1. Indeed, there is defective inhibiting of AP-1 in response to glucocorticoids in mononuclear cells of steroid-resistant patients.[45] This may be due to increased activation of AP-1 due to excessive activation of the JNK pathway, which has been demonstrated in the cells of steroid-resistant asthma patients.[50]

Defective histone acetylation

Mononuclear cells from asthmatic patients who are steroid-dependent or steroid-resistant show reduced suppression of cytokine release and a reduction in histone H4 acetylation in the nucleus following treatment with a high concentration of dexamethasone (1 μM).[51] In one group of patients nuclear localization of GR in response to a high concentration of glucocorticoids is impaired, and this accounts for the reduced histone acetylation, since there is a direct correlation between the degree of histone acetylation and the GR nuclear localization.[51] This may be a result of GR nitrosylation leading to reduced dissociation of GR from HSP90.[52] However, in another group of patients the defect in histone acetylation is found despite normal nuclear localization of GR. This may be a result of GR phosphorylation within the nucleus due to the activation of p38 MAP kinase,[46] which may result in a failure to recruit a distinct coactivator(s). This may result in failure of glucocorticoid receptors to *trans*-activate steroid-responsive genes.[53] In this group of patients specific acetylation of histone H4 lysine-5 by glucocorticoids is defective.[51] This presumably means that glucocorticoids are not able to activate certain genes that are critical to the anti-inflammatory action of high doses of glucocorticoids, but whether this is a rare genetic defect is not yet known.

Smoking asthmatics

Asthmatic patients who smoke have more severe disease and are also resistant to the anti-inflammatory effects of glucocorticoids.[54] A plausible explanation for this steroid resistance is the combined effect of asthma and cigarette smoking on HDAC, resulting

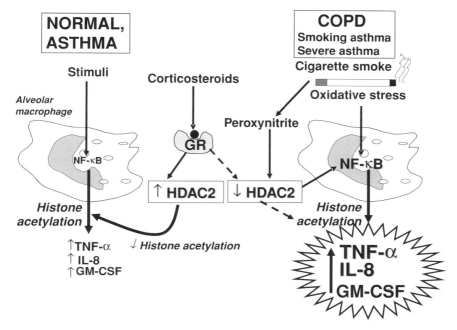

Figure 2.8 Proposed mechanism of glucocorticoid resistance in COPD, severe asthma and smoking asthma. Stimulation of normal and asthmatic alveolar macrophages activates nuclear factor-κB (NF-κB) and other transcription factors to switch on histone acetyltransferase leading to histone acetylation and subsequently to transcription of genes encoding inflammatory proteins, such as tumour necrosis factor-α (TNF-α), interleukin-8 (IL-8) and granulocyte-macrophage colony stimulating factor (GM-CSF). Glucocorticoids reverse this by binding to glucocorticoid receptors (GR) and recruiting histone deacetylase-2 (HDAC2). This reverses the histone acetylation induced by NF-κB and switches off the activated inflammatory genes. In COPD and smoking asthmatic patients cigarette smoke generates oxidative stress (acting through the formation of peroxynitrite) to impair the activity of HDAC2. This amplifies the inflammatory response to NF-κB activation, but also reduces the anti-inflammatory effect of glucocorticoids, as HDAC2 is now unable to reverse histone acetylation. A similar mechanism may operate in severe asthma where increased oxidative stress is generated by airway inflammation.

in a marked reduction in effect comparable to that seen in COPD patients, and this is confirmed by our preliminary data[55,56] (Figure 2.8).

Steroid resistance in COPD

Although inhaled glucocorticoids are highly effective in asthma, they provide relatively little therapeutic benefit in COPD, despite the fact that active airway and lung inflammation is present. This may reflect the fact that the inflammation in COPD is not suppressed by glucocorticoids, with no reduction in inflammatory cells, cytokines or proteases in induced sputum even with oral glucocorticoids. Furthermore, histological analysis of peripheral airways of patients with severe COPD shows an intense inflammatory response, despite treatment with high doses of inhaled glucocorticoids.[57] There is increasing evidence for an active steroid resistance mechanism in COPD, as glucocorticoids fail to inhibit cytokines (such as IL-8 and TNF-α) that they normally suppress.[58,59] *In vitro* studies show that cytokine release from alveolar macrophages is markedly resistant to the anti-inflammatory effects of glucocorticoids, compared to cells from normal smokers, and these in turn are more resistant than alveolar macrophages from non-smokers.[60] This lack of response to glucocorticoids may be explained, at least in part, by an inhibitory effect of cigarette smoking and oxidative stress on HDAC function, thus interfering with the critical anti-inflammatory action of glucocorticoids.[61] As discussed above, HDAC2 is required for the deacetylation of activated nuclear GR in order for GR to inhibit NF-κB activity and therefore the expression of inflammatory genes. The reduced activity of HDAC2 in COPD patients is associated with increased acetylation of GR, which may be a major mechanism accounting for corticosteroid resistance in COPD[33] (Figure 2.8). In addition, the increased level of acetylated GR may promote gene activation and gene suppression by binding to GR recognition sequences (GRE) in steroid-sensitive genes, such as genes involved in side effects of corticosteroids.

It is likely that oxidative and nitrative stress in COPD specifically impairs HDAC2,[62] resulting in steroid resistance.[63] Although this is seen in all stages of COPD it is most marked in patients with the most severe disease.[64] Even in patients with COPD who have stopped smoking the steroid resistance persists and these patients are known to have continuing oxidative stress. Oxidative stress is also increased in patients with severe asthma and during exacerbations, so that a reduction in HDAC may also account for the reduced responsiveness to glucocorticoids in these patients and the relative unresponsiveness of an acute exacerbation of asthma to glucocorticoids.[65]

2.9   Interaction with β_2-adrenergic receptors

Inhaled β_2-agonists and glucocorticoids are frequently used together in the control of asthma, and it is now recognized that there are important molecular interactions between these two classes of drug.[66] As discussed above, glucocorticoids increase the gene transcription of β_2-receptors, resulting in increased expression of cell surface receptors. This has been demonstrated in human lung *in vitro*[67] and nasal mucosa *in vivo* after topical application of a glucocorticoid.[68] In this way glucocorticoids protect against the downregulation of β_2-receptors after long-term administration.[69] This may be important for the non-bronchodilator effects of β_2-agonists, such as mast cell stabilization. Glucocorticoids may also enhance the coupling of β_2-receptors to G-proteins, thus enhancing β_2-agonist effects and reversing the uncoupling of β_2-receptors that may occur in response to inflammatory mediators, such as interleukin-1β, through a stimulatory effect on a G-protein coupled receptor kinase.[70]

There is also evidence that β_2-agonists may affect GR and thus enhance the anti-inflammatory effects of glucocorticoids. β_2-agonists increase the translocation of GR from cytoplasm to the nucleus after activation by glucocorticoids.[71] This effect has now been demonstrated in sputum macrophages of asthmatic patients after an inhaled glucocorticoid and inhaled long-acting β_2-agonist.[72] This suggests that β_2-agonists and glucocorticoids enhance each other's beneficial effects in asthma therapy.

2.10   Conclusions

There is now a much better understanding of how glucocorticoids act so effectively in asthma and also why they are relatively ineffective in COPD, based on a better understanding of their molecular mechanisms. Glucocorticoids exert their anti-inflammatory effects through influencing multiple signal transduction and gene expression pathways. Their most important action is switching off multiple activated inflammatory genes through inhibition of HAT and recruitment of HDAC2 activity to the inflammatory gene transcriptional complex. In addition, glucocorticoids may activate several anti-inflammatory genes and increase the degradation of mRNA encoding certain inflammatory proteins. This broad array of actions may account for the striking efficacy of glucocorticoids in complex inflammatory diseases such as asthma and the difficulty in finding alternative anti-inflammatory drugs. There is now a better understanding of how the responsiveness to glucocorticoids is reduced in severe asthma, asthmatic patients who smoke and in patients with COPD. An important mechanism now emerging is a reduction in HDAC2 activity as a result of oxidative stress. There is a two-way interaction between GR and β_2-adrenoceptors since glucocorticoids increase the expression of β_2-receptors, whereas β_2-agonists increase GR nuclear translocation and may thereby enhance the anti-inflammatory effects of glucocorticoids. These new insights into glucocorticoid action may lead to new approaches to treating inflammatory lung diseases and in particular to increasing efficacy of steroids in situations where they are less effective.

References

1. Barnes PJ. New drugs for asthma. Nat Rev Drug Discov 2004;3:831–44.
2. Rhen T, Cidlowski JA. Antiinflammatory action of glucocorticoids – new mechanisms for old drugs. New Engl J Med 2005;353:1711–23.
3. Barnes PJ. How corticosteroids control inflammation. Br J Pharmacol 2006;148:245–54.
4. Barnes PJ. Immunology of asthma and chronic obstructive pulmonary disease. Nat Immunol Rev 2008;8:183–92.
5. Barnes PJ, Chung KF, Page CP. Inflammatory mediators of asthma: an update. Pharmacol Rev 1998;50:515–96.
6. Barnes PJ. Transcription factors in airway diseases. Lab Invest 2006;86:867–72.
7. Kouzarides T. Chromatin modifications and their function. Cell 2007;128:693–705.
8. Barnes PJ, Adcock IM, Ito K. Histone acetylation and deacetylation: importance in inflammatory lung diseases. Eur Respir J 2005;25:552–63.
9. Adcock IM, Ford P, Barnes PJ, Ito K. Epigenetics and airways disease. Respir Res 2006;7:21.

10. Ito K, Barnes PJ, Adcock IM. Glucocorticoid receptor recruitment of histone deacetylase 2 inhibits IL-1β-induced histone H4 acetylation on lysines 8 and 12. Mol Cell Biol 2000;20:6891–903.

11. de Ruijter AJ, van Gennip AH, Caron HN, Kemp S, van Kuilenburg AB. Histone deacetylases (HDACs): characterization of the classical HDAC family. Biochem J 2003;370:737–49.

12. Thiagalingam S, Cheng KH, Lee HJ, Mineva N, Thiagalingam A, Ponte JF. Histone deacetylases: unique players in shaping the epigenetic histone code. Ann N Y Acad Sci 2003;983:84–100.

13. Peterson CL. HDACs at work: everyone doing their part. Mol Cell 2002;9:921–2.

14. Ito K, Caramori G, Lim S, et al. Expression and activity of histone deacetylases (HDACs) in human asthmatic airways. Am J Respir Crit Care Med 2002;166:392–6.

15. Lonard DM, Lanz RB, O'Malley BW. Nuclear receptor coregulators and human disease. Endocr Rev 2007;28:575–87.

16. Wu B, Li P, Liu Y, et al. 3D structure of human FK506-binding protein 52: implications for the assembly of the glucocorticoid receptor/Hsp90/immunophilin heterocomplex. Proc Natl Acad Sci U S A 2004;101:8348–53.

17. Lu NZ, Cidlowski JA. The origin and functions of multiple human glucocorticoid receptor isoforms. Ann N Y Acad Sci 2004;1024:102–23.

18. Lewis-Tuffin LJ, Cidlowski JA. The physiology of human glucocorticoid receptor beta (hGRbeta) and glucocorticoid resistance. Ann N Y Acad Sci 2006;1069:1–9.

19. Ismaili N, Garabedian MJ. Modulation of glucocorticoid receptor function via phosphorylation. Ann N Y Acad Sci 2004;1024:86–101.

20. Dostert A, Heinzel T. Negative glucocorticoid receptor response elements and their role in glucocorticoid action. Curr Pharm Des 2004;10:2807–16.

21. Kurihara I, Shibata H, Suzuki T, et al. Expression and regulation of nuclear receptor coactivators in glucocorticoid action. Mol Cell Endocrinol 2002;189:181–9.

22. Hall SE, Lim S, Witherden IR, et al. Lung type II cell and macrophage annexin I release: differential effects of two glucocorticoids. Am J Physiol 1999;276:L114–L121.

23. Newton R, Hart LA, Stevens DA, et al. Effect of dexamethasone on interleukin-1β-IL-1β)-induced nuclear factor-kB (NF-kB) and kB-dependent transcription in epithelial cells. Eur J Biochem 1998;254:81–9.

24. Mittelstadt PR, Ashwell JD. Inhibition of AP-1 by the glucocorticoid-inducible protein GILZ. J Biol Chem 2001;276:29603–10.

25. Lasa M, Abraham SM, Boucheron C, Saklatvala J, Clark AR. Dexamethasone causes sustained expression of mitogen-activated protein kinase (MAPK) phosphatase 1 and phosphatase-mediated inhibition of MAPK p38. Mol Cell Biol 2002;22:7802–11.

26. Reichardt HM, Tuckermann JP, Gottlicher M, et al. Repression of inflammatory responses in the absence of DNA binding by the glucocorticoid receptor. EMBO J 2001;20:7168–73.

27. Hart L, Lim S, Adcock I, Barnes PJ, Chung KF. Effects of inhaled corticosteroid therapy on expression and DNA-binding activity of nuclear factor-kB in asthma. Am J Respir Crit Care Med 2000;161:224–31.

28. Ito K, Adcock IM, Barnes PJ. Knockout of histone deacetylase-2 by RNA interference enhances inflammatory gene expression and reduces glucocorticoid sensitivity in human epithelial cells. Am J Respir Crit Care Med 2004;169:A847.

29. Peterson CL, Laniel MA. Histones and histone modifications. Curr Biol 2004;14:R546–R551.

30. Kagoshima M, Wilcke T, Ito K, et al. Glucocorticoid-mediated transrepression is regulated by histone acetylation and DNA methylation. Eur J Pharmacol 2001;429:327–34.

31. Wang Y, Fischle W, Cheung W, Jacobs S, Khorasanizadeh S, Allis CD. Beyond the double helix: writing and reading the histone code. Novartis Found Symp 2004;259:3–17.
32. Popov VM, Wang C, Shirley LA, et al. The functional significance of nuclear receptor acetylation. Steroids 2007;72:221–30.
33. Ito K, Yamamura S, Essilfie-Quaye S, et al. Histone deacetylase 2-mediated deacetylation of the glucocorticoid receptor enables NF-κB suppression. J Exp Med 2006;203:7–13.
34. Anderson P, Phillips K, Stoecklin G, Kedersha N. Post-transcriptional regulation of proinflammatory proteins. J Leukoc Biol 2004;76:42–7.
35. Dean JL, Sully G, Clark AR, Saklatvala J. The involvement of AU-rich element-binding proteins in p38 mitogen-activated protein kinase pathway-mediated mRNA stabilisation. Cell Signal 2004;16:1113–21.
36. Bergmann M, Barnes PJ, Newton R. Molecular regulation of granulocyte macrophage colony-stimulating factor in human lung epithelial cells by interleukin (IL)-1β, IL-4, and IL-13 involves both transcriptional and post-transcriptional mechanisms. Am J Respir Cell Mol Biol 2000;22:582–9.
37. Newton R, Staples KJ, Hart L, Barnes PJ, Bergmann MW. GM-CSF expression in pulmonary epithelial cells is regulated negatively by posttranscriptional mechanisms. Biochem Biophys Res Commun 2001;287:249–53.
38. Bergmann MW, Staples KJ, Smith SJ, Barnes PJ, Newton R. Glucocorticoid inhibition of GM-CSF from T cells is independent of control by NF-κB and CLE0. Am J Respir Cell Mol Biol 2004;30:555–63.
39. Barnes PJ. Corticosteroid effects on cell signalling. Eur Respir J 2006;27:413–26.
40. Barnes PJ. Cortoicosteroid effects on cell signalling. Eur Respir J 2006;27(2):413–26.
41. Clark AR. MAP kinase phosphatase 1: a novel mediator of biological effects of glucocorticoids? J Endocrinol 2003;178:5–12.
42. Engelbrecht Y, de Wet H, Horsch K, Langeveldt CR, Hough FS, Hulley PA. Glucocorticoids induce rapid up-regulation of mitogen-activated protein kinase phosphatase-1 and dephosphorylation of extracellular signal-regulated kinase and impair proliferation in human and mouse osteoblast cell lines. Endo 2003;144:412–22.
43. Adcock IM, Lane SJ. Corticosteroid-insensitive asthma: molecular mechanisms. J Endocrinol 2003;178:347–55.
44. Leung DY, Bloom JW. Update on glucocorticoid action and resistance. J Allergy Clin Immunol 2003;111:3–22.
45. Adcock IM, Lane SJ, Brown CA, Lee TH, Barnes PJ. Abnormal glucocorticoid receptor/AP-1 interaction in steroid resistant asthma. J Exp Med 1995;182:1951–8.
46. Irusen E, Matthews JG, Takahashi A, Barnes PJ, Chung KF, Adcock IM. p38 Mitogen-activated protein kinase-induced glucocorticoid receptor phosphorylation reduces its activity: Role in steroid-insensitive asthma. J Allergy Clin Immunol 2002;109:649–57.
47. Hamid QA, Wenzel SE, Hauk PJ, et al. Increased glucocorticoid receptor beta in airway cells of glucocorticoid-insensitive asthma. Am J Respir Crit Care Med 1999;159:1600–4.
48. Gagliardo R, Chanez P, Vignola AM, et al. Glucocorticoid receptor alpha and beta in glucocorticoid dependent asthma. Am J Respir Crit Care Med 2000;162:7–13.
49. Torrego A, Pujols L, Roca-Ferrer J, Mullol J, Xaubet A, Picado C. Glucocorticoid receptor isoforms alpha and beta in in vitro cytokine-induced glucocorticoid insensitivity. Am J Respir Crit Care Med 2004;170:420–5.
50. Sousa AR, Lane SJ, Soh C, Lee TH. In vivo resistance to corticosteroids in bronchial asthma is associated with enhanced phosphorylation of JUN N-terminal kinase and failure of

prednisolone to inhibit JUN N-terminal kinase phosphorylation. J Allergy Clin Immunol 1999; 104:565–74.

51. Matthews JG, Ito K, Barnes PJ, Adcock IM. Defective glucocorticoid receptor nuclear translocation and altered histone acetylation patterns in glucocorticoid-resistant patients. J Allergy Clin Immunol 2004;113:1100–8.

52. Galigniana MD, Piwien-Pilipuk G, Assreuy J. Inhibition of glucocorticoid receptor binding by nitric oxide. Mol Pharmacol 1999;55:317–23.

53. Szatmary Z, Garabedian MJ, Vilcek J. Inhibition of glucocorticoid receptor-mediated transcriptional activation by p38 mitogen-activated protein (MAP) kinase. J Biol Chem 2004;279: 43708–15.

54. Thomson NC, Spears M. The influence of smoking on the treatment response in patients with asthma. Curr Opin Allergy Clin Immunol 2005;5:57–63.

55. Murahidy A, Ito M, Adcock IM, Barnes PJ, Ito K. Reduction in histone deacetylase expression and activity in smoking asthmatics: a mechanism of steroid resistance. Proc Amer Thorac Soc 2005;2:A889.

56. Ahmad T, Barnes PJ, Adcock IM. Overcoming steroid insensitivity in smoking asthmatics. Curr Opin Investig Drugs 2008;9:470–7.

57. Hogg JC, Chu F, Utokaparch S, et al. The nature of small-airway obstruction in chronic obstructive pulmonary disease. N Engl J Med 2004;350:2645–53.

58. Keatings VM, Jatakanon A, Worsdell YM, Barnes PJ. Effects of inhaled and oral glucocorticoids on inflammatory indices in asthma and COPD. Am J Respir Crit Care Med 1997;155: 542–8.

59. Culpitt SV, Nightingale JA, Barnes PJ. Effect of high dose inhaled steroid on cells, cytokines and proteases in induced sputum in chronic obstructive pulmonary disease. Am J Respir Crit Care Med 1999;160:1635–9.

60. Culpitt SV, Rogers DF, Shah P, et al. Impaired inhibition by dexamethasone of cytokine release by alveolar macrophages from patients with chronic obstructive pulmonary disease. Am J Respir Crit Care Med 2003;167:24–31.

61. Ito K, Lim S, Caramori G, Chung KF, Barnes PJ, Adcock IM. Cigarette smoking reduces histone deacetylase 2 expression, enhances cytokine expression and inhibits glucocorticoid actions in alveolar macrophages. FASEB J 2001;15:1100–2.

62. Ito K, Tomita T, Barnes PJ, Adcock IM. Oxidative stress reduces histone deacetylase (HDAC)2 activity and enhances IL-8 gene expression: role of tyrosine nitration. Biochem Biophys Res Commun 2004;315:240–5.

63. Barnes PJ, Ito K, Adcock IM. A mechanism of corticosteroid resistance in COPD: inactivation of histone deacetylase. Lancet 2004;363:731–3.

64. Ito K, Ito M, Elliott WM, et al. Decreased histone deacetylase activity in chronic obstructive pulmonary disease. N Engl J Med 2005;352:1967–76.

65. Bhavsar P, Hew M, Khorasani N, et al. Relative corticosteroid insensitivity of alveolar macrophages in severe asthma compared to non-severe asthma. Thorax 2008;63(9):784–90.

66. Barnes PJ. Scientific rationale for inhaled combination therapy with long-acting beta-2-agonists and corticosteroids. Eur Respir J 2002;19:182–91.

67. Mak JCW, Nishikawa M, Barnes PJ. Glucocorticosteroids increase β_2-adrenergic receptor transcription in human lung. Am J Physiol 1995;12:L41–L46.

68. Baraniuk JN, Ali M, Brody D, et al. Glucocorticoids induce β_2-adrenergic receptor function in human nasal mucosa. Am J Respir Crit Care Med 1997;155:704–10.

69. Mak JCW, Nishikawa M, Shirasaki H, Miyayasu K, Barnes PJ. Protective effects of a glucocorticoid on down-regulation of pulmonary β_2-adrenergic receptors in vivo. J Clin Invest 1995;96:99–106.

70. Mak JC, Chuang TT, Harris CA, Barnes PJ. Increased expression of G protein-coupled receptor kinases in cystic fibrosis lung. Eur J Pharmacol 2002;436:165–72.

71. Roth M, Johnson PR, Rudiger JJ, et al. Interaction between glucocorticoids and beta-2-agonists on bronchial airway smooth muscle cells through synchronised cellular signalling. Lancet 2002;360:1293–9.

72. Usmani OS, Ito K, Maneechotesuwan K, et al. Glucocorticoid receptor nuclear translocation in airway cells following inhaled combination therapy. Am J Respir Crit Care Med 2005;172: 704–12.

3

Inhaled corticosteroids: clinical effects in asthma and COPD

Paul M. O'Byrne and Desmond M. Murphy

Firestone Institute for Respiratory Health, St Joseph's Hospital, Department of Medicine, McMaster University, Ontario, Canada

3.1 Introduction

Corticosteroids have been used to treat a variety of lung diseases since the early 1950s, when the benefits of oral cortisone were first reported both for hay fever and asthma induced by ragweed pollen, and the benefits of inhaled cortisone were reported in a small group of patients who had allergic or non-allergic asthma.[1] Subsequently, a placebo-controlled, multi-centre trial run by the Medical Research Council in the UK in 1956, demonstrated improvement in acute, severe asthma[2] with steroids, and a report at that time also described clinical benefit with their use in chronic asthmatics.[3] Subsequently, both oral and inhaled corticosteroids have evolved into the most important drugs currently available to treat many lung diseases, but especially asthma.[4,5] Inhaled corticosteroids are currently the most effective treatment for asthma and the most widely used regular treatment for airway disease.

3.2 Anti-inflammatory activity of corticosteroids

Most of the actions of corticosteroids, and almost certainly their anti-inflammatory activity, occur through activation of the glucocorticosteroid receptor (GR), which is found in virtually all of the body's cells. The GR, in the resting state, is bound to two molecules of heat shock protein-90 (HSP90) and one molecule of immunophilin p59. Binding of the corticosteroid to the receptor dissociates the receptor from HSP90, causing a conformational change in the receptor complex. This in turn facilitates corticosteroid–receptor complex binding to the promoter-enhancer regions of target genes, the glucocorticosteroid response elements, with resultant upregulation or downregulation of the gene, and thereby of the gene product.

Advances in Combination Therapy for Asthma and COPD, First Edition. Edited by Jan Lötvall.
© 2012 John Wiley & Sons, Ltd. Published 2012 by John Wiley & Sons, Ltd.

The corticosteroid–receptor complex can regulate gene product in a variety of different ways. First, the complex can bind directly (by protein–protein interaction) with transcription factors, such as activator protein-1 (AP-1) (which is unregulated during inflammation), and thereby inhibit the proinflammatory effects of a variety of cytokines. Second, the complex can bind to glucocorticoid response elements that overlap with the upregulatory site for another proinflammatory product (i.e. a cytokine), thereby causing downstream anti-inflammatory effects. Third, the complex is known to reduce the availability of another important transcription factor for cytokine production, nuclear factor-κB (NF-κB). Fourth, glucocorticosteroids can increase the levels of cell ribonucleases, and thereby reduce the levels of messenger RNA of potential inflammatory mediators. However, the main mode by which corticosteroids suppress inflammation is probably through switching off the ability of transcription factors such as NF-κB, AP-1, signal transducer and activation of transcription (STAT), and nuclear factor of activated T-cells (NF-AT) to induce inflammatory genes by effects downstream of DNA binding, thereby reducing the ability of these factors to induce histone modifications and chromatin remodelling. Modification of core histones, around which DNA is wound within the chromosomes, plays a critical role in determining which genes are activated and which genes are repressed. Histone acetylation affects gene transcription and is controlled by histone acetyltransferases (HATs). In contrast, histone deacetylases (HDACs), which remove the acetyl groups from hyperacetylated histones, counteract the effects of HATs and return histone to its basal state, with the concomitant suppression of gene transcription.[6] Thus, inflammatory genes, activated by inflammatory stimuli, result in increased levels of I-κB kinase-2 (IKK2), which in turn activates NF-κB. This results in acetylation of lysines in core histone H4, resulting in increased expression of genes encoding proinflammatory proteins. After activation by corticosteroids, GRs translocate to the nucleus and bind to coactivators to directly inhibit HAT activity, and histone deacetylases (HDAC) are recruited. This causes histone acetylation reversal, thereby shifting the balance of the system towards the suppression of inflammatory genes[7] (Figure 3.1a). By contrast, high doses of corticosteroids can activate genes, by binding to GRs, which then translocate to the nucleus, where they bind to glucocorticoid response elements (GRE) in the promoter region of steroid-sensitive genes and also directly or indirectly to coactivator molecules, such as CREB-binding protein (CBP), p300/CBP activating factor (PCAF) or steroid receptor coactivator-1 (SRC-1). These coactivator molecules have intrinsic histone acetyltransferase (HAT) activity, which causes acetylation of lysines on histone H4, and ultimately leads to activation of genes encoding anti-inflammatory proteins (Figure 3.1b).

3.3 Routes of administration

Corticosteroids are administered either systemically (orally or intravenously) or by inhalation to treat lung diseases. Systemic administration is generally reserved for patients who have severe asthma, as a trial of therapy in an attempt to optimize lung

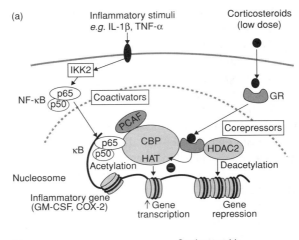

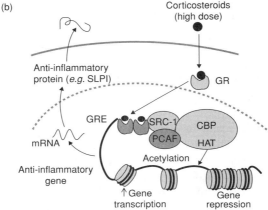

Figure 3.1   (a) Inflammatory gene suppression by corticosteroids. Inflammatory genes are activated by inflammatory stimuli, such as interleukin-1β (IL-1β) or tumour necrosis factor-α (TNF-α), resulting in activation of inhibitor of κB kinase-2 (IKK2), which activates the transcription factor nuclear factor-κB (NF-κB). A heterodimer composed of p50 and p65 NF-κB proteins translocates to the nucleus and binds to specific κB recognition sites and also to coactivators, such as CREB-binding protein (CBP) or p300/CBP-activating factor (PCAF), which have intrinsic histone acetyltransferase (HAT) activity. This causes acetylation of lysines in core histone H4, resulting in increased expression of genes encoding inflammatory proteins, such as granulocyte-macrophage colony-stimulating factor (GM-CSF). After activation by corticosteroids, glucocorticoid receptors (GR) translocate to the nucleus and bind to coactivators to directly inhibit HAT activity, and histone deacetylases (HDAC) are recruited, thus resulting in histone acetylation reversal leading to the suppression of inflammatory genes. (b) Gene activation by corticosteroids. Corticosteroids bind to cytoplasmic GR, which translocate to the nucleus, where they bind to glucocorticoid response elements (GRE) in the promoter region of steroid-sensitive genes and also directly or indirectly to coactivator molecules, such as CBP, PCAF or steroid-receptor coactivator-1 (SRC-1), which have intrinsic HAT activity. This causes acetylation of lysines on histone H4, leading to activation of genes encoding anti-inflammatory proteins, such as secretory leukoprotease inhibitor (SLPI). COX-2, cyclo-oxygenase-2. Reproduced with permission from Adcock IM, Ito K, Barnes PJ. Histone deacetylation: an important mechanism in inflammatory lung diseases. COPD 2005;2(4):445–455.

function in patients thought to have a component of fixed airflow obstruction, or in patients with a predominantly peripheral lung disease such as sarcoidosis.

Corticosteroids, such as prednisone or methylprednisolone, are rapidly and completely absorbed across the gastrointestinal tract and thus have a very high oral bioavailability. Therefore, intravenous glucocorticosteroids need only be used to treat airway diseases in exceptional circumstances, such as for patients who cannot swallow or who are vomiting. The majority of severe exacerbations of asthma can be treated adequately with oral prednisone (0.5–1 mg/kg/day, or its equivalent).

Inhaled corticosteroids are the preferred route to treat airway diseases because of the availability of topically potent corticosteroids, which are very effective and have a far more favourable side-effect profile than systemically administered corticosteroids. Toogood et al. showed this best in studies that compared clinically equivalent doses of inhaled and oral corticosteroids.[8] These studies suggest that, in patients with moderate to severe asthma, inhaled corticosteroids, such as beclometasone dipropionate (BDP) or budesonide,[9] are as effective as much higher doses of oral corticosteroids, with much less risk of systemic side effects.

3.4   Absorption and fate of corticosteroids

In the 1960s, modification of the hydrocortisone skeleton produced corticosteroids with topical selectivity for dermal application and the treatment of skin diseases. These compounds, betametasone valerate and BDP (highly lipophilic compounds, as are dexamethasone and triamcinolone), were administered by inhalation in the treatment of asthma in the early 1970s, and inhaled corticosteroids have been a mainstay of asthma treatment since. Later, other lipophilic glucocorticosteroids (flunisolide, budesonide, fluticasone propionate, mometasone, ciclesonide) were developed for the treatment of asthma and allergic rhinitis.

The main advantage of lipophilic glucocorticosteroids compared to their hydrophilic counterparts is a very high binding affinity for GR (at least 100 times greater than that of hydrocortisone). In addition, they have a very efficient first-pass hepatic metabolism, which results in an extremely low oral bioavailability, making the inhaled route of drug delivery preferable for these agents. The clearance rates for budesonide and fluticasone propionate (FP), for example, are very close to maximal hepatic clearance, and thus entirely limited by hepatic blood flow (approximately 1.5 L/min); the resultant oral bioavailability via gut absorption for budesonide is 11%,[10] and for fluticasone <1%[10] (Table 3.1). Thus, the systemic bioavailability of these compounds results almost entirely from absorption across the lung epithelium, rather than from the gut epithelium.

3.5   Currently available inhaled corticosteroids

Currently, seven topically active, inhaled corticosteroids are available for the treatment of asthma – BDP, triamcinolone, flunisolide, budesonide, fluticasone, mometasone, and ciclesonide (Table 3.1).

Table 3.1 Pharmacological properties of inhaled corticosteroids.

Corticosteroid	Relative binding affinity[a]	Half-life (h)	Volume of distribution (L/kg)	Clearance (L/min)	Water solubility (mg/mL)	Oral bioavailability (%)	Protein binding (%)
Beclometasone dipropionate (BDP)	0.5–13	NA	NA	NA	0.1–10	NA	87
Budesonide	9.4	2–3	2.7–4.3	0.9–1.3	14	11	88
Flunisolide	1.9	1.6	1.8	10	100	21	80
Fluticasone	18	4–14	3.7–8.9	0.9–1.3	4	<1	90
Triamcinolone	3.6	1.5	1.5	7	40	23	71
Mometasone	12.4	4.5	4.5	0.9	NA	<1	NA
Ciclesonide	12	3.4	10	3.8	1.7	<1	99

NA, not available.
[a] Dexamethasone = 1.

Beclometasone dipropionate (BDP)

Since 1972, BDP has been available by inhalation for the treatment of asthma. It has all of the properties of the other lipophilic corticosteroids; however, because of its early development, very little pharmacokinetic information is available on this compound. Initially, BDP is biotransformed into its active metabolite, beclometasone monopropionate, in the liver, but further metabolism of beclometasone monopropionate appears to be slower than that of the newer, topically active corticosteroids.

Triamcinolone

Triamcinolone has also not been fully characterized with regard to its pharmacokinetics. Its oral bioavailability is 22%, and plasma half-life is 1.5 hours after intravenous administration. Triamcinolone has a moderate affinity for GR (four times that of dexamethasone).

Flunisolide

Flunisolide has an oral bioavailability of 21%, but a lower affinity for GR, being five times lower than budesonide and 10 times lower than FP in human lung tissues. Its plasma half-life after intravenous administration is 1.6 hours, which is almost identical to the half-life of a single inhaled dose, indicating that flunisolide, and indeed all ICS, have no lung metabolism.

Budesonide

The pharmacokinetics of budesonide are the most extensively studied among the ICS to date.[10] Its oral bioavailability is 6–13%, indicating a high first-pass hepatic metabolism, and its plasma clearance of 1.3 L/min is close to the maximal liver clearance. The plasma half-life after intravenous administration is 3 hours. Budesonide has a high binding affinity for GR, being 10 times that of dexamethasone. Budesonide also forms long-chain fatty acid conjugates (through esterification) intracellularly, which provides a 'depot' of budesonide and ensures a prolonged clinical efficacy, allowing the potential for once-daily dosing regimens in some patients.

Fluticasone propionate (FP)

The oral bioavailability of fluticasone is <1%, which is the lowest of the available inhaled corticosteroids. This is due not only to its rapid first-pass liver metabolism (0.87 L/min per 1.73 m^2), but also to its poor absorption across the gut epithelium. The plasma half-life after intravenous administration varies from 3.7 to 14.4 h. This prolonged plasma half-life may be due to its highly lipophilic nature, causing its retention in lipid stores. Also, FP has the highest binding affinity to the GR yet measured, being 18 times that of dexamethasone.

Mometasone

Mometasone is a newer ICS, whose oral bioavailability is <1%. It has a high receptor binding, being 12.4 times that of dexamethasone. Its plasma half-life is 4.5 hours, and it has a volume of distribution of 4.5 L/kg. It has a long duration of clinical activity and is therefore effective in many patients with once-daily dosing.

Ciclesonide

Ciclesonide is the most recently available ICS. It has the unique property among the ICS in being a prodrug, which becomes activated by the actions of esterases in the airways. Its oral bioavailability is <1%, with a receptor affinity 12 times that of dexamethasone. It is the most lipophilic of the ICS and also has the highest serum protein binding (>99%).

3.6   Efficacy in asthma

Inhaled corticosteroids are the mainstay of modern asthma treatment.[4,5] They improve all of the symptoms and physiological abnormalities that characterize asthma, as well as markedly reducing the risks for patients experiencing severe asthma exacerbations.[11] The physiological aspects that benefit from ICS include airflow obstruction and airway hyperresponsiveness.[12] The changes in these parameters occur because of the anti-inflammatory effects of ICS, and in particular their ability to resolve eosinophilic airway inflammation[13] and airway oedema.[14] Also, ICS improve many of the pathological abnormalities that characterize asthma, including the structural changes that occur within the airway epithelium[15] and the observed increased deposition of subepithelial collagen;[16] they also cause a reduction in the airway neovascularization seen in asthma.[17]

Inhaled corticosteroids provide clinical benefit in all categories of asthma severity. Mild intermittent and persistent asthma constitutes the majority of asthmatic patients. Patients with even mild persistent asthma are often not well controlled.[18] Low doses of ICS can often provide ideal asthma control and reduce the risks of severe asthma exacerbations in both children and adults with mild persistent asthma. Intermittent ICS therapy at the time of an exacerbation has also been suggested to be an effective treatment strategy for mild persistent asthma,[19] but is less effective than low-dose regular therapy for most outcomes, both in adults[20,21] and children.[22] Patients who are not ideally controlled on low-dose ICS therapy can be considered to have moderate persistent asthma. In adult patients, the combination of ICS and LABA (usually in a single inhaler) is better than doubling the dose of ICS to improve asthma control and reduce exacerbation risks.[21] If asthma control is not achieved despite the patient taking effective therapy, measurement of the inflammatory response in the airway, using sputum indices as a surrogate, may be helpful in guiding further therapy.[23,24]

Dose–response characteristics of ICS in asthma

To establish the dose–response characteristics of ICS has been very difficult, mainly because these vary greatly between patients, and even vary in the same patient when the disease is mild and more severe. Also, the optimal outcome variable to measure is unclear, as is the time interval to allow between initiation of treatment at any specific dose and measurement of the response (Figure 3.2).[25] The maximal clinical benefit for symptoms or lung function for an ICS can take 6–8 weeks to be achieved,[26] and for some physiological parameters, such as improvements in airway hyperresponsiveness, improvements can continue for up to 1–2 years.[27]

Most studies demonstrate a statistically significant and clinically useful benefit from increasing the inhaled doses of ICS four-fold.[11,28] However, no large and well-designed study has been able to demonstrate a difference between two-fold incremental doses for those outcome variables most often measured in clinical asthma studies (i.e. symptoms and lung function) in the type of patients (those who have mild or moderate asthma) most often studied.[29,30] It appears that patients who have mild-to-moderate asthma have a very steep dose–response curve, and achieve maximal benefit from doses of ICS, such as budesonide or BDP, as low as 200 μg/day. By contrast, patients who have more severe asthma often receive clinical benefit from higher inhaled doses of 800–1600 μg/day.

3.7 Efficacy in COPD

In contrast to the compelling evidence supporting the early use of ICS in persistent asthma, there is much more debate on the balance between the efficacy and safety of ICS in COPD. This is probably because of the different inflammatory mechanisms that operate in asthma and COPD, where COPD is believed to develop because of

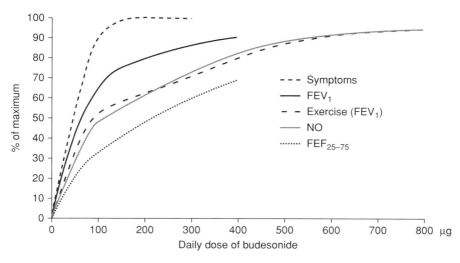

Figure 3.2 Steroid dose–response relationships for various outcome parameters in asthma. The shape of the dose–response curve varies for different outcomes. The dose–response curve for normalization of chronic inflammatory changes in the airways or for maintaining normal growth of lung function is not known. FEF_{25-75}, forced expiratory flow; FEV_1, forced expiratory volume in 1 second; NO, nitric oxide. Reproduced with permission from Barnes PJ, Pedersen S, Busse WW. Efficacy and safety of inhaled corticosteroids. New developments. Am J Respir Crit Care Med 1998;157(3Pt2): S1–53 © American Thoracic Society.

pulmonary inflammation involving predominantly neutrophils and macrophages,[11] with eosinophils playing a much less obvious role than in asthma.

Inhaled corticosteroids have been demonstrated to reduce acute exacerbations of COPD[31,32] and improve health status[33] in patients with severe and very severe COPD (GOLD stages III and IV). For this reason, the Global Initiative for Chronic Obstructive Lung Disease (GOLD) guidelines recommend ICS as add-on treatment to long-acting bronchodilator therapy for stage III and IV COPD.[34] ICS do not, however, reduce the inexorable decline in lung function that occurs in patients with COPD who continue to smoke. This lack of efficacy has been shown in COPD patients at varying stages of their disease.[35–37]

Several studies have demonstrated that the combination of ICS and long-acting inhaled β_2-agonists (LABA) is more effective in reducing COPD exacerbations, improving lung function and health status than either of these components administered alone.[32,38,39] Also, the combination of ICS and LABA reduces lung hyperinflation and improves exercise performance in COPD.[40] A recent large study has evaluated whether the benefits of combination therapy in COPD also extend to a reduction in patient mortality.[41] The study concluded that while there was a reduction in all-cause mortality in the patients treated with the combination of fluticasone and salmeterol, this did not reach statistical significance. The combination therapy significantly improved lung function, and health status (Figure 3.3); however, the hazard ratio for death in the combination therapy group, when compared with the placebo group, was 0.83, with

95% confidence intervals 0.681 to 1.002 (Figure 3.3). This represented a reduction in the risk of death of 17.5%. Thus, it is likely that a real benefit, albeit small, does exist. This effect on mortality was not seen with ICS treatment alone.

3.8   Side effects of ICS

Inhaled corticosteroids are absorbed across the lung into the systemic circulation, and do have effects beyond the lungs. Concerns about their systemic unwanted effects have greatly limited their use, especially in children. The side effects of ICS are dose related, with little or no evidence of clinically relevant, systemic side effects at doses of <400 μg/day of beclometasone or budesonide in children and of <1000 μg/day in adults.[42]

Local side effects

The main side effects that occur with lower doses of ICS are oral candidiasis and dysphonia, because of the oropharyngeal deposition of the inhaled corticosteroid. Clinically obvious oral candidiasis occurs in 5–10% of adult asthmatics treated with inhaled corticosteroids,[43] but in only 1% of children. However, positive oropharyngeal cultures for *Candida* spp. have been demonstrated in up to 45% of children and 70% of adults using corticosteroids.[44] The risk of clinically obvious oral candidiasis is increased by the concomitant use of antibiotics and inhaled corticosteroids, and is greatly reduced by the use of a spacer device to deliver the ICS, and by mouth rinsing after use. Dysphonia is a more common topical side effect of inhaled corticosteroids, which may occur in up to 30% of patients.[45]

Systemic side effects

Doses of inhaled glucocorticosteroids of >400 μg/day in children and of >1000 μg/day in adults may result in unwanted systemic side effects, such as changes in growth velocity in children, and biochemical changes suggesting effects on bone and the adrenal glands in adults. While the clinical significance of these changes is probably unimportant, all physicians who use ICS to treat asthmatics must be aware that these types of adverse effects may develop in their patients.

Effects on the hypothalamic-pituitary-adrenal (HPA) axis

Different ICS are not equal in their effects on the HPA axis. For example, in children a dose-dependent effect of urinary cortisols has been demonstrated with doses of BDP from 200 to 800 μg/day.[46] By contrast, doses of budesonide up to 800 μg/day do not have any effect on urinary cortisols, even when used for up to 1 year.[47] In adults, many studies have examined the effects of ICS on HPA axis function, and no evidence convincingly shows any measurable effect on the HPA axis of doses of BDP

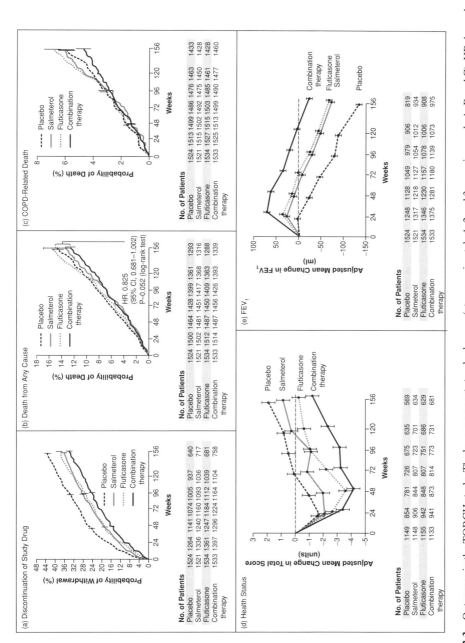

Figure 3.3 Outcomes in the TORCH study. The bars represent standard errors (at approximately 1, 2 and 3 years in panels A, B and C). HR, hazard ratio. Reproduced with permission from Calverley PM, Anderson JA, Celli B et al. Salmeterol and fluticasone propionate and survival in chronic obstructive pulmonary disease. N Engl J Med 2007;356(8):775–789 © Massachusetts Medical Society.

<1500 µg/day and budesonide <1600 µg/day. The measurable effects seen at higher doses[48] indicate systemic activity of ICS, but are of questionable clinical significance.

Osteoporosis

Inhaled corticosteroids can affect bone metabolism, but little evidence indicates that they cause osteoporosis at the conventionally used doses, and no evidence suggests they cause an increased risk of fractures. Bone densitometry has been carried out in adult asthmatic patients taking moderate doses of inhaled BDP,[49] and in COPD patients taking budesonide (800 µg/day).[35] These patients had no increase in bone loss. However, high doses of ICS (>1000 µg/day) are associated with a slight increased risk of non-vertebral fractures in older adults (12% for each 1000 µg/day increase in the dose of BDP or equivalent), but the magnitude of this risk is considerably less than other common risk factors for fracture in older adults.[50]

Posterior subcapsular cataracts

Posterior subcapsular cataracts occur more frequently in patients who take oral corticosteroids, which complicates the issue of whether they occur with greater frequency in patients who use ICS. Once the confounding effect of oral corticosteroids is removed, most studies in adults and children suggest no evidence that ICS increase the risk of developing posterior subcapsular cataracts.[51] One study has, however, indicated that high inhaled doses of BDP are associated with a slightly greater risk of posterior subcapsular cataracts in older patients.[52] This study did not, however, stratify for the confounding risk of allergy for cataract development in this population.

Growth retardation in children

Growth retardation in children as a result of ICS is a major reason for the spared use of these agents (perhaps even under-utilization) in the treatment of paediatric asthma. There is little doubt that systemic corticosteroids can stunt growth in children and that this effect can be permanent. To resolve this issue for ICS in asthmatic children has been exceedingly difficult, in part because asthmatic children do not have the same growth patterns as non-asthmatic children. Many asthmatic children have delayed onset of puberty, which appears more marked in children who have severe asthma.[53] However, eventually these children do catch up with their non-asthmatic peers and achieve normal height.[53] Thus, comparing asthmatic children with non-asthmatic controls may not be entirely appropriate. Also, studies that examine growth in children need to be continued over several years, as individual children have very different growth patterns. ICS do reduce growth velocity in children, even when administered at low doses.[20,22] This effect is maximal during the first year of treatment, and is gone by the third year. This, however, does not result in reduced final height in asthmatic children treated with ICS.[54]

Risks of lung infection

The use of ICS in asthmatic patients does not increase the risk of lung infection, nor the risk of reactivation of pulmonary tuberculosis. In patients with COPD, however, there is evidence that ICS treatment does increase the risk of pneumonia,[41,55] and this risk seems to be greatest in elderly patients with COPD receiving high doses of ICS (>1000 μg/day BDP equivalents).

Skin bruising

Skin bruising does occur as a dose-dependent side effect of ICS use. It is rare at daily doses of <1000 μg/day, and its incidence increases with age and duration of treatment. In one study of older patients on high doses of ICS, the prevalence of easy bruising was 11% for those on ICS and 3.5% for those who were not.[56]

3.9   Conclusions

Inhaled corticosteroids are the mainstay of asthma treatment in all patients with persistent asthma. Their pharmacokinetics, pharmacodynamics and systemic side-effect profile have been the focus of extensive research since their introduction in 1972. The availability of topically potent corticosteroids, with effective first-pass metabolism in the liver, has ensured that efficacy is obtained in almost all patients at doses not associated with clinically relevant, undesired effects. ICS also provide important clinical benefits in COPD, but only when taken together with LABAs and in patients with more severe disease. ICS use in COPD seems to be associated with an additional (albeit small) risk of pneumonia.

References

1. Gelfand ML. Administration of cortisone by the aerosol method in the treatment of bronchial asthma. N Engl J Med 1951;245:293–4.
2. Medical Research Council. Controlled trial of effects of cortisone acetate in status asthmaticus. Lancet 1956;2:803–6.
3. Foulds GS, Greaves DP, Herxheimer H, Kingdom LG. Hydrocortisone in treatment of allergic conjunctivitis, allergic rhinitis, and bronchial asthma. Lancet 1955;1:234–5.
4. Bateman ED, Hurd SS, Barnes PJ et al. Global strategy for asthma management and prevention: GINA executive summary. Eur Respir J 2008;31:143–78.
5. Expert Panel Report 3 (EPR-3): Guidelines for the Diagnosis and Management of Asthma – Summary Report 2007. J Allergy Clin Immunol 2007;120(5 Suppl.):S94–138.
6. Adcock IM, Ito K, Barnes PJ. Histone deacetylation: an important mechanism in inflammatory lung diseases. COPD 2005;2:445–55.
7. Barnes PJ, Adcock IM, Ito K. Histone acetylation and deacetylation: importance in inflammatory lung diseases. Eur Respir J 2005;25:552–63.

8. Toogood JH, Lefcoe NM, Haines DS et al. A graded dose assessment of the efficacy of beclomethasone dipropionate aerosol for severe chronic asthma. J Allergy Clin Immunol 1977;
   59(4):298–308.
9. Toogood JH, Baskerville J, Jennings B, Lefcoe NM, Johansson SA. Bioequivalent doses of budesonide and prednisone in moderate and severe asthma. J Allergy Clin Immunol 1989;84:688–700.
10. Ryrfeldt A, Andersson P, Edsbacker S, Tonnesson M, Davies D, Pauwels R. Pharmacokinetics and
    metabolism of budesonide, a selective glucocorticoid. Eur J Respir Dis Suppl 1982;122:86–95.
11. Pauwels RA, Lofdahl CG, Postma DS et al. Effect of inhaled formoterol and budesonide on exac-
    erbations of asthma. Formoterol and Corticosteroids Establishing Therapy (FACET) International
    Study Group. N Engl J Med 1997;337:1405–11.
12. Juniper EF, Kline PA, Vanzieleghem MA, Ramsdale EH, O'byrne PM, Hargreave FE. Long-
    term effects of budesonide on airway responsiveness and clinical asthma severity in inhaled
    steroid-dependent asthmatics. Eur Respir J 1990;3:1122–7.
13. Brightling CE, Green RH, Pavord ID. Biomarkers predicting response to corticosteroid therapy
    in asthma. Treat Respir Med 2005;4:309–16.
14. Horvath G, Wanner A. Inhaled corticosteroids: effects on the airway vasculature in bronchial
    asthma. Eur Respir J 2006;27:172–87.
15. Laitinen LA, Laitinen A, Haahtela T. A comparative study of the effects of an inhaled corticos-
    teroid, budesonide, and a beta 2-agonist, terbutaline, on airway inflammation in newly diagnosed
    asthma: a randomized, double-blind, parallel-group controlled trial. J Allergy Clin Immunol
    1992;90:32–42.
16. Laitinen A, Altraja A, Kampe M, Linden M, Virtanen I, Laitinen LA. Tenascin is increased in
    airway basement membrane of asthmatics and decreased by an inhaled steroid. Am J Respir Crit
    Care Med 1997;156:951–8.
17. Wilson JW, Stewart AG. Airway vascularity in asthma. Clin Exp Allergy 1999;29:1295–7.
18. Rabe KF, Adachi M, Lai CK et al. Worldwide severity and control of asthma in children and
    adults: the global asthma insights and reality surveys. J Allergy Clin Immunol 2004;114:40–7.
19. Boushey HA, Sorkness CA, King TS et al. Daily versus as-needed corticosteroids for mild
    persistent asthma. N Engl J Med 2005;352:1519–28.
20. Pauwels RA, Pedersen S, Busse WW et al. Early intervention with budesonide in mild persistent
    asthma: a randomised, double-blind trial. Lancet 2003;361:1071–6.
21. O'Byrne PM, Barnes PJ, Rodriguez-Roisin R et al. Low dose inhaled budesonide and for-
    moterol in mild persistent asthma: the OPTIMA randomized trial. Am J Respir Crit Care Med
    2001;164:1392–7.
22. Long-term effects of budesonide or nedocromil in children with asthma. The Childhood Asthma
    Management Program Research Group. N Engl J Med 2000;343:1054–63.
23. Green RH, Brightling CE, McKenna S et al. Asthma exacerbations and sputum eosinophil counts:
    a randomised controlled trial. Lancet 2002;360:1715–21.
24. Jayaram L, Pizzichini MM, Cook RJ et al. Determining asthma treatment by monitoring sputum
    cell counts: effect on exacerbations. Eur Respir J 2006;27:483–94.
25. Barnes PJ, Pedersen S, Busse WW. Efficacy and safety of inhaled corticosteroids. New develop-
    ments. Am J Respir Crit Care Med 1998;157:S1–53.
26. O'Byrne PM, Cuddy L, Taylor DW, Birch S, Morris J, Syrotiuk J. The clinical efficacy and cost
    benefit of inhaled corticosteroids as therapy in patients with mild asthma in primary care practice.
    Can Resp J 1996;3:169–75.
27. van Essen-Zandvliet EE, Hughes MD, Waalkens HJ, Duiverman EJ, Pocock SJ, Kerrebijn KF.
    Effects of 22 months of treatment with inhaled corticosteroids and/or beta-2-agonists on lung

function, airway responsiveness, and symptoms in children with asthma. The Dutch Chronic Non-specific Lung Disease Study Group. Am Rev Respir Dis 1992;146:547–54.

28. Busse WW, Chervinsky P, Condemi J et al. Budesonide delivered by Turbuhaler is effective in a dose-dependent fashion when used in the treatment of adult patients with chronic asthma. J Allergy Clin Immunol 1998;101:457–63.

29. Pedersen S, Hansen OR. Budesonide treatment of moderate and severe asthma in children: a dose-response study. J Allergy Clin Immunol 1995;95:29–33.

30. Dahl R, Lundback B, Malo JL et al. A dose-ranging study of fluticasone propionate in adult patients with moderate asthma. International Study Group. Chest 1993;104:1352–8.

31. Jones PW, Willits LR, Burge PS, Calverley PM. Disease severity and the effect of fluticasone propionate on chronic obstructive pulmonary disease exacerbations. Eur Respir J 2003;21:68–73.

32. Calverley P, Pauwels R, Vestbo J et al. Combined salmeterol and fluticasone in the treatment of chronic obstructive pulmonary disease: a randomised controlled trial. Lancet 2003;361:449–56.

33. Spencer S, Calverley PM, Burge PS, Jones PW. Impact of preventing exacerbations on deterioration of health status in COPD. Eur Respir J 2004;23:698–702.

34. Rabe KF, Hurd S, Anzueto A et al. Global strategy for the diagnosis, management, and prevention of chronic obstructive pulmonary disease: GOLD executive summary. Am J Respir Crit Care Med 2007;176:532–55.

35. Pauwels RA, Lofdahl CG, Laitinen LA et al. Long-term treatment with inhaled budesonide in persons with mild chronic obstructive pulmonary disease who continue smoking. European Respiratory Society Study on Chronic Obstructive Pulmonary Disease. N Engl J Med 1999;340:1948–53.

36. Vestbo J, Sorensen T, Lange P, Brix A, Torre P, Viskum K. Long-term effect of inhaled budesonide in mild and moderate chronic obstructive pulmonary disease: a randomised controlled trial. Lancet 1999;353:1819–23.

37. Burge PS, Calverley PM, Jones PW, Spencer S, Anderson JA, Maslen TK. Randomised, double blind, placebo controlled study of fluticasone propionate in patients with moderate to severe chronic obstructive pulmonary disease: the ISOLDE trial. Brit Med J 2000;320:1297–303.

38. Szafranski W, Cukier A, Ramirez A et al. Efficacy and safety of budesonide/formoterol in the management of chronic obstructive pulmonary disease. Eur Respir J 2003;21:74–81.

39. Mahler DA, Wire P, Horstman D et al. Effectiveness of fluticasone propionate and salmeterol combination delivered via the Diskus device in the treatment of chronic obstructive pulmonary disease. Am J Respir Crit Care Med 2002;166:1084–91.

40. O'Donnell DE, Sciurba F, Celli B et al. Effect of fluticasone propionate/salmeterol on lung hyperinflation and exercise endurance in COPD. Chest 2006;130:647–56.

41. Calverley PM, Anderson JA, Celli B et al. Salmeterol and fluticasone propionate and survival in chronic obstructive pulmonary disease. N Engl J Med 2007;356:775–89.

42. Pedersen S, O'Byrne P. A comparison of the efficacy and safety of inhaled corticosteroids in asthma. Allergy 1997;52(39 Suppl.):1–34.

43. Lefcoe NM, Toogood JH, Blennerhassett G, Baskerville J, Paterson NA. The addition of an aerosol anticholinergic to an oral beta agonist plus theophylline in asthma and bronchitis. A double-blind single dose study. Chest 1982;82:300–5.

44. Toogood JH. Side effects of inhaled corticosteroids. J Allergy Clin Immunol 1998;102:705–13.

45. Toogood JH, Jennings B, Greenway RW, Chuang L. Candidiasis and dysphonia complicating beclomethasone treatment of asthma. J Allergy Clin Immunol 1980;65:145–53.

46. Bisgaard H, Damkjaer NM, Andersen B et al. Adrenal function in children with bronchial asthma treated with beclomethasone dipropionate or budesonide. J Allergy Clin Immunol 1988;81:1088–95.

47. Bisgaard H, Pedersen S, Damkjaer NM, Osterballe O. Adrenal function in asthmatic children treated with inhaled budesonide. Acta Paediatr Scand 1991;80:213–17.

48. Brown PH, Greening AP, Crompton GK. Hypothalamo-pituitary-adrenal axis suppression in asthmatic adults taking high dose beclomethasone dipropionate. Br J Clin Pract 1992;46:102–4.

49. Matsumoto H, Ishihara K, Hasegawa T, Umeda B, Niimi A, Hino M. Effects of inhaled corticosteroid and short courses of oral corticosteroids on bone mineral density in asthmatic patients : a 4-year longitudinal study. Chest 2001;120:1468–73.

50. Weatherall M, James K, Clay J et al. Dose-response relationship for risk of non-vertebral fracture with inhaled corticosteroids. Clin Exp Allergy 2008;38:1451–8.

51. Toogood JH, Markov AE, Baskerville J, Dyson C. Association of ocular cataracts with inhaled and oral steroid therapy during long-term treatment of asthma. J Allergy Clin Immunol 1993;91:571–9.

52. Cumming RG, Mitchell P, Leeder SR. Use of inhaled corticosteroids and the risk of cataracts. N Engl J Med 1997;337:8–14.

53. Balfour-Lynn L. Effect of asthma on growth and puberty. Pediatrician 1987;14:237–41.

54. Agertoft L, Pedersen S. Effect of long-term treatment with inhaled budesonide on adult height in children with asthma. N Engl J Med 2000;343:1064–9.

55. Ernst P, Gonzalez AV, Brassard P, Suissa S. Inhaled corticosteroid use in chronic obstructive pulmonary disease and the risk of hospitalization for pneumonia. Am J Respir Crit Care Med 2007;176:162–6.

56. Tashkin DP, Murray HE, Skeans M, Murray RP. Skin manifestations of inhaled corticosteroids in COPD patients: results from Lung Health Study II. Chest 2004;126:1123–33.

4

LABAs: pharmacology, mechanisms and interaction with anti-inflammatory treatments

Gary P. Anderson

Departments of Pharmacology and Medicine, University of Melbourne, Parkville, Australia

The long-acting β_2-adrenoceptor agonists (LABAs), salmeterol and formoterol (Figure 4.1) were introduced into clinical practice as monotherapies in the closing decade of the twentieth century at a time of great concern about the safety of their antecedents, the short-acting β_2-adrenoceptor agonists (SABAs), and concern they would mask deteriorations of asthma.[1–3] In the ensuing decades a definitive body of very high quality basic and clinical data has supported the progressive introduction of LABAs into evidence-based-medicine clinical guidelines for the treatment of asthma and, in more recent years, of chronic obstructive pulmonary disease (COPD).

Whereas LABAs were originally positioned as tertiary therapy for refractory disease their use, especially as fixed combinations with an inhaled glucocorticosteroid (combination products), has proven to be exceptionally effective, and has seen LABA combinations emerge as the most efficacious therapy currently available for moderate to severe asthma.[4–10] This may not be true of LABAs used alone, a practice not recommended in current international treatment guidelines, although LABAs remain available as mono-products in many countries.[11] More recent data support the use of LABAs in COPD as single agents, in combination with steroids or as part of a triple therapy regime including antimuscarinic agents. Broadly, combinations provide excellent control of most moderately severe asthma and substantially reduce the future risk of exacerbations of all severity grades. The degree of benefit in COPD is less, reflecting the largely irreversible structural basis of airflow limitation and disease-related suppression of human glucocorticosteroid receptor (hGR)-mediated response transduction.

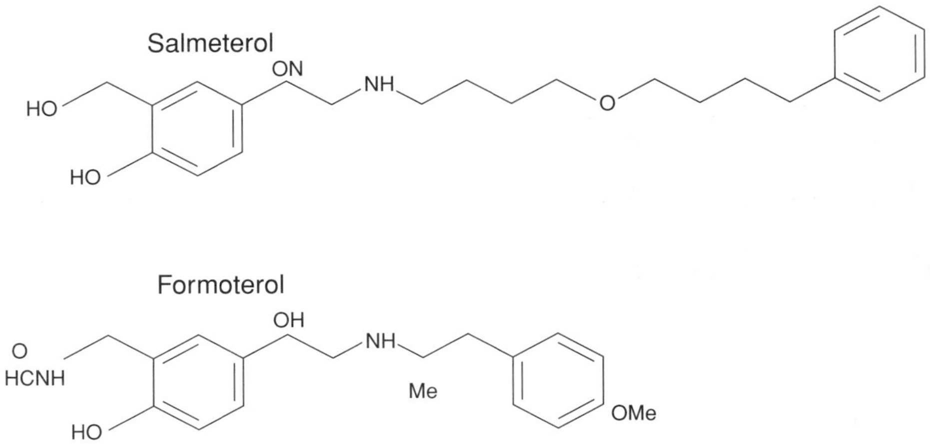

Salmeterol

Formoterol

Figure 4.1   The structure of the classical long-acting β_2-adrenoceptor agonists salmeterol and formoterol.

In asthma, combinations have now accrued more than 70 million patient treatment years and comprehensive analysis of their safety in clinical trial data sets with more than 30 000 patients enrolled, and have demonstrated safety and lack of adverse effect on mortality in asthma. Much less is known about safety in COPD although the data so far indicate no overt LABA-associated adverse safety signals. It is therefore very likely that the number of patients treated with LABAs, especially as combinations, will rise sharply in the coming decades as new generic reformulations become available, thereby further reducing treatment costs.

The clinical effectiveness, safety and attendant commercial success of formoterol and salmeterol used as combinations has been a great spur to the development of other LABAs with once-daily administration profiles, some of which have advanced to phase 3 clinical trials and which, therefore, are likely to be introduced into clinical practice. Carmoterol (formerly TA2005, in development under Chiesi but created by Takeda), has a pharmacological profile comparable with its contemporary formoterol, shows an approximately 10-fold higher potency reflecting highly avid receptor binding, and is lipid membrane avid – the role of membrane interactions is peculiar to LABA pharmacology and is discussed in detail below. Carmoterol binds very avidly to the receptor, possibly preferentially discriminating a particularly effective coupling state.[12–14] Indacaterol (Novartis) is a newly created molecule that has formoterol-like clinical properties but lower efficacy, and interacts with lipid membranes in an analogous manner but works twice as long.[15–20] GlaxoSmithKline (GSK) alone and in partnership with Theravance has been advancing a series of once-daily compounds (including GSK-159797, GSK-597901, GSK-159802, GSK-642444 and GSK-678007) but is yet to disclose the preferred development candidate(s). These compounds are also being developed as combination agents for asthma and also in some cases as combinations with a very-long-acting antimuscarinic agent for the COPD sector.

Given the striking effectiveness of combinations in asthma and growing evidence in COPD, this chapter focuses predominantly on LABAs and the underlying science thought to account for their benefits. While LABAs have classically been viewed as simply longer-acting version of short-acting drugs, there are now definitive data to support the concept that their mode of action, while mediated via the β_2-adrenoceptor, differs substantially from SABAs. Furthermore, there is evidence that LABAs exert beneficial interactions with steroids at the molecular level. LABAs also differ from each other in their fundamental pharmacology.

Clinically the most important properties that need to be understood and compared are:

- onset of action speed;
- duration of action;
- bronchodilation and bronchoprotection profile;
- propensity to induce tachyphylaxis (tolerance);
- influence of polymorphic receptor variants;
- mode of interaction with co-medication, especially steroids, and side-effect profile.

Scientifically, it is important to understand selectivity, efficacy, the mode of onset and duration, 'reassertion' behaviour, physicochemical properties with special reference to cell membrane interactions, receptor downregulation/desensitization and the molecular basis of interaction with anti-inflammatory agents especially steroids.

It is therefore appropriate to review the fundamental pharmacology of LABAs in this chapter. The similarities and differences in the pharmacology of the two LABAs, formoterol and salmeterol, are discussed and the next generation of ultralong-acting LABAs, such as indacaterol, is briefly introduced where it advances our understanding of basic mechanisms. Recent advances in understanding the molecular nature of the β_2-adrenoceptor, its variants and its signalling complexities, including controversial concepts of heterotypical coupling and adverse transduction, are considered. The molecular mechanisms underlying interactions with glucocorticosteroid signalling pathways and interactions with other anti-inflammatory agents are also briefly considered. In addition, a perspective is given on the limits of LABA and combination therapy.

4.1 Galenical forms of LABAs: formulations, isomers, enantiomers, diasteriomers and salts

The clinically marketed formulations of the LABAs formoterol and salmeterol are enantiomeric mixtures of optical isomers with the greatest pharmacological activity residing in the (R)-isomer and (RR)-isomer. Formoterol exists as a pure diasteriomer of (RR)-formoterol and (SS)-formoterol in a 1:1 ratio, and salmeterol comprises an equal mix of (R)- and (S)-isomers. Based on results with the components of the SABA salbutamol (albuterol), concern has been raised about possible adverse effects of (S/SS)-isomers but to date there is no convincing evidence that these have any meaningful effect at all.[21,22] The (S/SS)-isomers of LABAs are approximately 1000-fold less potent than the (R/RR)-isomers but do not inhibit or impair the activity of the (R/RR)-isomers or exert any beneficial or detrimental effects at clinically meaningful concentrations.[23] Arformoterol, which is pure (RR)-formoterol, has no known properties different from formoterol. Advances in chiral synthesis/purification and changes in regulatory requirements anticipated that novel LABAs will be developed as pure optical isomers. As part of patent life cycle management it is not unusual that new salt forms of LABAs are introduced often with exaggerated claims of benefits. While subtle and potentially clinically meaningful pharmacokinetic effects are not precluded, the degree of difference does not warrant separate discussion of the galenical salt forms of LABAs.

4.2   Absolute and functional β_2-adrenoceptor selectivity

β_2-Adrenoceptor agonists are classified by their selectivity, potency and pharmacological efficacy. Potency is less relevant to understanding their *in vivo* pharmacology than selectivity or efficacy because differences in potency are easily compensated for by adjusting inhaled doses whereas efficacy – the maximum effect observed in a given system – is separate from potency.

Three subtypes of human β-adrenoceptors have been unequivocally identified and cloned. For some time it was inferred from receptor binding studies that there might be a fourth subtype,[24] but this is now believed to represent an affinity state variant of the β_1-adrenoceptor. In humans *in vivo* the contemporary LABAs and newer agents in clinical development are so highly selective (>1000-fold) for the β_2-adrenoceptor subtype (Figure 4.2) at the molecular level that they have no clinically discernible or meaningful interaction with other β-adrenoceptors. Formoterol and salmeterol are at least 1000-fold selective for β_2-adrenoceptors compared to β_1-adrenoceptors, which means at clinically used doses they behave as pure β_2-agonists In binding or functional studies they have no discernible activity on any other G-protein-coupled receptor (GPCR) at clinically relevant concentrations. β_3-Adrenoceptors are not expressed in human lung, although they are present in the cardiac atrioventricular conducting system and on adipose tissue. *In vitro* at very high concentrations, formoterol and salmeterol activate the β_3-adrenoceptors although this effect cannot be demonstrated *in vivo*. Neither agent has any discernible β_1 activity *in vivo* at clinically relevant concentrations but interactions can be observed at high concentrations in model systems. The discussion will therefore focus entirely on the β_2-adrenoceptors in relation to LABA action.

Before they were cloned, notional β_1- and β_2-adrenoceptors were defined functionally from difference in activity at the heart (presumptive β_1) and lung (presumptive β_2). It is important to note that very pure molecular β_2-adrenoceptor selectivity does not always equate with classical functional selectivity because both β_1- and β_2-adrenoceptors are found in the human heart and lung. The most important locations relevant to the safety and tolerability profile of LABAs are populations mediating relaxation of peripheral arteriolar resistance vessels (and hence compensatory reflex tachycardia) and a subdominant β_2-adrenoceptor population in the heart mediating both increased rate

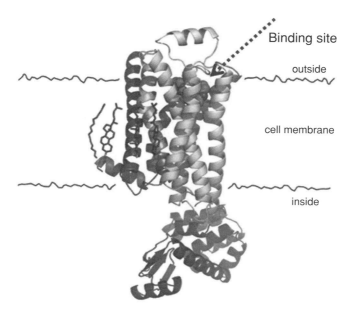

Figure 4.2   The β_2-adrenoceptor subtype structure. Molecules, such as β_2-adrenoceptor agonists, enter the receptor from outside the cell and trigger changes in the receptor structure that lead to a cascade of events inside the cell. Reproduced from http://www.aps.anl.gov/Science/Highlights/2007/20071203.html with permission.

and force of contraction. It is therefore possible for even a pure β_2-adrenoceptor agonist to increase the rate and force of the heartbeat and therefore the heart's workload and oxygen consumption. All β_2-selective adrenoceptor agonists are theoretically arrythmogenic but such disturbances have not been observed in humans during extensive rising dose tolerability and Holter monitoring safety studies.

β_2-Adrenoceptors are not only found on airway smooth muscle but also are very widely expressed elsewhere in the lung including stromal cells, in the vasculature, microcirculation and on the epithelium.[25] β_2-Adrenoceptors are expressed on leucocytes that traffic to the diseased lung, including eosinophils, mast cells, macrophages and lymphocyte subsets, where they mediate suppression of effector functions. β_2-Adrenoceptors are less abundant and less well coupled on these cells than in airway smooth muscle. Outside the lung β_2-adrenoceptors are very widely expressed, including in the brain (where they mediate antidepressive and antinociceptive activity) and on autonomic and sensory peripheral nerve terminals where they can mediate presynaptic suppression of neurotransmitter release. β_2-Adrenoceptors are present on skeletal muscle, where they mediate tremor and uptake of K^+. In experimental animals, but not in humans, high-dose systemic LABAs cause anabolic growth of skeletal muscle, which would be potentially advantageous in COPD. However, the net effect on muscle in humans of inhaled LABAs is to slightly decrease muscle performance by inducing dose-proportional tremor and increasing oxygen consumption without anabolic increases in mass. The hypokalaemia induced by β_2 agonists is compounded by up-take into erythrocytes. In susceptible individuals, β_2-adrenoceptor agonists may affect diabetes and thyroid function, reflecting well-known cautions and contraindications in diabetes and thyroid disease.

As β_2-adrenoceptors are present in the periphery, the detailed pharmacokinetics of LABAs is therefore central to understanding their safety and side-effect profiles. As developed below, it is also essential to consider their microkinetics, that is, partition into cell membranes.

4.3   Cellular organization of receptor clusters: functional structure of the β_2-adrenoceptor and mode of signalling

In receptor visualization studies β_2-adrenoceptor mRNA shows as rather evenly dis-tributed within an individual tissue type in the lung, appearing brightly over epithelium and sparsely but evenly over airway smooth muscle. It is important to note, how-ever, that at the cellular level protein visualization of actual receptor protein reveals a punctuate pattern because the receptors cluster into highly specialized functional membrane domains that are co-enriched for their transduction intermediates. These domains, called 'rafts' or 'lipid rafts', also contain specialized lipid compositions; hence, it is fundamentally important that LABAs are lipophilic/membrane avid and, unlike SABAs, are able to partition into lipid membranes, especially into lipid rafts, as discussed below.

Most textbooks and reviews present a very simple model of β_2-adrenoceptor action using a 'classical key-in-lock' model where the agonist 'turns on' the receptor by occupying a binding pocket. This representation of the β_2-adrenoceptor obscures how this GPCR system actually functions, which is more subtle and complex. A large body of evidence has advanced our understanding of this receptor system, and understanding the specific details of receptor conformation, formation of complexes and disposition in the cell membrane are particularly important to understanding the clinical properties of LABAs and the differences that exist between them.

The β_2-adrenoceptor was the first GPCR to be cloned, and its sequence led to rapid advances in conceptualizing the functional structure of the receptor. In partic-ular, it was immediately apparent from sequence homology that the β_2-adrenoceptor would resemble the 'heptahelical', or seven-transmembrane (7TM), domain structure of bacteriorhodopsin, which had been visualized by electron microscopy and X-ray diffraction in bacterial purple membrane. Accordingly, adrenoceptors belong to the class A 'rhodopsin like' GPCRs.

In receptors of this class the alpha helices formed by the primary amino acid chain intrinsically span the cell membrane and cluster creating an architecture of helical coils loosely bundled to form a central ligand-binding pocket that is open to the extra-cellular aqueous phase.[26, 27] This architecture is not static but rather flexible, moving spontaneously and in response to drugs. Extensive mutagenesis, mapping and specialized ligand-binding studies greatly refined the model and predicted a ligand-binding domain located within the binding core about 11 Å from the surface. This research identified the key amino acid residues that formed the binding topology for agonists and also revealed the unexpected finding that the binding of β-antagonists shows only partial overlap with agonist binding. In addition to classical binding in the ligand core, it is known that the receptor can be pushed into a signalling state by experimental allosteric modulators, which bind to the receptor away from the classical ligand-binding pocket, and also by some chemical reagents, such as reducing agents that attack disulphide bonds, but there are no clinically relevant drugs that work by either of these mechanisms. However, since the β_2-adrenoceptor can form homo- and heterodimers and oligomers, it is possible that the receptor may also exert self-allosterism.

Whereas bacteriorhodopsin was amenable to X-ray diffraction and electron micrographic structural studies, the β_2-adrenoceptor has proved elusive, entirely resisting all efforts to be enriched and crystallized for X-ray diffraction studies in its native state.[28] In 2007 a breakthrough occurred when derivatives of the receptor were created that were genetically engineered with large linking moieties that allowed an artificial extended lattice to form and then to be crystallized in complex with an antagonist, that is, in an inactive state.[29,30] These studies unequivocally validated and confirmed the earlier model, described above, in almost every detail.[31] The studies also suggested (by inference because the receptor was complexed with an antagonist not an agonist and was therefore in an inactive state) the molecular nature of receptor activation and the conformational changes that enable coupling of its intracellular G-protein components with adenylate cyclase and other transduction intermediates.

This model is very close to that originally conceptualized for activation of the β_2-adrenoceptor. A reasonable synthesis of current understanding is as follows: when agonists bind to the active sites of the β_2-adrenoceptor core they change the conformational shape of the receptor, allowing activation of cytoplasmic G proteins, which are signalling intermediates. Classically, this G protein is a stimulatory G protein (G_s), a heterotrimeric protein complex. It is likely that inactive G_s is bound to the inactive β_2-adrenoceptor. Activation occurs when the conformation change in the receptor caused by ligand binding promotes guanosine 5'-diphosphate (GDP) bound to the G_s heterotrimer to be exchanged for GTP. The G_s heterotrimer dissociates into its βγ dimer subunit and an α-subunit. The α-subunit binds and activates effector molecules, typically the enzyme adenylate cyclase. The latter increases cyclic adenosine monophosphate (cAMP) concentrations, activating protein kinase A (PKA), which in turn promotes decreased contractility of airway smooth muscle by reducing calcium levels and inhibiting the activity of myosin light chain kinase (MLCK), the master regulator of contractility. G_s may also activate bronchodilation by activating large-conductance potassium channels (maxi-K channels). However, salmeterol, which is an effective bronchodilator in humans, lacks this property,[32] and the role of maxi-K channels remains disputed. The activation cycle is halted when GTP is converted to GDP, which is a rapid reaction. The rates of activation-deactivation of adenylate cyclase are therefore important determinants of effect. cAMP is hydrolysed by phosphodiesterases.

This model is very consistent with the known properties of formoterol and salmeterol including differential binding to discrete activation states of the receptor that may also relate to differences in efficacy.[33]

It should also be noted that whereas the $\beta\gamma$ subunit was initially considered an inactive chaperone, there is now good evidence that it is active in its own right, and its effects, which include activation of MAP kinases, may not necessarily be advantageous in disease. While it is not a major pathway there is direct evidence that the β_2-adrenoceptor can also, in special circumstances, couple to inhibitory G protein (G_i) entraining the phosphatidyl inositol pathway known to lead to functional antagonism (see below) of G_s signalling.[34] Desensitized receptors that are uncoupled from G_s may also directly activate extracellular signal-regulated kinase (ERK) kinases. The β_2-adrenoceptor may also directly couple to L-type calcium channels, modulating their activity, although the lack of effect of calcium blockers in asthma argues against this as an important bronchodilator pathway.

The system is extremely efficient under normal conditions: when the first definitive ligand binding studies with matched cAMP accumulation measurements were made, researchers were astonished that complete relaxation required <3% fractional receptor occupancy (although this fraction changes in disease).

4.4   Dimers and oligomers: homo- and heterodimerism/oligomerism

One of the most intriguing areas of recent research has been the realization that the β_2-adrenoceptor most likely forms dimer and more complex oligomers. These complexes can be composed of copies of the β_2-adrenoceptor (homomers) but it is also predicted that the β_2-adrenoceptor can form heterodimers with other receptors – complexing with opioid receptors and prostaglandin EP1 receptors has been demonstrated.[35] Very recent studies in which purified monomeric β_2-adrenoceptors labelled with photon-emitting tags that are sensitive to molecular proximity were recomposed into liposomes suggest that the β_2-adrenoceptor has a natural tendency to form homotetramers.

Some models suggest that homodimers are formed when β_2-adrenoceptors exchange transmembrane domains leading to interwoven receptor complexes. Other models suggest that the receptors associate in close proximity but retain their discrete integrity. How signalling functions in these complexes remains uncertain. The existence of heterodimers raises the possibility that a β_2-agonist might bind to the β_2-adrenoceptor but cause an atypical signal via the partner receptor. This, together with the information that the β_2-adrenoceptor can couple to G_i under special conditions,[36] raises the possibility of detrimental, even proinflammatory effects, *in vivo* although in clinical studies the opposite seems true. In studies on the tendency to form tetramers it is currently proposed that the monomeric version of the receptor is a signalling entity and that the complexes may be less able to signal. This inference is based on the observation that the pure β_2 inverse agonist ICI 118 551, which reduces basal cAMP levels, promoted oligomerization of receptors into macrocomplexes, and this may help in understanding the somewhat bizarre 'reassertion' behaviour of LABAs discussed below.

4.5   Pharmacogenomics of the β₂-adrenoceptor and adenylate cyclase polymorphism in relation to LABAs

It has also been known for many years now that the gene encoding the β_2-adrenoceptor is polymorphic, and five variants of the receptor, each with one amino acid altered, have been defined. In theory these five variants predict around 1000 possible combinations, which would be impossible to study systematically in the clinic. The promoter is also polymorphic. However, Liggett and others have demonstrated that the variants are almost invariably inherited in haplotype patterns so that the problem of studying the effects of these polymorphisms is tractable. Genetic defects in β_2-adrenoceptors (and steroid responsiveness) are risk factors for severe asthma.[37] While there is a large body of evidence pointing to effects of these variants on cell trafficking and signalling *in vitro*, any effects that occur in humans and affect LABAs must be subtle and beyond detection or of a nature that is not yet understood. This is because there is very strong evidence based on large studies that β_2-adrenoceptor polymorphisms have no effect on bronchodilation elicited by salmeterol or formoterol, or affect asthma control by LABAs, as we currently understand it today.[38–41] Adenylate cyclase (ADCY) has nine known main isoforms. An AI772M polymorphism affecting the catalytic domain of ADCY9 was associated with a positive beneficial interaction between a SABA and budesonide, but data are lacking on interactions with LABAs.[42]

4.6   Understanding the 'reassertion' paradox, 'exosites' and relative speed of onset: the membrane diffusion microkinetic model of LABA action

All LABAs are by definition long acting and they also, to differing degrees, display a phenomenon called reassertion. 'Reassertion' is where the relaxing effect of the drug can be reversed by a water-soluble β-antagonist, such as sotolol, but reappears (reasserts) after the blocker is washed from the tissue indicating some form of persistence. In the case of salmeterol the duration of reassertion is strikingly long and largely independent of concentration, whereas formoterol displays a shorter and concentration-dependent reassertion behaviour.[43–50]

It is important to note that identification of a novel mechanism of action can offer lucrative patent and reimbursement advantages that may be worth billions of dollars, and there is accordingly intense activity to create and support such concepts. As manufacturers largely finance the evidence base for drug mechanism studies (and the clinical evidence base) this context should be considered when interpreting evidence although there is no doubt that, in the case of LABAs, the scientific standard and integrity of such studies is beyond reproach.

It is clear from the earliest studies that salmeterol was designed as a structural analogue of salbutamol, preserving the active head group and extending a long side-chain with the hope it might bind to a notional 'exosite' – analogous notions had been expressed even in the 1950s. At the time salmeterol was first made (the patent was granted in 1976) this was a brilliant intellectual visualization, but when the drug was introduced and promoted in the 1990s it was already a scientifically untenable concept. The understanding that the β_2-adrenoceptor was rhodopsin-like came in 1986, and a simple comparison of receptor size, position of the binding pocket and the length of salmeterol (about 25 Å) precluded the existence of an exosite external to the β_2-adrenoceptor on first principles. For an exosite to work it would have to bind the aromatic side-chain with high affinity, but the pharmacological evidence precludes this.[51] Despite early evidence of sustained adenylate cyclase activation,[52] subsequent dissociated signalling complex reassembly experiments showed that salmeterol has properties precluding an exosite.[53] Systematic receptor chimerization and molecule arrangement studies did, however, suggest that salmeterol binds to the ligand-binding core of the receptor in an unusual manner and the binding is largely irreversible. Whether these data support the concept of an exosite within the receptor (an intro-exo-site) is more an argument of semantics than science.[45]

The exosite concept was also not adequate to explain other properties of salmeterol or other LABAs. The most widely accepted model of LABA action that accounts for all known properties of LABAs is the membrane diffusion microkinetic model.[16, 27] This model proposes that LABAs do not remain solely in the aqueous phase, the classical diffusion route to the ligand-binding core, but rather incorporate into, to variable degrees, the cell membrane.[54–56] From here they may diffuse to the receptor via lipid or water. Salmeterol, for example, is profoundly membrane avid, because of its long aliphatic side-chain, and adopts a highly specific orientation in the outer plasmalemma layer.[57] Indacaterol has an avidity for lipid raft lipids twice that of salmeterol. Formoterol has a very unusual behaviour in that it is only membrane avid in high concentrations, such as those achieved topically after inhalation, when it then is readily partitioned into lipid membranes. This helps to explain the paradox that formoterol-induced bronchodilation is long acting whereas peripheral side effects, if they occur, are of short duration. Very recent data have refined this concept by showing that the specialized lipids in the rafts where the receptors and their transduction intermediates are clustered are especially avid acceptors of LABAs such as indacaterol. When membrane microkinetics was first proposed it was postulated that some form of functional coupling might help to explain reassertion such that an antagonist bound to one receptor might suppress signalling from a receptor bound with agonist. The existence of receptor dimers and oligomers now provides a structural basis for this concept, which together with competition with LABA in membrane reserves, accounts for 'reassertion'. In fact, reassertion behaviour can be used to find new types of LABAs in screening studies.[58]

Another oddity is that in isolated cells and in dissociated receptor binding studies the rate of onset of action of salmeterol is actually very fast but *in vivo* its action develops very slowly, precluding the use of salmeterol for rescue bronchodilation. Microkinetics helps explain this by simply pointing out that diffusion deep into the bundles of cells that comprise airway smooth muscle is a slow process for profoundly lipid-loving molecules as they cannot permeate into the bundle via the water in the cellular interstices but must rather diffuse laterally within the membrane compartment. This also accounts for the excellent smooth bronchodilator characteristics of salmeterol *in vivo* that make it so well suited for sustained maintenance bronchodilation.[45,53]

4.7 Regulation and desensitization

The β_2-adrenoceptor gene is unusual in that it lacks introns. The promoter has positive response elements for both glucocorticosteroids and cAMP.[59] The promoter is polymorphic suggesting variation in primary transcript levels that might relate to disease, but promoter polymorphism alone or in extended haplotypes does not affect receptor expression or coupling in asthma.[60]

Prolonged exposure to β_2-adrenoceptor agonist leads to desensitization of the response. While the same mechanisms are thought to operate in any cell type where desensitization occurs it is critically important to understand that the mix of effects and the maximal degree of desensitization varies with cell types. Airway smooth muscle in particular is refractory to complete desensitization, which explains why LABAs maintain their bronchodilator effect over years of regular treatment. Activation of cAMP-dependent protein kinases, for example protein kinase A (PKA), also causes feedback phosphorylation of the β_2-adrenoceptor itself. The receptor can also be phosphorylated by G-protein-coupled receptor kinases (GRKs) that recognize activated receptors. Phosphorylation of the receptor has two main consequences. Firstly, the receptor can be quite rapidly translocated into an intracellular vesicle. From here it can either be recycled to the cell surface or targeted for degradation. Phosphorylation also promotes β-arrestin binding, which has two major known effects: it blocks G_s activation and also helps target β_2-adrenoceptors into vesicles by serving as a scaffold for the trafficking adaptor clathrin.[61,62] Very long-term exposure also downregulates β_2-adrenoceptor mRNA leading to reduced surface receptor expression. As the B2ADR gene has a positive cAMP response element mediating increased mRNA transcription after activation the reduction is thought to reflect a translational block and/or an induced instability. It is not clear if this also involves regulation of micro (regulatory) RNAs.

Heterotypical desensitization can also occur when cAMP levels are raised via a different adenylate cyclase coupled GCRP, notably the prostaglandin E_2 (PGE$_2$) receptor. As PGE$_2$ levels spike in infections and are induced by inflammatory cytokines this mechanism has been proposed as a reason for the dampening of beta-agonist responses after disease exacerbation. The process is prevented by steroids and the degree of protected functional relaxation is greater for LABAs with higher efficacy.[63]

Cells such as mast cells, eosinophils and macrophages having fewer β_2-adrenoceptors that may also be less well coupled to signalling, may undergo near complete loss of responsiveness during sustained exposure. In contrast bronchodilation is always preserved. Airway smooth muscle is, however, not entirely privileged as initial exposure also results in a step function decrease in receptor number and probably a decrease in functional coupling. However, this is minor in relation to the very small fraction of receptors that need to be activated to cause bronchodilation. It is therefore important always to study the net effect after regular LABA treatment rather than rely on short-term studies, which appear to overstate the degree of change. While it is a subtle difference, bronchodilation is not the same as bronchoprotection, and it is apparent from clinical studies that loss of protection from methacholine-induced bronchoconstriction, and from exercise-induced bronchoconstriction, is more prominent than changes in the forced expiratory volume in 1 second (FEV_1).[64] Both changes in bronchodilation and bronchoprotection are ameliorated, but not entirely abolished, by concomitant steroid administration. While it is 'intuitive' that more potent LABAs or those with higher efficacy to stimulate signalling (see below) should cause more desensitization, this is not the case. Salmeterol, which has low efficacy, readily downregulates receptors and in several systems its effect is greater than formoterol, a behaviour that may relate to its lipid properties.[65] Salmeterol and formoterol both maintain clinical effect even after years of regular treatment.

In addition to direct homotypical desensitization in response to an agonist active at the β_1-adrenoceptor, this system can also be desensitized indirectly by a process called heterotypical or heterologous desensitization. Here any agent, such as PGE_2 or phosphodiesterase inhibitors that elevate intracellular cAMP, can cause a reciprocal decrease in β_2-adrenoceptor number or function in the same cell. This effect is readily demonstrable *in vitro*,[66] where it can also be linked to PKA activation, but whether it occurs *in vivo* in humans remains highly controversial. A further and extremely intellectually interesting problem is that the β_2-adrenoceptor has been demonstrated to form heterodimers with the PGE_2 receptor EP_1 subtype.

4.8   Full versus partial agonism (pharmacological efficacy)

All currently known synthetic β_2-adrenoceptor agonists are partial agonists, which means they activate signal transduction (e.g. via cAMP) less efficiently and to a lower maximal extent than the natural catecholamine, adrenaline (epinephrine), or the synthetic derivative catecholamine isoprenaline, which are full agonists.[67] Efficacy is a pharmacological term that describes the maximum functional effect seen in a system and therefore varies with the properties of that system (Figure 4.3). The degree of efficacy varies markedly among β_2-agonists but is less discernible in cell types with large numbers of β_2-adrenoceptors or where signal transduction coupling is highly efficient.[68, 69] For this reason, in humans, the spectrum of low to high efficacies is not detectable when direct bronchodilation is measured. However, less efficacious agents do not protect as well against induced bronchoconstriction and are less able to inhibit responses in some inflammatory cells with low surface numbers of receptors, such as the eosinophil.[69] Formoterol has been shown to better protect against methacholine-induced bronchoconstriction in asthmatic humans than salmeterol.[70]

While the new receptor modelling studies are relatively easy to understand in terms of receptor activation, the concept of partial agonism – which to many is incorrectly inferred to be a 'partial' activation of an individual receptor – seems impossible to comprehend since the signal to adenylate cyclase is quantal (caused by an

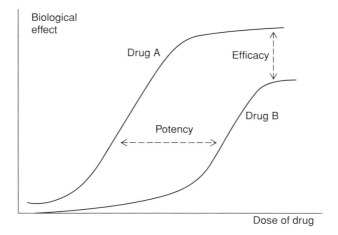

Figure 4.3 Principles of potency and efficacy. Potency reflects the dose of a drug that is required to achieve a certain effect, whereas pharmacological efficacy is related to the maximal effect that can be induced with high doses of the drug. Some β_2-adrenoceptor agonists are highly potent and have greater efficacy than others (see text).

alpha-subunit binding) not continuous. However, the problem is easier to understand when the behaviour of the entire receptor population is considered rather than that of an isolated receptor.

The reason why the β_2-adrenoceptor may never be crystallized in its native state is central to understanding the nature of signal transduction and drug action in relation to receptor function, especially to the concept of partial agonism. It is now understood that the receptor, while having a recognizable architecture, has a fluid conformation and remains spontaneously flexible, alternating between discrete structural/activation states. Formoterol and salmeterol differentially discriminate between these states, and this may reflect differences in their pharmacological efficacy. This has very important implications for understanding drug action because it is the ability of the beta-adrenoceptor to move continually between discrete structural states that determines its affinity for ligands and its ability to signal. It is therefore best to understand drug effects by considering the system as a population of receptors that can be shifted wholly or partly into different net functional affinity and signalling states. Under basal conditions at any instant, even in the absence of ligand, a small fraction of the population will be in the active signalling state. This explains why there is a small spontaneous generation of cAMP and why 'inverse agonists', which freeze the receptor in an inactive conformation, can reduce basal cAMP. It also explains why many cell biology experiments that overexpress the receptor in cell lines are almost worthless for understanding the clinical mode of action of LABAs: expression of an unnaturally high receptor number will automatically increase the apparent effects of these drugs. It is possible, for example, to stimulate a full cellular response in the complete absence of agonist if sufficient receptors are overexpressed artificially, and to convert a weak partial agonist into an apparently full agonist. Indeed, the behaviour of all beta-agonists is strongly affected by receptor number on a cell type and the efficiency with which these receptors are coupled to transduction pathways. For the same degree of fractional occupancy, full agonists can stimulate the maximal functional effects in a given system, partial agonists will hold on a fraction of the receptors in a signalling state, antagonists will have no net effect, and inverse agonists will freeze receptors out of an active state causing basal transduction to fall.

The net effect is not only a function of the intrinsic receptor properties but also profoundly influenced by the nature of individual cells and tissues. For example, when studied objectively under physiological conditions with human airway smooth muscle, formoterol has a higher system efficacy (ability to entrain cAMP signalling and relax the muscle) than salmeterol, which behaves as a 'partial agonist', able to relax the muscle to a lesser extent than formoterol. However, in cell lines where the receptor has been overexpresssed, salmeterol can be made to behave as a full agonist. Whereas salmeterol is a partial agonist on airway smooth muscle *in vitro* it has no efficacy mediated by β_2-adrenoceptors on cells such as eosinophils and macrophages because these cells have lower receptor numbers and/or less effective coupling. In strictly pharmacological terms, with reference to degree of relaxation of human airway smooth muscle *in vitro*, although formoterol and salmeterol are both very potent, formoterol is a strong partial agonist whereas salmeterol is less efficacious. However, while this effect is discernible on isolated tissue it is not readily apparent in humans *in vivo*, where both formoterol and salmeterol produce near equivalent bronchodilating changes in FEV_1. This means that human airway smooth muscle *in situ* need only lengthen a small degree to induce full bronchodilation.

There are two important functional corollaries of partial agonism. The first is that weak partial agonists also behave as beta-antagonists to an extent inverse to their efficacy. This is because they occupy but do not activate a substantial fraction of receptors at any instant. *In vitro* studies of salmeterol show exactly this behaviour, progressively blocking the effects of a second β_2-agonist as its own concentration increases. Several groups have estimated a formal pA2 (a measure of antagonist potency) for salmeterol. Whereas salmeterol used at clinically relevant doses does not impede rescue bronchodilation by a second beta-agonist, controversy surrounds effects on inflammation as salmeterol blocks the effect of formoterol as a suppressor of inflammatory cytokine release in human monocyte derived macrophages.

The second functional corollary is the degree to which the benefits of individual LABAs are reduced by functional antagonism, especially during disease exacerbations. LABAs appear approximately equivalent in the degree of control of disease they provide when used as combinations. Addition of LABAs to regular steroid therapy produces a striking reduction in the absolute number and severity of disease exacerbations, which is preserved over time. The cause of these exacerbations was not known. Based on epidemiological studies it is probable that a sizeable fraction was due to viral infections, the most important cause of such changes.

There is very good evidence for beneficial molecular interactions between steroids and LABAs, as detailed below. As many of these effects are subtle, albeit the reduction in exacerbations is striking, it is prudent firstly to consider possible strong effects. On current evidence asthmatics are no more likely than non-asthmatics to suffer viral upper respiratory tract infections (URTIs), but are much more likely to have lung symptoms. It seems unlikely that the combinations or their components fundamentally alter antiviral immunity to decrease the 'hit rate' of such infections. It is therefore more likely that combinations decrease the amplitude of lung function in such events, resulting in fewer symptomatic episodes including fewer severe episodes. As uncontrolled asthma and inflammation is a major predictor of future risk of a symptomatic exacerbation it must be considered that patient adherence to combinations is much higher than to steroids prescribed alone, and that combinations effectively reduce underlying lung inflammation by promoting steroid exposure. While a number of apparent acute 'anti-inflammatory' effects can be demonstrated for both salmeterol and formoterol, neither agent has any impressive effect after regular use in asthmatics when assessed in bronchial biopsies.[71,72] LABAs alone do not reduce the frequency of disease exacerbations, have no ability to suppress controlled exacerbations in volunteers, and may mask patient perception of deteriorating lung function.[2,3] Balanced against this is the now clear evidence that combinations produce better suppression of inflammation than steroids alone in both asthma and COPD. The effect in COPD is of particular interest as smoking or ex-smoking strongly suppresses the activity of steroids in the lungs, and steroids alone have no or very weak anti-inflammatory effects in this disease (and in asthmatics who smoke, who comprise about 30% of the total patient population). The capacity of combinations to suppress neutrophilic inflammation may be of particular importance in both COPD and exacerbations,[73,74] particularly as steroids promote neutrophil survival rather than induce their apoptosis.

Further, if an exacerbation occurs in an inflamed lung it is apparent that bronchoconstriction is more intense because the degree of decline in lung function is greater. Hence, simply by promoting adherence and therefore stabilizing the airway milieu, combinations reduce the chance of strong functional antagonism occurring where the ability of the LABA to relax airway smooth muscle is biochemically impeded.

4.9 Beta-blockers not LABAs?

In a series of studies that are as provocative as they are contrived, Bond and colleagues have advanced the concept of treating asthmatics with beta-antagonists (specifically inverse agonists).[75–77] This concept is based on the idea of reverting decompensated transduction pathways to a more basal or natural state. In mouse asthma models benefits have been shown for some aspects of inflammation and reduction of mucus (induction of mucus is not an adverse effect of LABAs). However, when human mild asthmatics were treated with nadolol in an open study the improvement in provocative concentration reducing FEV_1 with 20% (PC20) was offset by an alarming 5% fall in FEV_1. Given that accidental exposure to beta-blockers in the form of eye drops has been documented as a cause of death there is a natural tendency to dismiss this line of research out of hand. The concept also possesses logical challenges given that salmeterol itself can behave as a beta-blocker on human and animal airway smooth muscle.[78] However, it does underscore the need to understand the β_2-adrenoceptor as a fluid system moving between discrete operational states – we have probably yet to identify the ideal LABA.

4.10   Non-receptor-mediated effects?

In early preclinical studies it was noted that salmeterol exerted non-specific inhibitory effects in the presence of saturating concentrations of beta-antagonists. Salmeterol may in part relax airway smooth muscle and stabilize mediator release in this manner.[43, 79] There are also several cases where the effects of formoterol and salmeterol are very similar but salmeterol produces no detectable change in cAMP or membrane polarity. As LABAs, especially salmeterol, are membrane avid, and this membrane partition has unequivocally been demonstrated to alter membrane physics and fluidity, non-receptor-mediated effects of LABA seem very likely. It should be remembered that the partition of LABAs into lipid is not random – they align in a highly ordered manner in the outer plasmalemma and have particular affinity for lipid rafts. These rafts are also essential for the activation events leading to assembly and function of so-called inflammasomes', especially the so-called NLRP3 (NOD-like receptor containing pyrin domain 3) inflammasome,[80] known to be important in the acute effectors arm of innate and adaptive immune defences and hence in early inflammation. While it is entirely speculative at present, it may be particularly important that the inflammasome is essential for induction of interleukin-1 (IL-1), a cytokine specifically linked with β_2-adrenoceptor uncoupling.

4.11   Biochemical basis of functional antagonism and its critical role in LABA action in disease and exacerbations

Functional antagonism in the context of airway smooth muscle is the ability of a strong contraction to impede the biochemistry of relaxation; this is a major, if not widely appreciated, determinant of responses to all β_2-adrenoceptor agonists. To understand this point it is import to know that even full agonists can be converted to partial agonists when airway smooth muscle is strongly contracted. As airway smooth muscle undergoes progressively stronger contractions, all β_2-adrenoceptor agonists lose potency and efficacy (but only in the lung, not systemically) and weaker partial agonists may entirely fail to relax airway smooth muscle. This is the ultimate basis of the additive interaction between LABAs and antimuscarinic agents or leukotriene modifiers in asthma and COPD.

The biochemistry of this impairment is the accumulation of inositol phosphate (IP). Many inflammatory mediators signal via GPCRs coupled by G_q to this pathway causing accumulation of IP that ultimately leads to activation of blocking pathways, such as activation of calmodulin kinase, which is able to impair adenylate cyclase activation, for example. G_s and G_q pathways are in constant exchange (cross-talk influencing muscle responsiveness).[36] IP levels are directly correlated with the loss of potency of β_2-adrenoceptor agonists. Decreases in β_2-adrenoceptor mRNA, deficient adenylate cyclase activity, and atypical coupling of the β_2-adrenoceptor to G_i rather than G_s and receptor uncoupling from G_s are all predicted to occur from animal models.[81] In severe asthma inhibitory cross-talk between G_i/G_q-coupled inflammatory and contractile mediators that signal via inositol 1,4,5-trisphosphate (IP$_3$)/PKC/diacylglycerol (DAG), such as cysteinyl leukotrienes, acetylcholine, substance P or histamine, can biochemically impair G_s-mediated signal transduction,[82,83] damaging the ability to sustain cAMP accumulation. Hence functional antagonism of this type causes a measurable fall in efficacy of all agonists and can convert near-full agonists to weak partial agonists.[67]

One more mechanism that can worsen still further this reduction in drug effect, especially in poorly controlled disease where there are high levels of inflammatory mediators such as IL-1, is receptor 'uncoupling' from adenylate cyclase. Bai and colleagues confirmed that severe airway inflammation fundamentally impairs the ability of β_2-adrenoceptor agonists to relax airway smooth muscle;[81,84] they demonstrated that the β_2-adrenoceptor uncouples from its transduction pathway in fatal asthma by an unknown mechanism. The molecular basis of uncoupling is incompletely understood but it is mimicked, at least in part, by mediators, notably IL-1 and tumour necrosis factor-(TNF-β),[85] which are likely to be overproduced during sudden exacerbations. This is likely to represent an extreme scenario, as transient exposure to inflammation does not adversely affect β_2-adrenoceptor signalling.[86]

Functional antagonism can be demonstrated clinically, with several studies underscoring its importance. In elegantly simple experiments in asthmatic volunteers, Palmqvist and colleagues have shown that rising doses of formoterol but not salmeterol more completely protect from methacholine-induced bronchoconstriction.[70] In a more disease-focused model, Duong et al. assessed the capacity of formoterol alone or with steroids given immediately after allergen challenge to prevent the late asthmatic response and the associated change in PC20 methacholine.[87] They found that the combination, but not its components alone, was effective. Most asthma exacerbations in which functional antagonism might play a role are triggered by viral infections. In viral exacerbations it is difficult to compare the absolute protection afforded by salmeterol compared to formoterol because the clinical protocols for optimal use of these drugs are quite different.

4.12 Molecular cooperativity between LABAs and steroids

The clinical success of combination products, used in maintenance or maintenance-plus-rescue protocols, has led to great interest in identifying possible molecular pathways that might help explain these somewhat unexpected benefits. The combination effect is particularly striking for reducing the chances of future exacerbations of all severity grades, and this effect is maintained over time. There is now considerable and accumulating evidence of bidirectional steroid–β_2-adrenoceptor cooperativity at the molecular level.[88–90]

Before examining these pathways it should be noted that steroids exert very context-specific effects in asthma, which are likely to vary over the natural history of the disease: steroids, for example, unequivocally strengthen the intensity of type 2 helper T-cell (Th2) immune deviation,[91–95] a defect linked to the early life diathesis as reviewed in detail elsewhere.[96] Steroids also do not exert uniform benefits in asthma or COPD. Steroids suppress basal and cyclo-oxygenase-2 (COX-2)-generated PGE_2 production. PGE_2, acting via G_s-coupled EP2 receptors, is a highly efficacious cAMP inducer.[97,98] In COPD, although suppression of PGE_2 might worsen airflow limitation, it might also reduce future lung cancer risk.

It should also be noted that while the mechanisms discussed below are essentially generic, and therefore should potentiate peripheral side effects as readily as lung benefits, the highly membrane-avid properties of LABAs largely restrict their action to the lung and there is no evidence whatsoever that LABA potentiate the systemic side effects of steroids in asthma or COPD.

It has been known for decades that steroids upregulate β_2-adrenoceptor numbers, and pharmacologists routinely add cortisol to organ bath studies to prevent extraneuronal uptake of catecholamines (modern LABAs are not substrates for this process). Steroids have also recently been shown to prevent inflammatory mediator-induced desensitization/uncoupling in airway smooth muscle. β_2-Adrenoceptors are transcriptionally upregulated by glucocorticosteroids via their positive glucocorticoid response element (GRE), and steroids can reverse, at least partially, the degree of loss of surface receptors that occurs during homologous desensitization to sustained agonist stimulation, even in the case of the weakest partial agonists.[99–103] Steroids increase the binding of agonists to the high-affinity state of the receptor and also promote G_s alpha expression.[104] Steroids also prevent and restore inflammatory mediator-induced uncoupling *in vitro*. In the clinic, in the case of formoterol, oral but not inhaled steroids were shown to protect against loss of protection to methacholine-induced bronchospasm.[105, 106] Inhaled beclometasone attenuated tolerance to the loss of protective effect of salmeterol against allergen challenge.[107]

Much recent work has been catalysed by the very unexpected results of Roth and of Eickenberg and colleagues, who showed that LABAs promote the translocation of hGR into the nucleus of smooth muscle cells in a kinase-dependent manner and, when translocated, induce transcription from a GRE-dependent reporter gene construct in a cell line.[108, 109] These findings raised the possibility of LABAs reinforcing the hGR signal, although there has been much subsequent work examining whether LABAs can directly promote transcription of steroid-sensitive genes from GREs in the absence of steroid. This seems mostly not to be the case, and LABAs are, on current evidence, best considered as agents that may augment or reinforce the action of steroids on some genes or gene families.

These effects are probably mediated by two major classes of action: (i) promoting transit of hGR to the nucleus and probably increasing its net residency time there; and (ii) augmenting GRE-dependent processes. Other effects are not precluded. The net effects are usually small and mostly additive, but sometimes truly synergistic effects have been clearly demonstrated. In general these effects have been cross-replicated for both salmeterol and formoterol, with some difference relating mostly to the lower system efficacy of salmeterol. No one effect seems compelling, and it is most likely that a cumulative net benefit accrues from the sum of individually small effects on many discrete process, none of which is dominant.

To best appreciate the current understanding of these interactions it is useful first to consider the multiple modes of action of glucocorticosteroids.

It is noteworthy that hGR is ancient and is known to have acquired multiple ways of exerting its regulatory effects over eons. hGR is almost ubiquitously expressed in cells and tissues relevant to asthma,[110] and is almost invariably coexpressed on cells bearing β_2-adrenoceptors. Only one hGR gene is known, the NR3C1 gene, consisting of seven core exons (exons 2–8). However, there is increasing awareness of how alternative splicing may give rise to tissue-specific variants including a truncated beta form that lacks the ability to modulate gene transcription but may affect the steroid activity. There are two major exon 8–9 splice variants and an upstream 5′-untranslated region holding 11 splice variants. Other variants are suspected.[111]

The hGR itself is an intracellular receptor, located in the cytoplasm, at rest complexed to heat shock protein (HSP90, HSP70, HSP56) chaperones. This means that steroids must diffuse through the cell membrane in order to bind – it is not known if they affect LABA microkinetics at the level of lipid rafts. While some effects of steroids are independent of receptors, and some hGR effects occur in the cytoplasm, the main biology of steroids is associated with regulation of gene expression at the transcriptional level in the cell nucleus. One level of action is to form a DNA-binding homodimer or bind to other nuclear transcription factors thereby enhancing or repressing their action, for example the proinflammatory transcription factors activator protein-1 (AP-1) (c-Jun/c-Jun homodimer or c-Fos/c-Jun heterodimer) and nuclear factor-κB (NF-κB). Ligand-occupied hGR has been shown to bind physically to AP-1, but this interaction is weak.[112] Alternatively, occupied hGR may competitively bind an essential cofactor needed for AP-1-regulated gene transcription.[113] The proinflammatory transcription factor NF-κB is held inactive in the cytoplasm by physical interaction with its endogenous inhibitor, I-κB.[114, 115] Occupied hGR are thought to inhibit NF-κB by two mechanisms: physical binding to the p65 NF-κB subunit,[116] and induction of I-κB gene transcription.[117] It is theoretically possible that β_2-agonists, via end-effector kinases, might increase the net efficiency of these processes, but the evidence for this is weak and unconvincing.

The human glucocorticoid receptor can also direct binding to DNA and GREs in a process termed 'transcriptional *trans*-activation'. GREs are classically positive regulators of transcription; however, examples of negative GREs are known. Three important examples of positively regulated genes are the β_2-adrenoceptor, anti-inflammatory lipocortin, and I-κB, the intrinsic inhibitor of the proinflammatory transcription factor NF-κB. hGR can therefore largely be considered as a ligand-activated transcription factor or cofactor that operates to alter gene transcription. The work of Eickenberg and colleagues suggested that LABAs might cause hGR translocation and activation of GREs in the absence of ligand. The translocation is unequivocal but GRE activation in the absence of ligand is not convincing and has not been demonstrated *in vivo* – LABAs do not have true steroid-like effects and are not truly steroid sparing. It seems that the major benefit here is promoting and increasing the net residence time of ligand-occupied hGR in the nucleus and thereby increasing the net probability that a given occupied hGR will bind to a GRE (or transcriptional complex) and also extending the net time of such interactions. Within this class of interaction, one of the most convincing mechanisms to date is that LABAs enhance steroid-induced induction of MAP kinase phosphatase (MKP, also called DUSP – dual specificity phosphatase), an enzyme able to broadly deactivate the major MAP family kinases that are powerful inducers of inflammation.[88] The reduced inflammation in turn leads to reduced functional antagonism and a reduced chance of inflammatory uncoupling as well as decreasing the chance of a catastrophic decline in lung function should an exacerbation occur.

Genes bearing both positive and negative GREs comprise only the minority of steroid-regulated genes. An emerging layer of complexity in steroid regulation of gene transcription is the likely effect of steroid receptor complexes as regulators of condensed chromatin structure and access of the initiation complex to genes.[118, 119] It is increasing clear that one of the major modes of action of steroids is to regulate transcription by influencing higher order transcriptional complexes and the architecture of DNA (and hence the physical access of the macromolecular machinery of transcriptional complexes to genes) at the level of histones via effects on histone acetylases (HATs) and histone deacetylases (HDACs). The finding that steroid subsensitivity in COPD (and also in smokers and smoking asthmatics) could be reversed in part with theophylline, which potentiates cAMP accumulation by suppressing the activity of phosphodiesterase, initially suggested that LABAs might also work in this manner. Repression of eotaxin expression has been linked to a shared effect on histone 4 acetylation.[120] However, subsequent research has established that the locus of action of theophylline in these systems is at the level of HDAC2 and mediated by phosphoinositide 3-kinase (PI3Kinase delta), not cAMP. HDAC2 is important for steroid-induced chromatin remodelling. The activity of HDAC2 is reduced by oxidative stress, and in long-standing more severe disease is specifically shuttled to the S28 proteosome for proteolytic destruction by E3-ligases. There is at present no convincing evidence for LABA-mediated effects in chromatin architecture, and by inference epigenetic regulatory mechanisms. Most recently, a still higher order of regulation has been inferred from studies on steroid effects mediated via regulatory microRNAs (miRNAs). Again there is no convincing evidence that LABAs exert interactions with steroids at this level but the field is in its infancy.

It is therefore likely that hGRs are able to exert extremely varied and complex effects on gene transcription. This subtlety may also explain why some inhibitory effects of steroids are cell type specific. Furthermore, glucocorticosteroid (GCS) decreases the stability of mRNA for a number of gene products, notably IL-1 and IL-6,[121, 122] by an unknown mechanism(s), presumably involving ribonuclease activity.

The GPCR also has multiple phosphorylation sites on serine and threonine residues and is a substrate for numerous kinases including proline-dependent kinase, p34 cdc2 kinase, casein kinase II and calmodulin. Phosphorylation seems not to affect *trans*-activation but does govern trafficking to and from the nucleus. While it was initially very controversial, the landmark study of Eickelberg and co-workers,[109] who observed that salmeterol promoted nuclear translocation and GRE binding of hGR in the absence of ligand, in human vascular endothelial smooth muscle cells and fibroblasts, has been repeatedly confirmed in multiple test systems. As hGR residence time in the nucleus is a key determinant of effect this is fundamentally important. It is currently thought that effects on both nuclear importins (IPO13, importin 13 is particularly implicated) and exportins may contribute. The consensus position from subsequent studies of multiple genes is that LABAs promote translocation but not transcriptional regulation in their own right whereas they have additive and sometimes synergistic effects when combined with steroids.

Thus in multiple test systems LABAs enhance the beneficial effects of steroids. It seems unavoidable to conclude that the clinical benefit of combining LABAs with steroids in fixed combination is the result of entrainment of multiple complementary pathways, in some cases with only weak effects but in aggregate exerting a clinically meaningful benefit.

4.13 Perspective

The challenges of current basic research are to improve our understanding of how such responses are functionally networked and also to define their limits at the molecular level in order to further refine and enhance drug therapy. There is a particular need to understand better how smoking history impedes these benefits and why these processes are much less effective in very severe, refractory asthma. Research in this direction should eventually determine whether these further pathogenetic mechanisms are tractable to therapeutic intervention. As well as current concepts of combining LABAs with steroids or anticholinergics, in the future it seems certain we will see LABAs combined with entirely novel agents that in themselves may have no discernible functional benefit but work to extend and reveal the full therapeutic potential of this class of drugs that have already transformed asthma management worldwide.

References

1. Haahtela T, Jarvinen M, Kava T, et al. Effects of reducing or discontinuing inhaled budesonide in patients with mild asthma. N Engl J Med 1994;331:700–5.
2. McIvor RA, Pizzichini E, Turner MO, Hussack P, Hargreave FE, Sears MR. Potential masking effects of salmeterol on airway inflammation in asthma. Am J Respir Crit Care Med 1998;158:924–30.
3. Turner MO, Johnston PR, Pizzichini E, Pizzichini MM, Hussack PA, Hargreave FE. Anti-inflammatory effects of salmeterol compared with beclomethasone in eosinophilic mild exacerbations of asthma: a randomized, placebo controlled trial. Can Respir J 1998;5:261–8.
4. Greening AP, Ind PW, Northfield M, Shaw G. Added salmeterol versus higher-dose corticosteroid in asthma patients with symptoms on existing inhaled corticosteroid. Allen & Hanburys Limited UK Study Group. Lancet 1994;344:219–24.

5. Woolcock A, Lundback B, Ringdal N, Jacques LA. Comparison of addition of salmeterol to inhaled steroids with doubling of the dose of inhaled steroids. Am J Respir Crit Care Med 1996;153:1481–8.

6. Pauwels RA, Lofdahl CG, Postma DS, et al. Effect of inhaled formoterol and budesonide on exacerbations of asthma. Formoterol and Corticosteroids Establishing Therapy (FACET) International Study Group. N Engl J Med 1997;337:1405–11.

7. Taylor DR, Town GI, Herbison GP, et al. Asthma control during long-term treatment with regular inhaled salbutamol and salmeterol. Thorax 1998;53:744–52.

8. Chervinsky P, Goldberg P, Galant S, et al. Long-term cardiovascular safety of salmeterol powder pharmacotherapy in adolescent and adult patients with chronic persistent asthma: a randomized clinical trial. Chest 1999;115:642–8.

9. Verberne AA, Frost C, Roorda RJ, van der Laag H, Kerrebijn KF. One year treatment with salmeterol compared with beclomethasone in children with asthma. The Dutch Paediatric Asthma Study Group. Am J Respir Crit Care Med 1997;156:688–95.

10. Vervloet D, Ekstrom T, Pela R, et al. A 6-month comparison between formoterol and salmeterol in patients with reversible obstructive airways disease. Respir Med 1998;92:836–42.

11. Taylor DR. The β-agonist saga and its clinical relevance: on and on it goes. Am J Respir Crit Care Med 2009;179:976–8.

12. Kikkawa H, Isogaya M, Nagao T, Kurose H. The role of the seventh transmembrane region in high affinity binding of a beta 2-selective agonist TA-2005. Mol Pharmacol 1998;53: 128–34.

13. Kikkawa H, Naito K, Ikezawa K. Tracheal relaxing effects and beta 2-selectivity of TA-2005, a newly developed bronchodilating agent, in isolated guinea pig tissues. Jpn J Pharmacol 1991;57:175–85.

14. Voss HP, Donnell D, Bast A. Atypical molecular pharmacology of a new long-acting beta 2-adrenoceptor agonist, TA 2005. Eur J Pharmacol 1992;227:403–9.

15. Battram C, Charlton SJ, Cuenoud B, et al. In vitro and in vivo pharmacological characterization of 5-[(R)-2-(5,6-diethyl-indan-2-ylamino)-1-hydroxyethyl]-8-hydroxy-1H-quino lin-2-one (indacaterol), a novel inhaled beta(2) adrenoceptor agonist with a 24-h duration of action. J Pharmacol Exp Ther 2006;317:762–70.

16. Lombardi D, Cuenoud B, Kramer SD. Lipid membrane interactions of indacaterol and salmeterol: do they influence their pharmacological properties? Eur J Pharm Sci 2009;38:533–47.

17. Pearlman DS, Greos L, LaForce C, Orevillo CJ, Owen R, Higgins M. Bronchodilator efficacy of indacaterol, a novel once-daily beta2-agonist, in patients with persistent asthma. Ann Allergy Asthma Immunol 2008;101:90–5.

18. Sayers I, Hawley J, Stewart CE, et al. Pharmacogenetic characterization of indacaterol, a novel beta2-adrenoceptor agonist. Br J Pharmacol 2009;158:277–86.

19. Sturton RG, Trifilieff A, Nicholson AG, Barnes PJ. Pharmacological characterization of indacaterol, a novel once daily inhaled 2 adrenoceptor agonist, on small airways in human and rat precision-cut lung slices. J Pharmacol Exp Ther 2008;324:270–5.

20. Yang WH, Martinot JB, Pohunek P, et al. Tolerability of indacaterol, a novel once-daily beta2-agonist, in patients with asthma: a randomized, placebo-controlled, 28-day safety study. Ann Allergy Asthma Immunol 2007;99:555–61.

21. Waldeck B. Enantiomers of bronchodilating beta2-adrenoceptor agonists: is there a cause for concern? J Allergy Clin Immunol 1999;103:742–8.

22. Mitra S, Ugur M, Ugur O, Goodman HM, McCullough JR, Yamaguchi H. (S)-Albuterol increases intracellular free calcium by muscarinic receptor activation and a phospholipase C-dependent mechanism in airway smooth muscle. Mol Pharmacol 1998;53:347–54.

23. Delmotte P, Sanderson MJ. Effects of formoterol on contraction and Ca^{2+} signaling of mouse airway smooth muscle cells. Am J Respir Cell Mol Biol 2010;42:373–381.

24. Kaumann AJ, Preitner F, Sarsero D, Molenaar P, Revelli JP, Giacobino JP. (–)–CGP 12177 causes cardiostimulation and binds to cardiac putative beta 4-adrenoceptors in both wild-type and beta 3-adrenoceptor knockout mice. Mol Pharmacol 1998;53:670–5.

25. Carstairs JR, Nimmo AJ, Barnes PJ. Autoradiographic visualization of beta-adrenoceptor subtypes in human lung. Am Rev Respir Dis 1985;132:541–7.

26. Isogaya M, Yamagiwa Y, Fujita S, Sugimoto Y, Nagao T, Kurose H. Identification of a key amino acid of the beta2-adrenergic receptor for high affinity binding of salmeterol. Mol Pharmacol 1998;54:616–22.

27. Anderson GP, Linden A, Rabe KF. Why are long-acting beta-adrenoceptor agonists long-acting? Eur Respir J 1994;7:569–78.

28. Grigorieff N, Ceska TA, Downing KH, Baldwin JM, Henderson R. Electron-crystallographic refinement of the structure of bacteriorhodopsin. J Mol Biol 1996;259:393–421.

29. Cherezov V, Rosenbaum DM, Hanson MA et al. High-resolution crystal structure of an engineered human beta2-adrenergic G protein-coupled receptor. Science 2007;318:1258–65.

30. Rosenbaum DM, Cherezov V, Hanson MA, et al. GPCR engineering yields high-resolution structural insights into beta2-adrenergic receptor function. Science 2007;318:1266–1273.

31. Rasmussen SG, Choi HJ, Rosenbaum DM, et al. Crystal structure of the human beta2 adrenergic G-protein-coupled receptor. Nature 2007;450:383–7.

32. Small RC, Chiu P, Cook SJ, Foster RW, Isaac L. Beta-adrenoceptor agonists in bronchial asthma: role of K+-channel opening in mediating their bronchodilator effects. Clin Exp Allergy 1993;23:802–11.

33. Roux FJ, Grandordy B, Douglas JS. Functional and binding characteristics of long-acting beta 2-agonists in lung and heart. Am J Respir Crit Care Med 1996;153:1489–95.

34. Chen-Izu Y, Xiao RP, Izu LT, et al. G(i)-dependent localization of beta(2)-adrenergic receptor signaling to L-type Ca(2+) channels. Biophys J 2000;79:2547–56.

35. McGraw DW, Mihlbachler KA, Schwarb MR, et al. Airway smooth muscle prostaglandin-EP1 receptors directly modulate beta2-adrenergic receptors within a unique heterodimeric complex. J Clin Invest 2006;116:1400–9.

36. McGraw DW, Elwing JM, Fogel KM, et al. Crosstalk between Gi and Gq/Gs pathways in airway smooth muscle regulates bronchial contractility and relaxation. J Clin Invest 2007;117:1391–8.

37. Weir TD, Mallek N, Sandford AJ, et al. beta2-Adrenergic receptor haplotypes in mild, moderate and fatal/near fatal asthma. Am J Respir Crit Care Med 1998;158:787–91.

38. Hawkins GA, Weiss ST, Bleecker ER. Clinical consequences of ADRbeta2 polymorphisms. Pharmacogenomics 2008;9:349–58.

39. Bleecker ER, Postma DS, Lawrance RM, Meyers DA, Ambrose HJ, Goldman M. Effect of ADRB2 polymorphisms on response to longacting beta2-agonist therapy: a pharmacogenetic analysis of two randomised studies. Lancet 2007;370:2118–25.

40. Wechsler ME, Kunselman SJ, Chinchilli VM, et al. Effect of beta2-adrenergic receptor polymorphism on response to longacting beta2 agonist in asthma (LARGE trial): a genotype-stratified, randomised, placebo-controlled, crossover trial. Lancet 2009;374:1754–64.

41. Yancey SW, Klotsman M, Ortega HG, Edwards LD, Anderson WH. Acute and chronic lung function responses to salmeterol and salmeterol plus fluticasone propionate in relation to Arg16Gly beta(2)-adrenergic polymorphisms. Curr Med Res Opin 2009;25:1011–18.

42. Tantisira KG, Small KM, Litonjua AA, Weiss ST, Liggett SB. Molecular properties and pharmacogenetics of a polymorphism of adenylyl cyclase type 9 in asthma: interaction between beta-agonist and corticosteroid pathways. Hum Mol Genet 2005;14:1671–7.

43. Ball DI, Brittain RT, Coleman RA, et al. Salmeterol, a novel, long-acting beta 2-adrenoceptor agonist: characterization of pharmacological activity in vitro and in vivo. Br J Pharmacol 1991;104:665–71.

44. Coleman RA. On the mechanism of the persistent action of salmeterol: what is the current position? Br J Pharmacol 2009;158:180–2.

45. Green SA, Spasoff AP, Coleman RA, Johnson M, Liggett SB. Sustained activation of a G protein-coupled receptor via "anchored" agonist binding. Molecular localization of the salmeterol exosite within the 2-adrenergic receptor. J Biol Chem 1996;271:24029–35.

46. Johnson M, Butchers PR, Coleman RA, et al. The pharmacology of salmeterol. Life Sci 1993;52:2131–43.

47. Nials AT, Ball DI, Butchers PR, et al. Formoterol on airway smooth muscle and human lung mast cells: a comparison with salbutamol and salmeterol. Eur J Pharmacol 1994;251:127–35.

48. Nials AT, Coleman RA, Johnson M, Vardey CJ. The duration of action of non-beta 2-adrenoceptor mediated responses to salmeterol. Br J Pharmacol 1997;120:961–7.

49. Nials AT, Sumner MJ, Johnson M, Coleman RA. Investigations into factors determining the duration of action of the beta 2-adrenoceptor agonist, salmeterol. Br J Pharmacol 1993;108:507–15.

50. Naline E, Zhang Y, Qian Y, et al. Relaxant effects and durations of action of formoterol and salmeterol on the isolated human bronchus. Eur Respir J 1994;7:914–20.

51. Bergendal A, Linden A, Skoogh BE, Gerspacher M, Anderson GP, Lofdahl CG. Extent of salmeterol-mediated reassertion of relaxation in guinea-pig trachea pretreated with aliphatic side chain structural analogues. Br J Pharmacol 1996;117:1009–15.

52. Clark RB, Allal C, Friedman J, Johnson M, Barber R. Stable activation and desensitization of beta 2-adrenergic receptor stimulation of adenylyl cyclase by salmeterol: evidence for quasi-irreversible binding to an exosite. Mol Pharmacol 1996;49:182–9.

53. Teschemacher A, Lemoine H. Kinetic analysis of drug–receptor interactions of long-acting beta2 sympathomimetics in isolated receptor membranes: evidence against prolonged effects of salmeterol and formoterol on receptor-coupled adenylyl cyclase. J Pharmacol Exp Ther 1999;288:1084–92.

54. Rubenstein LA, Zauhar RJ, Lanzara RG. Molecular dynamics of a biophysical model for beta2-adrenergic and G protein-coupled receptor activation. J Mol Graph Model 2006;25:396–409.

55. Kramer SD, Lombardi D, Primorac A, Thomae AV, Wunderli-Allenspach H. Lipid-bilayer permeation of drug-like compounds. Chem Biodivers 2009;6:1900–16.

56. Lombardi D, Cuenoud B, Wunderli-Allenspach H, Kramer SD. Interaction kinetics of salmeterol with egg phosphatidylcholine liposomes by surface plasmon resonance. Anal Biochem 2009;385:215–23.

57. Rhodes DG, Newton R, Butler R, Herbette L. Equilibrium and kinetic studies of the interactions of salmeterol with membrane bilayers. Mol Pharmacol 1992;42:596–602.

58. Summerhill S, Stroud T, Nagendra R, Perros-Huguet C, Trevethick M. A cell-based assay to assess the persistence of action of agonists acting at recombinant human beta(2) adrenoceptors. J Pharmacol Toxicol Methods 2008;58:189–97.

59. Collins S, Altschmied J, Herbsman O, Caron MG, Mellon PL, Lefkowitz RJ. A cAMP response element in the beta 2-adrenergic receptor gene confers transcriptional autoregulation by cAMP. J Biol Chem 1990;265:19330–5.

60. Lipworth B, Koppelman GH, Wheatley AP, et al. Beta2 adrenoceptor promoter polymorphisms: extended haplotypes and functional effects in peripheral blood mononuclear cells. Thorax 2002;57:61–6.

61. Laporte SA, Oakley RH, Holt JA, Barak LS, Caron MG. The interaction of beta-arrestin with the AP-2 adaptor is required for the clustering of beta 2-adrenergic receptor into clathrin-coated pits. J Biol Chem 2000;275:23120–6.

62. Laporte SA, Oakley RH, Zhang J, et al. The beta2-adrenergic receptor/betaarrestin complex recruits the clathrin adaptor AP-2 during endocytosis. Proc Natl Acad Sci U S A 1999;96:3712–17.

63. Adner M, Larsson B, Safholm J, Naya I, Miller-Larsson A. Budesonide prevents cytokine-induced decrease of the relaxant responses to formoterol and terbutaline, but not to salmeterol, in mouse trachea. Pharmacol Exp Ther 2010;333:273–80.

64. Bhagat R, Kalra S, Swystun VA, Cockcroft DW. Rapid onset of tolerance to the bronchoprotective effect of salmeterol. Chest 1995;108:1235–9.

65. Duringer C, Grundstrom G, Gurcan E, et al. Agonist-specific patterns of beta2-adrenoceptor responses in human airway cells during prolonged exposure. Br J Pharmacol 2009;158:169–79.

66. Hu A, Nino G, Grunstein JS, Fatma S, Grunstein MM. Prolonged heterologous beta2-adrenoceptor desensitization promotes proasthmatic airway smooth muscle function via PKA/ERK1/2-mediated phosphodiesterase-4 induction. Am J Physiol Lung Cell Mol Physiol 2008;294:L1055–67.

67. Lemoine H, Overlack C. Highly potent beta-2 sympathomimetics convert to less potent partial agonists as relaxants of guinea pig tracheae maximally contracted by carbachol. Comparison of relaxation with receptor binding and adenylate cyclase stimulation. J Pharmacol Exp Ther 1992;261:258–70.

68. Molimard M, Naline E, Zhang Y, Le Gros V, Begaud B, Advenier C. Long- and short-acting beta2 adrenoceptor agonists: interactions in human contracted bronchi. Eur Respir J 1998;11:583–8.

69. Munoz NM, Rabe KF, Vita AJ, et al. Paradoxical blockade of beta adrenergically mediated inhibition of stimulated eosinophil secretion by salmeterol. J Pharmacol Exp Ther 1995;273:850–4.

70. Palmqvist M, Ibsen T, Mellen A, Lötvall J. Comparison of the relative efficacy of formoterol and salmeterol in asthmatic patients. Am J Respir Crit Care Med 1999;160:244–9.

71. Roberts JA, Bradding P, Britten KM, et al. The long-acting beta2-agonist salmeterol xinafoate: effects on airway inflammation in asthma. Eur Respir J 1999;14:275–82.

72. Howarth PH, Beckett P, Dahl R. The effect of long-acting beta2-agonists on airway inflammation in asthmatic patients. Respir Med 2000;94(Suppl. F):S22–5.

73. Bourbeau J, Christodoulopoulos P, Maltais F, Yamauchi Y, Olivenstein R, Hamid Q. Effect of salmeterol/fluticasone propionate on airway inflammation in COPD: a randomised controlled trial. Thorax 2007;62:938–43.

74. Bloemen PG, van den Tweel MC, Henricks PA, et al. Increased cAMP levels in stimulated neutrophils inhibit their adhesion to human bronchial epithelial cells. Am J Physiol 1997;272:L580–7.

75. Hanania NA, Singh S, El-Wali R, et al. The safety and effects of the beta-blocker, nadolol, in mild asthma: an open-label pilot study. Pulm Pharmacol Ther 2008;21:134–41.

76. Nguyen LP, Lin R, Parra S, et al. Beta2-adrenoceptor signaling is required for the development of an asthma phenotype in a murine model. Proc Natl Acad Sci U S A 2009;106:2435–40.

77. Nguyen LP, Omoluabi O, Parra S, et al. Chronic exposure to beta-blockers attenuates inflammation and mucin content in a murine asthma model. Am J Respir Cell Mol Biol 2008;38:256–62.

78. Advenier C, Qian Y, Koune JD, Molimard M, Candenas ML, Naline E. Formoterol and salbutamol inhibit bradykinin- and histamine-induced airway microvascular leakage in guinea-pig. Br J Pharmacol 1992;105:792–8.

79. Chong LK, Cooper E, Vardey CJ, Peachell PT. Salmeterol inhibition of mediator release from human lung mast cells by beta-adrenoceptor-dependent and independent mechanisms. Br J Pharmacol 1998;123:1009–15.

80. Shio MT, Eisenbarth SC, Savaria M, et al. Malarial hemozoin activates the NLRP3 inflammasome through Lyn and Syk kinases. PLoS Pathog 2009;5:e1000559.

81. Bai TR. Abnormalities in airway smooth muscle in fatal asthma. Am Rev Respir Dis 1990;141:552–7.

82. Van Amsterdam RG, Meurs H, Ten Berge RE, Veninga NC, Brouwer F, Zaagsma J. Role of phosphoinositide metabolism in human bronchial smooth muscle contraction and in functional antagonism by beta-adrenoceptor agonists. Am Rev Respir Dis 1990;142:1124–8.

83. Chilvers ER, Lynch BJ, Challiss RA. Dissociation between beta-adrenoceptor-mediated cyclic AMP accumulation and inhibition of histamine-stimulated phosphoinositide metabolism in airways smooth muscle. Biochem Pharmacol 1997;53:1565–8.

84. Bai TR. Abnormalities in airway smooth muscle in fatal asthma. A comparison between trachea and bronchus. Am Rev Respir Dis 1991;143:441–3.

85. Wills-Karp M, Uchida Y, Lee JY, Jinot J, Hirata A, Hirata F. Organ culture with proinflammatory cytokines reproduces impairment of the beta-adrenoceptor-mediated relaxation in tracheas of a guinea pig antigen model. Am J Respir Cell Mol Biol 1993;8:153–9.

86. Penn RB, Shaver JR, Zangrilli JG, et al. Effects of inflammation and acute beta-agonist inhalation on beta 2-AR signaling in human airways. Am J Physiol 1996;271:L601–8.

87. Duong M, Gauvreau G, Watson R et al. The effects of inhaled budesonide and formoterol in combination and alone when given directly after allergen challenge. J Allergy Clin Immunol 2007;119:322–7.

88. Kaur M, Chivers JE, Giembycz MA, Newton R. Long-acting beta2-adrenoceptor agonists synergistically enhance glucocorticoid-dependent transcription in human airway epithelial and smooth muscle cells. Mol Pharmacol 2008;73:203–14.

89. Korn SH, Jerre A, Brattsand R. Effects of formoterol and budesonide on GM-CSF and IL-8 secretion by triggered human bronchial epithelial cells. Eur Respir J 2001;17:1070–7.

90. Korn SH, Wouters EF, Wesseling G, Arends JW, Thunnissen FB. Interaction between glucocorticoids and beta2-agonists: alpha and beta glucocorticoid-receptor mRNA expression in human bronchial epithelial cells. Biochem Pharmacol 1998;56:1561–9.

91. Coyle AJ, Le Gros G, Bertrand C, et al. Interleukin-4 is required for the induction of lung Th2 mucosal immunity. Am J Respir Cell Mol Biol 1995;13:54–9.

92. Gavett SH, O'Hearn DJ, Li X, Huang SK, Finkelman FD, Wills-Karp M. Interleukin 12 inhibits antigen-induced airway hyperresponsiveness, inflammation, and Th2 cytokine expression in mice. J Exp Med 1995;182:1527–36.

93. Bruselle GG, Kips JC, Peleman RA, et al. Role of IFN-gamma in the inhibition of the allergic airway inflammation caused by IL-12. Am J Respir Cell Mol Biol 1997;17:767–71.

94. Hasko G, Szabo C, Nemeth ZH, Salzman AL, Vizi ES. Stimulation of beta-adrenoceptors inhibits endotoxin-induced IL-12 production in normal and IL-10 deficient mice. J Neuroimmunol 1998;88:57–61.

95. Panina-Bordignon P, Mazzeo D, Lucia PD, et al. Beta2-agonists prevent Th1 development by selective inhibition of interleukin 12. J Clin Invest 1997;100:1513–19.

96. Anderson GP. Interactions between corticosteroids and beta-adrenergic agonists in asthma disease induction, progression, and exacerbation. Am J Respir Crit Care Med 2000;161:S188–96.

97. Vlahos R, Stewart AG. Interleukin-1alpha and tumour necrosis factor-alpha modulate airway smooth muscle DNA synthesis by induction of cyclo-oxygenase-2: inhibition by dexamethasone and fluticasone propionate. Br J Pharmacol 1999;126:1315–24.

98. Kujubu DA, Herschman HR. Dexamethasone inhibits mitogen induction of the TIS10 prostaglandin synthase/cyclooxygenase gene. J Biol Chem 1992;267:7991–4.

99. Mak JC, Nishikawa M, Barnes PJ. Glucocorticosteroids increase beta 2-adrenergic receptor transcription in human lung. Am J Physiol 1995;268:L41–6.

100. January B, Seibold A, Allal C, et al. Salmeterol-induced desensitization, internalization and phosphorylation of the human beta2-adrenoceptor. Br J Pharmacol 1998;123:701–11.

101. Hauck RW, Harth M, Schulz C, Prauer H, Bohm M, Schomig A. Effects of beta 2-agonist- and dexamethasone-treatment on relaxation and regulation of beta-adrenoceptors in human bronchi and lung tissue. Br J Pharmacol 1997;121:1523–30.

102. Mak JC, Nishikawa M, Shirasaki H, Miyayasu K, Barnes PJ. Protective effects of a glucocorticoid on downregulation of pulmonary beta 2-adrenergic receptors in vivo. J Clin Invest 1995;96:99–106.

103. Mak JC, Chuang TT, Harris CA, Barnes PJ. Increased expression of G protein-coupled receptor kinases in cystic fibrosis lung. Eur J Pharmacol 2002;436:165–72.

104. Kalavantavanich K, Schramm CM. Dexamethasone potentiates high-affinity beta-agonist binding and g(s)alpha protein expression in airway smooth muscle. Am J Physiol Lung Cell Mol Physiol 2000;278:L1101–6.

105. Tan KS, Grove A, McLean A, Gnosspelius Y, Hall IP, Lipworth BJ. Systemic corticosteriod rapidly reverses bronchodilator subsensitivity induced by formoterol in asthmatic patients. Am J Respir Crit Care Med 1997;156:28–35.

106. Boulet LP, Cartier A, Milot J, Cote J, Malo JL, Laviolette M. Tolerance to the protective effects of salmeterol on methacholine-induced bronchoconstriction: influence of inhaled corticosteroids. Eur Respir J 1998;11:1091–7.

107. Giannini D, Bacci E, Dente FL, et al. Inhaled beclomethasone dipropionate reverts tolerance to the protective effect of salmeterol on allergen challenge. Chest 1999;115:629–34.

108. Roth M, Johnson PR, Rudiger JJ, et al. Interaction between glucocorticoids and beta2 agonists on bronchial airway smooth muscle cells through synchronised cellular signalling. Lancet 2002;360:1293–9.

109. Eickelberg O, Roth M, Lorx R, et al. Ligand-independent activation of the glucocorticoid receptor by beta2-adrenergic receptor agonists in primary human lung fibroblasts and vascular smooth muscle cells. J Biol Chem 1999;274:1005–10.

110. Vachier I, Chiappara G, Vignola AM, et al. Glucocorticoid receptors in bronchial epithelial cells in asthma. Am J Respir Crit Care Med 1998;158:963–70.

111. Turner JD, Schote AB, Keipes M, Muller CP. A new transcript splice variant of the human glucocorticoid receptor: identification and tissue distribution of hGR Delta 313-338, an alternative exon 2 transactivation domain isoform. Ann N Y Acad Sci 2007;1095:334–41.

112. Yang-Yen HF, Chambard JC, Sun YL, et al. Transcriptional interference between c-Jun and the glucocorticoid receptor: mutual inhibition of DNA binding due to direct protein–protein interaction. Cell 1990;62:1205–15.

113. Konig H, Ponta H, Rahmsdorf HJ, Herrlich P. Interference between pathway-specific transcription factors: glucocorticoids antagonize phorbol ester-induced AP-1 activity without altering AP-1 site occupation in vivo. EMBO J 1992;11:2241–6.

114. Diamond MI, Miner JN, Yoshinaga SK, Yamamoto KR. Transcription factor interactions: selectors of positive or negative regulation from a single DNA element. Science 1990;249:1266–72.

115. Baeuerle PA, Baltimore D. I kappa B: a specific inhibitor of the NF-kappa B transcription factor. Science 1988;242:540–6.

116. Ray A, Prefontaine KE. Physical association and functional antagonism between the p65 subunit of transcription factor NF-kappa B and the glucocorticoid receptor. Proc Natl Acad Sci U S A 1994;91:752–6.

117. Auphan N, DiDonato JA, Rosette C, Helmberg A, Karin M. Immunosuppression by glucocorticoids: inhibition of NF-kappa B activity through induction of I kappa B synthesis. Science 1995;270:286–90.

118. Wolffe AP, Wong J, Li Q, Levi BZ, Shi YB. Three steps in the regulation of transcription by the thyroid hormone receptor: establishment of a repressive chromatin structure, disruption of chromatin and transcriptional activation. Biochem Soc Trans 1997;25:612–15.

119. Beato M, Sanchez-Pacheco A. Interaction of steroid hormone receptors with the transcription initiation complex. Endocr Rev 1996;17:587–609.

120. Nie M, Knox AJ, Pang L. beta2-Adrenoceptor agonists, like glucocorticoids, repress eotaxin gene transcription by selective inhibition of histone H4 acetylation. J Immunol 2005;175:478–86.

121. Tobler A, Meier R, Seitz M, Dewald B, Baggiolini M, Fey MF. Glucocorticoids downregulate gene expression of GM-CSF, NAP-1/IL-8, and IL-6, but not of M-CSF in human fibroblasts. Blood 1992;79:45–51.

122. Lee SW, Tsou AP, Chan H, et al. Glucocorticoids selectively inhibit the transcription of the interleukin 1 beta gene and decrease the stability of interleukin 1 beta mRNA. Proc Natl Acad Sci U S A 1988;85:1204–8.

5

Long- and ultra-long-acting β$_2$-agonists

Mario Cazzola[*] and Maria Gabriella Matera[†]

[*]Unit of Respiratory Clinical Pharmacology, Department of Internal Medicine, University of Rome 'Tor Vergata', Rome, Italy
[†]Unit of Pharmacology, Department of Experimental Medicine, Second University of Naples, Naples, Italy

5.1   Introduction

β$_2$-Agonists have been the mainstay bronchodilator agents used for the treatment of asthma and chronic obstructive pulmonary disease (COPD) since the development of inhaled isoprenaline (isoproterenol) preparations in the 1960s. They bind to the β$_2$-adrenoceptor (AR), which is present in the cell membrane of a number of airway cell types, including airway smooth muscle, airway epithelial cells, inflammatory cells including mast cells, vascular endothelium and vascular smooth muscle. However, the major site of action of β$_2$-agonists in the airways is the airway smooth muscle cell. Following binding of β$_2$-agonist to the β$_2$-AR on airway smooth muscle, a signalling cascade is triggered that results in a number of events, all of which contribute to relaxation of airway smooth muscle.[1,2]

Traditionally, β-agonists are divided into three broad groups according to duration of action following inhalation of conventional doses:

1. the catecholamines, isoprenaline and rimiterol, which have a very short action of 1–2 h;
2. those conventionally described as short acting, such as salbutamol and terbutaline, which are active for 3–6 h, although fenoterol may be slightly shorter acting;
3. the long-acting β-agonists (LABAs) salmeterol and formoterol, which cause bronchodilation for at least 12 h.

The relatively short duration of action of compounds such as salbutamol and terbutaline, which after inhalation elicit a prompt effect lasting between 3 and 5 h, has been

Advances in Combination Therapy for Asthma and COPD, First Edition. Edited by Jan Lötvall.
© 2012 John Wiley & Sons, Ltd. Published 2012 by John Wiley & Sons, Ltd.

seen as a disadvantage particularly for patients with nocturnal asthma, although they are effective in the treatment of severe attacks of asthma and as rescue medications in COPD. The development of longer-acting β_2-agonists has, therefore, been heralded as a major new development in the treatment of airway obstructive disorders.[1]

5.2   Long-acting β_2-agonists

Long-acting β_2-agonists, including salmeterol and formoterol, are central both in asthma and COPD. The extended duration of action of the long-acting β_2-agonists – which were designed specifically for regular use – of at least 12 h, depends on several factors including lipophilicity, affinity and selectivity.[1] Adequate water solubility and moderate lipophilicity of formoterol ensures rapid diffusion to the β_2-AR on the smooth muscle and rapid bronchodilating activity.[3] Salmeterol diffuses more slowly to the β_2-AR because of its high lipophilicity, and this finding explains the slower onset of action.[3] Unlike salbutamol, which is hydrophilic and has a rapid onset and short duration of action, both formoterol and salmeterol possess adequate lipophilic properties to remain in the airway tissues as a depot in close vicinity to the β_2-AR, explaining their long duration of effect.[3] The long duration of salmeterol has also been suggested to depend on an anchored binding within the β_2-AR.[3]

The intended use of LABAs is protective, to prevent symptoms, whether spontaneous or due to some environmental or activity-related airway insult. As well as being more convenient for the patient, there are increased benefits in terms of lung function, exercise performance and health status with regular treatment with LABAs.

Asthma

The regular use of LABAs is now established in asthma guidelines as the preferred option for second-line controller therapy in addition to inhaled corticosteroids (ICSs).[4,5] This has been driven by data showing beneficial effects of LABAs on exacerbation rates, at the same time suggesting a putative corticosteroid-sparing effect. As LABAs are devoid of any clinically meaningful anti-inflammatory activity *in vivo*, their effects on exacerbations are presumably due to a diurnal stabilizing effect on airway smooth muscle, as well as possibly enhancing anti-inflammatory effects of ICSs. The study called Salmeterol Off Corticosteroids, or 'SOCS',[6] showed that asthma control deteriorated in those treated with placebo, but there was no difference between those continuing on ICSs and those receiving monotherapy with salmeterol, for conventional clinical outcomes such as morning and evening peak flows, symptom scores, rescue salbutamol use, or quality of life. However, markers of airway inflammation remained controlled in patients on ICSs, whereas those treated with salmeterol alone showed an increase in sputum eosinophils, eosinophil cationic protein, exhaled nitric oxide and methacholine sensitivity, similar to the changes seen in the placebo group. Moreover, there was an increased rate of treatment failures and asthma exacerbations in those patients on salmeterol monotherapy, again similar to those subjects who had been switched to placebo. Thus, LABAs have marked effects on symptoms and lung function, and this may make it difficult to clinically assess anti-inflammatory control with ICSs when used in a combination inhaler.[7]

The use of LABAs for asthma as monotherapy without concomitant use of ICSs is associated with increased adverse events including exacerbations and asthma deaths.[8,9] However, a direct physiological or pharmacological mechanism for LABAs worsening asthma pathology has not been established, although it seems likely that continuous, twice-daily exposure to an exogenous LABA such as salmeterol or formoterol results in reduced β_2-AR numbers (i.e. downregulation) on bronchial smooth muscle and inflammatory cells, together with uncoupling of the β_2-AR from the G protein adenylyl cyclase.[10] It is possible that the untoward effects of LABAs might be due to β_2-AR polymorphism. In fact, polymorphisms of the β_2-AR can affect regulation of the receptor.[11] There is a growing body of evidence that β_2-AR genotype (position 16) is a marker for adverse clinical outcomes with chronic β_2-agonist exposure.[12,13] In particular, an impaired therapeutic response to salmeterol seems to be present both with and without concurrent ICS use.[13] A retrospective analysis of genotype data from steroid-treated asthmatics exposed to regular LABAs or placebo showed loss of bronchoprotection between first and last doses in Gly16 and Arg16 genotypes, with the degree of protection being significantly less in Arg16 than in Gly16 genotypes.[14] Approximately 15% of the population is homozygous for Arg16, but it has been documented that African-Americans have an increased frequency of B16 Arg/Arg.[15] The overall evidence for any strong association between genotype at the level of the β_2-AR is, however, weak.

The U.S. Food and Drug Administration (FDA) recommended that salmeterol and formoterol no longer be used to treat asthma as monotherapy, because of one study that showed a small but significant increase in mortality in a group treated with salmeterol,[16] and a meta-analysis largely based on this study that seemed to support the contention that LABAs produce excess serious asthma exacerbations.[17] However, the FDA later decided that the combination inhalers containing fluticasone propionate and salme-terol or budesonide and formoterol remain available. This is important, because not only of the extensive clinical use of these combinations, but also the evidence both *in vitro* and *in vivo* to suggest that there is a favourable interaction between LABAs and ICSs at the receptor level, leading to an enhanced steroid effect if LABAs are given concomitantly.[18] The addition of a LABA to an ICS also increases patient adherence to ICS therapy, probably both by providing a sensation of immediate symptom im-provement as well as allowing the use of a lower dose of ICS.[4,5] In any case, a large Cochrane systematic review for the effectiveness and safety of LABAs[19] has provided evidence that LABAs are safe and beneficial in control of asthma, and intriguingly the benefit was reported to be present both with and without concomitant ICS use. Two other Cochrane systematic reviews have found that regular treatment with LABAs is more effective than regular treatment with short-acting β_2-agonists,[20] and is at least as effective as theophylline with clearly fewer side effects.[21] These reviews support the use of LABAs as additional therapy when asthma is inadequately controlled by ICS at moderate dose, as recommended in current guidelines.[4,5]

COPD

Long-acting β_2-agonists, being long-acting bronchodilators, are the mainstay of COPD therapy.[22,23] They work through their direct relaxation effect on airway smooth muscle cells, although many have non-bronchodilator activities that may contribute to their beneficial effects in COPD.[24] The acute response to short-acting bronchodilators does not predict long-term response to maintenance therapy with LABAs.[25]

The two LABAs that have been clinically available for many years, salmeterol and formoterol, have been shown to significantly improve symptoms in COPD patients.[26] In fact, several prospective randomized trials and a high-quality meta-analysis[27,28] have shown that LABAs improve lung function and health status-related quality of life, and reduce exacerbations in symptomatic patients with moderate-to-severe COPD. The improvement in lung function, measured by means of the baseline change in FEV_1 (forced expiratory volume in 1 second) is rather small, amounting on average to 100–150 mL.[29] However, this improvement is highly statistically significant and it is associated with an improvement in the patient's condition and health status perception. Moreover, LABAs have at least the hypothetical potential to improve the mucociliary clearance in patients with COPD.

The studies on LABAs up to one year failed to show any effect of the treatment on the progression of COPD, measured by means of the rate of decline of FEV_1, although the TORCH study has revealed that salmeterol reduced the rate of FEV_1 decline by 13 mL/year compared with placebo.[30] Interestingly, all trials also failed to find any correlation between the improvement in symptoms and in FEV_1.[29]

When optimized monotherapy is insufficient, combined treatment with a β_2-agonist and an antimuscarinic agent may be useful.[31] There is evidence that long-acting β_2-agonists may represent the most effective option for combined treatment with ipratropium.[32]

Considering that formoterol provides a greater degree of early bronchodilation (in the first 2 h) than tiotropium and comparable bronchodilation over 12 h,[33] the possibility of combining these two agents seems to be helpful in stable COPD patients.[34,35] These two studies[34,35] excluded the once-daily co-administration of the two drugs, as formoterol is given on a twice-daily basis. Interestingly, the additive effect of a second long-acting bronchodilator in patients receiving a first long-acting bronchodilator does not depend on which type of bronchodilator is given first.[36] Also the combination of tiotropium + salmeterol has a greater bronchodilator effect than either agent individually.[37] Also, it was observed that the onset of action of the two drugs combined was faster than when they were given alone, which is worthy of attention since both agents elicit a slow onset of action.

It is now widely accepted that the aim of managing COPD is to target both the symptoms and the inflammatory process. While ICSs are employed to reduce inflammation in more severe patients, their role as stand-alone medication in COPD is not very well documented. However, since LABAs and ICSs have complementary and synergistic effects, when delivered as combination therapy from a single inhaler, it is no surprise that a one-year study investigating the effect of a combination of LABA + ICS showed a sustained improvement in lung function to significantly greater levels compared with either component alone, and a parallel decrease in the rate of exacerbations, improved health status and decreased dyspnoea.[38–40] Another large trial was designed and powered to investigate the effect of three years' treatment with the salmeterol/fluticasone combination, salmeterol alone, fluticasone alone or placebo on all-cause mortality as the primary outcome in patients with COPD.[41] The difference in mortality rates narrowly failed to reach statistical significance, although treatment was associated with a numerically lower risk of dying than placebo; the respective mortality rates were 12.6% in the combination therapy group and 15.2% in the placebo group, giving an absolute risk reduction in all-cause mortality of 2.6% ($P = 0.052$). The risk of mortality was significantly lower with the combined therapy compared with fluticasone, but not in comparison with salmeterol. Data from this study on the secondary outcomes are consistent with and extend previous observations in studies using combinations of LABA + ICS,[38–40] showing that the combination regimen reduced exacerbations significantly, as compared with placebo, including those exacerbations requiring hospitalization. The combination regimen was also significantly better than each of its components alone in preventing exacerbations, and these benefits were accompanied by sustained improvements in health status and lung function measured as FEV_1, and the values for both were better at the end of the trial than at baseline.

It must be mentioned that a meta-analysis[42] has argued that β₂-agonist use does not affect the frequency of severe exacerbations, but rather results in an increased rate of respiratory deaths compared with placebo. In this analysis, there was a two-fold increased risk for severe exacerbations associated with β₂-agonists compared with anticholinergics in COPD. Intriguingly, according to this meta-analysis, the addition of β₂-agonist to anticholinergic use did not improve any clinical outcomes. It has been suggested that a worsening of disease control could be explained by some degree of tolerance to the bronchodilator effect of β₂-agonists.[42] Another explanation of a negative effect by β₂-agonists on some health variables is that they can induce increased heart rate, increased contractile force and decreased peripheral vascular resistance, leading to increased pulse pressure and an increase in cardiac output. Together with changes in serum potassium and magnesium levels, which are factors that may affect conduction pathways in the heart, β₂-agonists could alter the risk of sudden cardiac death especially in COPD patients with cardiac comorbidities.[43]

Unfortunately, the administration of LABAs to patients with airway obstruction often results in a transient decrease in partial pressure of oxygen in arterial blood (P_aO_2) despite concomitant bronchodilation.[44] This decrease in P_aO_2 with beta-agonists has been attributed to the pulmonary vasodilation induced by these agents, due to the activation of β-ARs that are present in pulmonary vessels, thereby increasing blood flow to poorly ventilated lung regions and thus increasing V/Q ratio (ventilation/perfusion) imbalance, inducing a shunt-like effect.[45,46] β₂-Agonists have been suggested to induce a fall in pulmonary vascular resistance also because of an increase in cardiac output and in right ventricular ejection.[47] Importantly, the addition of an ICS reduces the acute effect of LABAs on blood-gas tensions.[48] This effect is likely linked to the documented potential of ICSs to cause an acute reduction in bronchial blood flow.[49]

5.3   Novel ultra-long-acting β_2-agonists

After the discovery of formoterol and salmeterol, new candidate LABAs emerged, but this research was neglected following the halt to the development of picumeterol in 1993.[50] In fact, this agent was able to induce long-lasting relaxation of the airway smooth muscle, both *in vitro* and *in vivo* in animal models, but its bronchodilation was not long-lasting in atopic asthmatics.[51] In addition, it did not improve provocative concentration (PC20) when compared with placebo.[51]

Nonetheless, considering the central role and extensive clinical efficacy of LABAs in both asthma and COPD, there has been renewed interest in the field in recent years, and now once-daily β_2-adrenoceptor agonists (ultra-LABAs) are in development in an attempt to simplify their administration to patients.[52–54] Thus, it is believed that adherence can be improved with prescribed therapy using a once-daily regimen to reduce the dose frequency to the minimum necessary to maintain disease control. Therefore, the incorporation of once-daily dosing is possibly an important strategy to improve compliance, and is certainly a regimen preferred by most patients.[55] A series of beta-agonists with longer duration, and sometimes longer half-lives, are currently under development with the hopes of achieving once-daily dosing.[52–54]

Indacaterol

Indacaterol (QAB-149), which has the structure (5-{(1R)-2-[(5,6-diethyl-2,3-dihydro-1H-inden-2-yl)amino]-1-hydroxyethyl}-8-hydroxyquinolin-2(1H)-one), is a once-daily LABA in development by Novartis, and has recently been approved for the treatment of COPD in Europe. Two doses are available, 150 and 300 µg, given once daily. So far, little clinical experience has been built up with indacaterol, and relatively few clinical studies are published, but this will expand extensively in the coming years.

Preclinical development

Indacaterol offers a relatively quick onset of action and clear quantifiable 24-hour duration of effect.[56] A study comparing the properties of indacaterol with salmeterol, formoterol and salbutamol, on small airways in precision-cut lung slices from human contracted with carbachol,[57] documented the rank order of potency as formoterol ≥ salmeterol > indacaterol > salbutamol. Indacaterol had similar intrinsic efficacy to formoterol, followed by salbutamol and salmeterol. The onset of action was fast for salbutamol, formoterol and indacaterol, whereas it was significantly slower for salmeterol. The duration of action ranking was indacaterol > salmeterol > formoterol >

salbutamol. In preclinical studies (relative to isoprenaline) indacaterol (73%) has more of a full agonist profile than the partial agonist salmeterol (38%).[58] This property could explain why it has also been shown that indacaterol does not induce tachyphylaxis,[56] and does not antagonize the bronchorelaxant effect of a short-acting β$_2$-agonist.[57] Preclinical data also suggest that, for a given degree of bronchodilator activity, indacaterol has a greater cardiovascular safety margin than formoterol or salmeterol.[56]

Considering this excellent pharmacological profile, several trials have evaluated the efficacy and safety of indacaterol in patients with asthma and COPD.

Asthma

In patients with intermittent or mild to moderate persistent asthma, single 200 μg and 400 μg doses of indacaterol provided effective and sustained 24-hour bronchodilator control with a rapid onset of action (<5 min) and a good tolerability and safety profile.[59,60] In particular, FEV$_1$ was significantly higher for the 400 μg dose compared with the 200 μg dose, from 15 minutes to 2 hours after dosing and from 5 hours onwards. Indacaterol was associated with good tolerability and safety.[60] The trough FEV$_1$ at 24 h post-dose, is significantly higher with all doses of indacaterol and formoterol compared with placebo, when comparing single-dose indacaterol morning dose of indacaterol 150, 300 or 600 μg, and formoterol 12 μg morning and evening via an Aerolizer®. For the two higher doses of indacaterol, the trough FEV$_1$ was higher than with formoterol.[61] The most frequent adverse events were transient cough and throat clearing upon inhalation, which were observed in 15% of subjects with the 300 and 600 μg doses of indacaterol.

Once-daily 100, 200, 300, 400 or 600 μg doses of indacaterol demonstrate sustained 24-hour bronchodilator efficacy, with similar efficacy on days 1 and 7.[62] For standardized FEV$_1$ AUC$_{22\text{-}24h}$ (area under the curve) on day 1, indacaterol doses ≥200 μg were superior to placebo and similar or greater than formoterol 12 μg twice daily. By day 7, mean differences from placebo in FEV$_1$ standardized AUC$_{22\text{-}24h}$ were 0.08, 0.16, 0.15, 0.11 and 0.16 L for indacaterol 100, 200, 300, 400, and 600 μg, respectively. Mean FEV$_1$ for indacaterol doses ≥200 μg on day 7 was higher than placebo ($P < 0.05$) pre-dose and at all post-dose time points. Adverse events (AEs) were generally mild and no serious AEs were reported.

In patients with persistent asthma on a stable regimen of ICSs randomized to treatment for 7 days with once-daily indacaterol 50, 100, 200 or 400 μg via metered dose dry powder inhaler (MDDPI) (Certihaler™), indacaterol 400 μg via single dose dry powder inhaler (SDDPI) or placebo,[63] all doses of indacaterol provided rapid-onset, sustained 24-hour bronchodilator efficacy on once-daily dosing from day 1, with no loss of efficacy after 7 days of treatment, although indacaterol 200 μg appeared to be the optimum dose, offering the best efficacy/safety balance. A randomized, open-label crossover study in adult subjects with asthma (FEV$_1$ ≥ 60% predicted) confirmed that indacaterol 200 μg provides effective 24-hour bronchodilation, with a longer duration than salmeterol 50 μg and a good overall safety profile.[64]

The results of a study that assessed the safety and tolerability of indacaterol 200, 400 or 600 μg or placebo once daily for 28 days in asthma patients suggested that indacaterol has a wide therapeutic index, is well tolerated and is neither associated with adverse cardiac effects nor clinically significant changes in β_2-mediated systemic effects.[65] This may be because doses used were simply not sufficiently high to have an impact on these safety variables despite all indacaterol doses achieving clinically relevant differences in FEV_1 of >200 mL versus placebo at most post-dose time points. Nonetheless, higher doses of indacaterol (800 μg) demonstrate effects on serum potassium and blood glucose, but these changes were considered not to be clinically important.[66] At a single dose of 1000 μg, indacaterol had a good safety profile and was not associated with sustained systemic adverse effects; mean heart rate and QTc interval remained within normal ranges following administration.[62]

COPD

Indacaterol has also been studied in COPD patients, demonstrating 24-hour bronchodilator efficacy, with a clinically meaningful bronchodilator effect by at least one hour post-dose and no evidence of tachyphylaxis.[67] Another trial assessed 24-hour bronchodilator efficacy and safety of single doses of indacaterol 150 μg, 300 μg, 600 μg, placebo or formoterol (12 μg b.i.d.) in patients with moderate-to-severe COPD.[68] The trough FEV_1 at 24 h post-dose was significantly higher with all doses of indacaterol compared with placebo, with clinically relevant differences of ≥140 mL. Also the 12-hour trough FEV_1 with formoterol was greater than placebo, and greater with indacaterol 300 and 600 μg versus formoterol. All indacaterol doses significantly ($P < 0.001$) increased FEV_1 and FVC (forced vital capacity) versus placebo at all time points. The most frequent adverse effect (AE) was transient cough (3.9–6.4%) and, in general, AEs were mild.

A larger trial enrolled 635 patients with moderate to severe COPD, and randomized patients to one of the following regimens: indacaterol 50, 100, 200 or 400 μg once daily via MDDPI, or indacaterol 400 μg once daily via SDDPI, or placebo. The trial showed that all doses of indacaterol were associated with statistically significant dose-dependent improvements in FEV_1 compared with placebo, starting from 5 min after the first dose on day 1 of the 7-day treatment period.[69] Dose-dependent FEV_1 increases were seen for indacaterol by the first time point (5 minutes) and at all time points on days 1 and 7 ($P < 0.05$ vs placebo, all doses). The treatment effect persisted throughout the 24-hour dosing interval, and increases in trough FEV_1 with the 200 and 400 μg/day dosages were classified as clinically relevant. FVC and forced expiratory flow at 25–75% of FVC (FEF_{25-75}) were also significantly improved by indacaterol versus placebo, and rescue medication use was reduced. During an open-label extension period involving 263 patients, the effects of indacaterol on FEV_1 were similar to those of tiotropium bromide. A large multi-centre study recruited 1683 patients with moderate to severe COPD, and randomized them to either indacaterol 150 or 300 μg or placebo, or open-label tiotropium 18 μg, all given once daily for a period of 26 weeks.[70] Trough FEV_1 was significantly higher after treatment with either dose of indacaterol versus both placebo and tiotropium (Figure 5.1). Furthermore, health-related quality

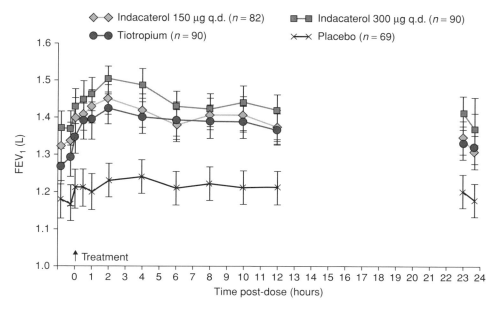

Figure 5.1   Twelve-hour serial measurements of FEV$_1$ (forced expiratory volume in 1 second) after 26 weeks of treatment with regular placebo, indacaterol 150 μg and 300 μg, and tiotropium. Reproduced with permission from Donohue JF, Fogarty C, Lötvall J, Mahler DA, Worth H, Yorgancioglu A, Iqbal A, Swales J, Owen R, Higgins M, Kramer B. INHANCE Study Investigators. Once-daily bronchodilators for chronic obstructive pulmonary disease: indacaterol versus tiotropium. Am J Respir Crit Care Med. 2010 Jul 15;182(2):155–62 © American Thoracic Society.

of life was also improved with indacaterol in this study, and there were no indications of differences in adverse effects. This study implies that indacaterol has higher clinical efficacy than tiotropium in patients with moderate to severe COPD.

The safety and tolerability of once-daily administration of two doses of indacaterol (400 and 800 μg) was assessed over a 28-day period in patients with moderate COPD.[71] It was documented that once-daily indacaterol was well tolerated at doses up to 800 μg with a good overall safety profile. As 800 μg represents two to four times the therapeutic dose suggested by earlier studies, these results imply that the therapeutic window for indacaterol may be wide, and that the doses that are available for clinical use are appropriate from a safety perspective.

Carmoterol

Carmoterol (CHF 4226, TA 2005; 8-hydroxy-5-[(1R)-1-hydroxy-2-[N-[(1R)-2-(p-methoxy-phenyl)-1-methylethyl]-amino]-ethyl]-carbostyril hydrochloride) is a non-catechol β₂-adrenoceptor agonist with a p-methoxyphenyl group on the amine side-chain and an 8-hydroxyl group on the carbostyril aromatic ring,[72] and possesses structural elements similar to both formoterol and procaterol. Carmoterol binds firmly to the β₂-AR,[73] a property shared by some other agonists that like carmoterol are based on a carbostyril skeleton.[74] In studies employing chimeric β₂-AR, the methoxyphenyl group in carmoterol has been found to be critical to the β_2-selectivity of the molecule.[75] Carmoterol is in development by Chiesi, under licence from Tanabe. Unfortunately, although carmoterol is the oldest of all ultra-LABAs under investigation, its development is substantially delayed.

Preclinical development

Carmoterol displays a fast onset and long duration of activity both in *in vitro* and *in vivo* experimental conditions.[72–74] It is clearly more potent than other LABAs, such as formoterol and salmeterol, requiring single inhaled doses to be as low as 1–4 μg, and has a onset of action similar to salbutamol and formoterol.[72,73,75–77] Furthermore, the duration of tracheal smooth muscle relaxation is longer for carmoterol compared to both formoterol and salmeterol.[77]

Asthma

The results obtained in healthy volunteers and asthmatic patients have provided evidence that the pharmacokinetics of carmoterol are proportional to the dose, and non-linear accumulation of the drug after repeated dosing treatments is negligible.[78] Interestingly, using Modulite™ technology that utilizes a hydrofluoroalkane (HFA) propellant, a lung deposition of carmoterol as high as 41% of the nominal dose can be achieved.[79] Because of the small particle size of the HFA pMDI (pressurized metered dose inhaler) aerosol (0.8 μm), no significant differences in lung deposition of carmoterol between healthy subjects, patients with asthma and patients with COPD have been documented.[79]

In patients with persistent asthma, carmoterol 2 μg administered once daily was as effective as formoterol 12 μg twice daily.[80] The trough FEV_1 values on the morning of day 8 were clinically and significantly greater in both active treatment groups compared with placebo, and the effect of carmoterol on trough FEV_1 was comparable to formoterol. Safety and tolerability are similar for carmoterol and formoterol.[81]

COPD

In patients with COPD,[82,83] a single 4 μg, but not a 1 or 2 μg, dose of carmoterol had an effect on 24-hour trough FEV_1 that was better than two 50 μg doses of salmeterol given 12 hours apart, suggesting that carmoterol may be useful as a once-daily bronchodilator in these patients. After 2 weeks of treatment, once-daily doses of 2 and 4 μg of carmoterol resulted in placebo-adjusted improvements compared to baseline in trough FEV_1 of 94 and 112 mL, respectively, whereas salmeterol 50 μg twice daily resulted in an increase of 78 mL. Similarly, doses of 2 and 4 μg carmoterol resulted in placebo-adjusted improvements compared to baseline in trough FVC of 133 and 123 mL, respectively. Subgroup evaluation of $FEV_1 AUC_{0-24}$ showed a significant dose–response relationship. All doses of carmoterol were deemed safe and well tolerated,[84] but Carmoterol 4 μg was associated with more headache and tremor than lower doses. Lower doses of carmoterol were associated with cough and dyspnoea. There were no significant changes in ECG, blood pressure, or serum potassium or glucose compared with salmeterol or placebo. Moreover, no tolerance to the bronchodilating effects of carmoterol or salmeterol was observed over the 2 weeks of treatment, as evidenced by the unchanged mean FEV$_1$ and the unchanged peak FEV$_1$.[85] A small and statistically insignificant reduction in the acute bronchodilation seen after dosing on day 14 was considered due to a significant increase in pre-dose trough FEV$_1$ rather than to the development of tolerance.

Milveterol

Milveterol (GSK-159797; TD-3327), *N*-{2-hydroxy-5-[(1*R*)-1-hydroxy-2-{[2-(4-{[(2*R*)-2-hydroxy-2-phenylethyl]amino}phenyl)ethyl]amino}ethyl]phenyl} formamide, is a once-daily LABA in development by GlaxoSmithKline (GSK) and Theravence.

Milveterol achieved the target increase in FEV$_1$ throughout the 25-hour evaluation period in a study of patients with mild asthma following single-dose inhalation. It was well tolerated, with no increase in heart rate.[52] A placebo-controlled crossover study tested the bronchodilatory effect, safety and tolerability of multiple dose levels of milveterol administered by a dry powder inhaler in patients with mild asthma, as referenced previously.[53] Doses in the anticipated clinical range produced clinically significant increases in FEV$_1$ through 24 hours, with little change in heart rate. At 24 hours, 10 and 20 μg doses of milveterol produced adjusted mean changes from baseline FEV$_1$ of 460 and 540 mL, respectively, compared to a change of 130 mL for placebo. The placebo-corrected mean maximum heart rate increase over the 26-hour period of measurement was 1.0 bpm for the 10 μg dose and 2.7 bpm for the 20 μg dose. In patients with asthma who were controlled on ICSs, all doses of milveterol studied (10, 15 and 20 μg), administered once a day, showed comparable bronchodilator activity to salmeterol 50 μg, dosed twice a day, at trough on the 14th day of treatment.[86] The lowest dose also produced a placebo-adjusted, weighted mean heart rate change over the first 4 hours after dosing on day 14 that was similar to that for salmeterol.

Although this is an interesting profile, it is likely that GSK and Theravance will continue to explore an optimized dose range for milveterol only as a backup because of the better therapeutic index of GSK-642444, another ultra-LABA in development by the two companies.

Vilanterol trifenatate

Vilanterol trifenatate (GSK-642444) is another ultra-LABA compound that GSK and Theravance have put into a pool for potential development for clinical use.

Asthma

All doses studied of GSK-642444 (25, 100 and 400 μg), dosed once a day over 14 days in patients with asthma, showed greater bronchodilator activity than salmeterol dosed twice a day, and produced placebo-adjusted, dose-dependent mean changes from baseline FEV_1 of over 200 mL at trough on the 14th day of treatment. The two lower doses also produced smaller changes than salmeterol in placebo-adjusted weighted mean heart rate over the first 4 hours after dosing on day 14.[86] Apparently, GSK-642444 presents a potentially greater therapeutic index than GSK-159797.[86]

One study evaluated the efficacy of five doses (3, 6.25, 12.5, 25 and 50 μg) of GSK-642444 administered once-daily for 4 weeks via a novel inhaler in patients with moderate to severe asthma who were receiving an ICS and short-acting β-agonist rescue medication as needed.[87] GSK-642444 induced dose-dependent improvements in lung function. All but the two lowest doses of GSK-642444 produced statistically significant improvements in FEV_1 measured 23–24 hours after the last dose. Efficacy was observed by a number of secondary endpoints including improvements in peak expiratory flow both in the morning and evening, and the percentage of symptom-free days and rescue-free days. Use of rescue medication was significantly lower in patients receiving the three highest doses of GSK-642444, compared to patients on placebo. Onset of action was dose-dependent, with the bronchodilator effect being sustained over 24 hours. Furthermore, improvements in lung function 24 hours after the first dose were maintained throughout the 28-day treatment period. Throughout the 4-week study period GSK-642444 was well tolerated at all doses and the frequency of adverse events was comparable to placebo. Headache was the most commonly observed adverse event in all arms and was comparable to placebo. The highest dose (50 μg) produced a small change in heart rate (a known effect of β-agonists) that did not exceed the predefined clinically relevant threshold. There were no serious adverse events reported in the study.

COPD

A trial that evaluated the dose–response, efficacy and safety of five doses (3, 6.25, 12.5, 25 and 50 μg) of GSK-642444 administered once-daily for 4 weeks in patients with moderate-to-severe COPD, showed a dose-dependent increase in lung function, with 25 and 50 μg exceeding a predefined threshold of 130 mL increase in FEV_1 at trough.[87] Favourable trends were also seen in morning and evening improvements in peak expiratory flow and reduced use of rescue medication. The drug was safe and well tolerated, with the most frequently reported adverse event being headache. There was no effect on average heart rate at any dose compared to placebo.

Olodaterol

Olodaterol, or BI-1744-CL, is under development by Boehringer Ingelheim as a potential inhaled $β_2$-agonist treatment for COPD and asthma.

Preclinical development

A study has compared the pharmacological profile of Olodaterol and formoterol in preclinical models.[88,89] *In vitro*, EC_{50} (effective concentration causing 50% of maximal effect) values for olodaterol against β_1, β_2 and β_3 in Chinese hamster ovary (CHO) cell membranes were 27, 0.1 and 199 nM (15, 0.2 and 26 nM for formoterol), respectively, with intrinsic activity scores of 53, 88 and 81% (96, 97 and 100% for formoterol), respectively. K_i (inhibition constant) values were 84, 0.9 and 2020 nM, respectively. The bronchoprotective potency of Olodaterol delivered by Respimat® inhaler in acetylcholine models of bronchospasm in both guinea pigs (dose range 0.1–3 µg/kg for bronchoprotection, 1–10 minutes for speed of onset) and dogs (0.15–0.6 µg/kg) showed equivalency to formoterol for speed of onset and a longer duration of protection. No difference was observed in serum potassium, lactate or heart rate compared with formoterol.

Asthma

The bronchoprotective effects of single doses (2, 5, 10 and 20 µg) of olodaterol (olodaterol) and placebo, administered using the Respimat® soft mist inhaler, against methacholine (MCH) provocation, were examined in 31 patients with intermittent asthma on separate days.[90] MCH challenges provocative concentration causing a 20% reeducation in FEV_1 (PC20 FEV_1) were performed at 30 min, and at 4, 8, 24 and 32 h following each single dose of medication. For olodaterol 20 µg, PC20 FEV_1 geometric mean ratios at other post-dose time points were also significantly increased compared with placebo (18.6 mg/mL at 30 min, 18.5 mg/mL at 4 h, 18.6 mg/mL at 8 h, and 6.3 mg/mL at 32 h). Similar time profiles were observed at all other doses.

COPD

The efficacy of different doses (2, 5, 10 or 20 µg) of olodaterol has also been examined in patients with stable COPD.[88,91] The maximum effect was produced by 20 µg, but was not noticeably different from 10 µg. FEV_1 was found to improve by 170 mL, and FVC by about 200 mL, an effect that waned and reached a nadir by 15 h. There was a slight recovery by 23 h but only to within the baseline. Olodaterol did increase FEV_1 and FVC over the values produced by placebo at all time points, and the plateau with a slight rise in lung function seen with olodaterol was replicated with placebo. No serious adverse events were reported, and only four minor adverse events were reported, with no changes detected in cardiovascular measurements or serum potassium. Further work will examine the effect of the 40 µg dose.

Saligenin or indole-containing and adamantyl-derived β_2-agonists

Pfizer is investigating a series of β_2-agonists for the potential treatment of respiratory disorders. The design and profile of saligenin-containing LABAs has been described.[92] Evaluation using a guinea-pig tissue model demonstrated that analogues within this series have significantly longer duration of action than salmeterol and have the potential for a once-daily profile in human.[93] Adamantyl-derived inhaled LABAs have also been described, and these may provide future opportunities.[94] A key design feature of these agents was to ensure that compounds would have low oral bioavailability compared to salmeterol to reduce systemic effects through the swallowed fraction after inhalation.

An amide derivative with an adamantyl group was found to be potent against the β_2-AR ($EC_{50} = 54\,nM$) and selective over the β_1 target showed 1300 times greater selectivity for β_2 than β_1 receptors.[95] In anaesthetized dogs, the compound had twice the duration of action of salmeterol and had comparable lung absorption rates. High clearance, a short half-life (1.6 h) and low oral bioavailability were seen in rat. It was predicted that in human the pharmacokinetics/pharmacodynamics dose projection was 7 to 70 mg once daily in a dry powder inhalant.

In vitro, the potency and selectivity were studied using CHO cell membranes expressing human β-ARs.[96] At β_2 receptors UK-503,590 had equivalent potency to salmeterol, was approximately six-fold weaker than formoterol and 243 times more potent than salbutamol. Moreover, it was 56 times more selective for β_1 and β_3 than salmeterol. UK-503,590 also demonstrated a duration of action that was equivalent to salmeterol but significantly longer than formoterol in the guinea-pig tracheal model. Salmeterol as well as UK-503,590, but not formoterol, exhibited reassertion in the guinea-pig trachea, indicating persistent activation of the receptors. Also the design and profile of a series of indole-containing long-acting β_2-adrenoceptor agonists has been described. Evaluation of these analogues using an *in vitro* guinea-pig tracheal tissue model demonstrates that analogues within this series have a salmeterol-like duration of action with potential for a long duration of action in humans.

In anaesthetized dogs, UK-503,590 was 10-fold more potent and has an improved therapeutic index compared to salmeterol, with a two-fold longer duration of action at the maximum tolerated dose.[97] Furthermore, UK-503,590 induced a doubling of duration of protection for bronchoconstriction (>8 h), and heart rate, blood pressure and ECG measures were unchanged over the dose range used (0.03–3 µg).

Compound X is a LABA being developed by Pfizer.[98] Selectivity was assessed using CHO cells that expressed recombinant human β_1, β_2 or β_3 receptors. The EC_{50} for increasing cyclic AMP at β_1-, β_2- and β_3-ARs was 28.6, 0.08 and 42.8 nM, respectively. The potency of compound X at β_2-ARs was similar to salmeterol, 100-fold more potent than salbutamol and nine-fold less potent than formoterol. Compound X had a duration of action of 4.3 h (3.4–6.1 h), which was significantly longer than formoterol (2.3 h; 2.0–2.7 h) but shorter than salmeterol. *In vivo*, in anaesthetized dogs, intratracheal administration of compound X provided dose-related inhibition of acetylcholine-induced bronchoconstriction ($ED_{50} = 1.0$ µg).[99] Cardiac parameters, including blood pressure, heart rate and cardiac contractility, were measured to determine the therapeutic index. Compound X has a potency and therapeutic index equivalent to those of salmeterol, with a two-fold longer duration of action at the maximum tolerated dose compared to both formoterol and salmeterol in the anaesthetized dog.

LAS-100977

Almirall Prodesfarma is developing LAS-100977, a once-daily LABA. Twenty-five asthma patients were treated once a day with placebo, 50 mg of salmeterol or one of several doses of LAS-100977.[100] The primary endpoint was change from pre-dose trough FEV_1. A significant increase in FEV_1 was seen in patients receiving all doses of LAS-100977 compared with those treated with either placebo or salmeterol. The drug was well tolerated, with tachycardia and tremor seen at the higher doses. A 24-hour duration of action was confirmed.

5.4   Conclusion

β₂-Agonists are still central to the symptomatic management of asthma and COPD, and as a second controller in asthma. It is likely that once-daily dosing of a LABA will lead to increased convenience for patients, which may also enhance compliance and may have advantages leading to improved overall clinical outcomes in patients with asthma and COPD. The majority of agents under development have a high intrinsic efficacy and a rapid onset of action. While a rapid onset of action and a prolonged 24-hour effect are desirable in the management of asthma and COPD, the use of agonists with high intrinsic efficacy may theoretically be associated with a rapid onset of tolerance, a fact that may limit their clinical use.[101] The only real limits set for the development of a LABA with a new product profile are the medical needs and marketing opportunities. Someone who is planning to develop a new ultra-LABA must consider very carefully the pharmacological characteristics of the β₂-agonist component to understand how it will fit into current treatment strategies, or even whether it should be used only in combination with other drugs. Most likely, this group of bronchodilating drugs is here for many decades to come.

References

1. van der Woude HJ, Aalbers R. Long-acting β₂-agonists: comparative pharmacology and clinical outcomes. Am J Respir Med 2002;1:55–74.
2. Hall IP. β2-Adrenoceptor agonists. In: Barnes PJ, Rennard SI, Drazen JM, Thomson NC (eds), *Asthma and COPD: Basic Mechanisms and Clinical Management*, 2nd edn. Academic Press, Oxford, 2009; pp. 609–14.
3. Lötvall J. Pharmacological similarities and differences between β₂-agonists. Respir Med 2001;95(Suppl. B):S7–11.
4. Expert Panel Report 3 (EPR–3). Guidelines for the Diagnosis and Management of Asthma – Summary Report 2007. J Allergy Clin Immunol 2007;120(5 Suppl.):S94–138.
5. Bateman ED, Hurd SS, Barnes PJ, et al. Global strategy for asthma management and prevention: GINA executive summary. Eur Respir J 2008;31:143–78.
6. Lazarus SC, Boushey HA, Fahy JV, et al. Long-acting β₂-agonist monotherapy vs continued therapy with inhaled corticosteroids in patients with persistent asthma: a randomized controlled trial. JAMA 2001;285:2583–93.

7. Jackson CM, Lipworth B. Benefit–risk assessment of long-acting β_2-agonists in asthma. Drug Safety 2004;27:243–70.

8. Cazzola M, Matera MG. Safety of long-acting β_2-agonists in the treatment of asthma. Ther Adv Respir Dis 2007;1:35–46.

9. Lipworth BJ. Long-acting β_2-adrenoceptor agonists: a smart choice for asthma? Trends Pharmacol Sci 2007;28:257–62.

10. Lipworth BJ, Hall IP, Tan S, Aziz I, Coutie W. Effects of genetic polymorphism on ex vivo and in vivo function of β_2-adrenoceptors in asthmatic patients. Chest 1999;115:324–8.

11. Israel E, Chinchilli VM, Ford JG, et al. Use of regularly scheduled albuterol treatment in asthma: genotype-stratified, randomised, placebo-controlled cross-over trial. Lancet 2004;364:1505–12.

12. Taylor DR, Drazen JM, Herbison GP, Yandava CN, Hancox RJ, Town GI. Asthma exacerbations during long term beta agonist use: influence of β_2 adrenoceptor polymorphism. Thorax 2000;55:762–7.

13. Wechsler ME, Lehman E, Lazarus SC, et al. β-Adrenergic receptor polymorphisms and response to salmeterol. Am J Respir Crit Care Med 2006;173:519–26.

14. Lee DK, Currie GP, Hall IP, Lima JJ, Lipworth BJ. The arginine-16 β_2-adrenoceptor polymorphism predisposes to bronchoprotective subsensitivity in patients treated with formoterol and salmeterol. Br J Clin Pharmacol 2004;57:68–75.

15. Ellsworth DL, Coady SA, Chen W, et al. Influence of the β_2-adrenergic receptor Arg16Gly polymorphism on longitudinal changes in obesity from childhood through young adulthood in a biracial cohort: the Bogalusa Heart Study. Int J Obes Relat Metab Disord 2002;26: 928–37.

16. Nelson HS, Weiss ST, Bleecker ER, Yancey SW, Dorinsky PM. The Salmeterol Multicenter Asthma Research Trial: a comparison of usual pharmacotherapy for asthma or usual pharmacotherapy plus salmeterol. Chest 2006;129:15–26.

17. Salpeter SR, Buckley NS, Ormiston TM, Salpeter EE. Meta-analysis: effect of long-acting β-agonists on severe asthma exacerbations and asthma-related deaths. Ann Intern Med 2006;144:904–12.

18. Sin DD, Man SF. Corticosteroids and adrenoceptor agonists: the complements for combination therapy in chronic airways diseases. Eur J Pharmacol 2006;533:28–35.

19. Walters EH, Walters J, Gibson P. Inhaled long acting β agonists for stable chronic asthma. Cochrane Database Syst Rev 2003;(4):CD001385.

20. Walters EH, Walters J, Gibson P. Regular treatment with long acting β agonists versus daily regular treatment with short acting beta agonists in adults and children with stable asthma. Cochrane Database Syst Rev 2002;(3):CD003901.

21. Shah L, Wilson A, Gibson P, Coughlan J. Long acting β-agonists versus theophylline for maintenance treatment of asthma. Cochrane Database Syst Rev 2003;(3):CD001281.

22. Celli BR, MacNee W. ATS/ERS Task Force. Standards for the diagnosis and treatment of patients with COPD: a summary of the ATS/ERS position paper. Eur Respir J 2004;23:932–46.

23. Rabe KF, Hurd S, Anzueto A, et al. Global strategy for the diagnosis, management, and prevention of chronic obstructive pulmonary disease: GOLD executive summary. Am J Respir Crit Care Med 2007;176:532–55.

24. Johnson M, Rennard S. Alternative mechanisms for long-acting beta(2)-adrenergic agonists in COPD. Chest 2001;120:258–70.

25. Cazzola M, Vinciguerra A, Di Perna F, Matera MG. Early reversibility to salbutamol does not always predict bronchodilation after salmeterol in stable chronic obstructive pulmonary disease. Respir Med 1998;92:1012–16.

26. Cazzola M, Hanania NA, Jones PW, et al. It's about time – directing our attention toward modifying the course of COPD. Respir Med 2008;102(Suppl. 1):S37–48.
27. Sin DD, McAlister FA, Man SF, Anthonisen NR. Contemporary management of chronic obstructive pulmonary disease: scientific review. JAMA 2003;290:2301–12.
28. Man SF, McAlister FA, Anthonisen NR, Sin DD. Contemporary management of chronic obstructive pulmonary disease; clinical applications. JAMA 2003;290:2313–16.
29. Rossi A, Khirani S, Cazzola M. Long-acting β₂-agonists (LABA) in chronic obstructive pulmonary disease: efficacy and safety. Intern J COPD 2008;3:521–9.
30. Celli BR, Thomas NE, Anderson JA, et al. Effect of pharmacotherapy on rate of decline of lung function in chronic obstructive pulmonary disease: results from the TORCH study. Am J Respir Crit Care Med 2008;178:332–8.
31. Cazzola M, Matera MG. The effective treatment of COPD: Anticholinergics and what else? Drug Discov Today: Ther Strat 2006;3:277–86.
32. D'Urzo AD, De Salvo MC, Ramirez–Rivera A, et al. In patients with COPD, treatment with a combination of formoterol and ipratropium is more effective than a combination of salbutamol and ipratropium: a 3-week, randomized, double-blind, within-patient, multicenter study. Chest 2001;119:1347–56.
33. Richter K, Stenglein S, Mücke M, et al. Onset and duration of action of formoterol and tiotropium in patients with moderate to severe COPD. Respiration 2006;73:414–19.
34. Vogelmeier C, Kardos P, Harari S, Gans SJ, Stenglein S, Thirlwell J. Formoterol mono– and combination therapy with tiotropium in patients with COPD: a 6-month study. Respir Med 2008;102:1511–20.
35. Tashkin D, Pearle J, Iezzoni D, Varghese ST. Treatment with formoterol plus tiotropium is more effective than treatment with tiotropium alone in patients with stable chronic obstructive pulmonary disease: Findings from a randomized, placebo-controlled trial. J COPD 2009;6:17–25.
36. Cazzola M, Noschese P, Salzillo A, De Giglio C, D'Amato G, Matera MG. Bronchodilator response to formoterol after regular tiotropium or to tiotropium after regular formoterol in COPD patients. Respir Med 2005;99:524–8.
37. Cazzola M, Centanni S, Santus P, et al. The functional impact of adding salmeterol and tiotropium in patients with stable COPD. Respir Med 2004;98:1214–21.
38. Calverley P, Pauwels R, Vestbo J, et al. Combined salmeterol and fluticasone in the treatment of chronic obstructive pulmonary disease: a randomised controlled trial. Lancet 2003;361:449–56.
39. Szafranski W, Cukier A, Ramirez A, et al. Efficacy and safety of budesonide/formoterol in the management of chronic obstructive pulmonary disease. Eur Respir J 2003;21:74–81.
40. Calverley PM, Boonsawat W, Cseke Z, Zhong N, Peterson S, Olsson H. Maintenance therapy with budesonide and formoterol in chronic obstructive pulmonary disease. Eur Respir J 2003;22:912–19.
41. Calverley PMA, Anderson JA, Celli B, et al. Salmeterol and fluticasone propionate and survival in chronic obstructive pulmonary disease. N Engl J Med 2007;356:775–89.
42. Salpeter SR, Buckley NS, Salpeter EE. Meta-analysis: anticholinergics, but not β-agonists, reduce severe exacerbations and respiratory mortality in COPD. J Gen Intern Med 2006;21:1011–19.
43. Cazzola M, Matera MG, Donner CF. Inhaled β₂-adrenoceptor agonists: cardiovascular safety in patients with obstructive lung disease. Drugs 2005;65:1595–610.
44. Santus P, Centanni S, Morelli N, Di Marco F, Verga M, Cazzola M. Tiotropium is less likely to induce oxygen desaturation in stable COPD patients compared to long-acting β₂-agonists. Respir Med 2007;101:1798–803.

45. Ingram RH Jr, Krumpe PE, Duffell GM, Maniscalco B. Ventilation-perfusion changes after aerosolized isoproterenol in asthma. Am Rev Respir Dis 1970;101:364–70.
46. Wagner PD, Dantzker DR, Iacovoni VE, Tomlin WC, West JB. Ventilation-perfusion inequality in asymptomatic asthma. Am Rev Respir Dis 1978;118:511–24.
47. MacNee W, Wathen CG, Hannan WJ, Flenley DC, Muir AL. Effects of pirbuterol and sodium nitroprusside on pulmonary haemodynamics in hypoxic cor pulmonale. Br Med J 1983;287:1169–72.
48. Cazzola M, Noschese P, De Michele F, D'Amato G, Matera MG. Effect of formoterol/budesonide combination on arterial blood gases in patients with acute exacerbation of COPD. Respir Med 2006;100:212–17.
49. Kumar SD, Brieva JL, Danta I, Wanner A. Transient effect of inhaled fluticasone on airway mucosal blood flow in subjects with and without asthma. Am J Respir Crit Care Med 2000;161:918–21.
50. Waldeck B. Some pharmacodynamic aspects on long-acting β-adrenoceptor agonists. Gen Pharmacol 1996;27:575–80.
51. Anonymous. Novel long-acting β_2 agonists; Glaxo Wellcome plc: WO02070490 & WO02076933. Current Opin Ther Patents 2003;13:273–7.
52. Cazzola M, Matera MG, Lötvall J. Ultra long-acting β_2 agonists in development for asthma and chronic obstructive pulmonary disease. Expert Opin Investig Drugs 2005;14:775–83.
53. Matera MG, Cazzola M. Ultra-long-acting β_2-adrenoceptor agonists: an emerging therapeutic option for asthma and COPD? Drugs 2007;67:503–15.
54. Cazzola M, Matera MG. Novel long-acting bronchodilators for COPD and asthma. Br J Pharmacol 2008;155:291–9.
55. Campbell LM. Once-daily inhaled corticosteroids in mild to moderate asthma: improving acceptance of treatment. Drugs 1999;58(Suppl. 4):25–33.
56. Battram C, Charlton SJ, Cuenoud B, et al. In vitro and in vivo pharmacological characterization of 5-[(R)-2-(5,6-diethyl-indan-2-ylamino)-1-hydroxy-ethyl]-8-hydroxy-1H-quinolin-2-one (indacaterol), a novel inhaled β_2 adrenoceptor agonist with a 24-h duration of action. J Pharmacol Exp Ther 2006;317:762–70.
57. Sturton RG, Trifilieff A, Nicholson AG, Barnes PJ. Pharmacological characterization of indacaterol, a novel once daily inhaled β_2 adrenoceptor agonist, on small airways in human and rat precision-cut lung slices. J Pharmacol Exp Ther 2008;324:270–5.
58. Naline E, Trifilieff A, Fairhurst RA, Advenier C, Molimard M. Effect of indacaterol, a novel long-acting β_2-adrenoceptor agonist, on human isolated bronchi. Eur Respir J 2007;29:575–81.
59. Beeh KM, Derom E, Kanniess F, Cameron R, Higgins M, van As A. Indacaterol, a novel inhaled β_2-agonist, provides sustained 24-h bronchodilation in asthma. Eur Respir J 2007;29:871–8.
60. Pearlman DS, Greos L, LaForce C, Orevillo CJ, Owen R, Higgins M. Bronchodilator efficacy of indacaterol, a novel once-daily β_2-agonist, in patients with persistent asthma. Ann Allergy Asthma Immunol 2008;101:90–5.
61. LaForce C, Korenblat P, Osborne P, Dong F, Owen R, Higgins M. 24-hour bronchodilator efficacy of single doses of indacaterol in patients with persistent asthma, and comparison with formoterol [abstract]. Eur Respir J 2008;32:516s.
62. Kanniess F, Boulet LP, Pierzchala W, Cameron R, Owen R, Higgins M. Efficacy and safety of indacaterol, a new 24-hour β_2-agonist, in patients with asthma: a dose-ranging study. J Asthma 2008;45:887–92.
63. LaForce C, Alexander M, Deckelmann R, et al. Indacaterol provides sustained 24 h bronchodilation on once-daily dosing in asthma: a 7-day dose-ranging study. Allergy 2008;63:103–11.

64. Brookman LJ, Knowles LJ, Barbier M, Elharrar B, Fuhr R, Pascoe S. Efficacy and safety of single therapeutic and supratherapeutic doses of indacaterol versus salmeterol and salbutamol in patients with asthma. Curr Med Res Opin 2007;23:3113–22.

65. Chuchalin AG, Tsoi AN, Richter K, et al. Safety and tolerability of indacaterol in asthma: a randomized, placebo-controlled 28-day study. Respir Med 2007;101:2065–75.

66. Yang W, Higgins M, Cameron R, Owen R. Indacaterol, a novel once-daily β_2-agonist, is well tolerated in persistent asthma [abstract]. Eur Respir J 2006;28:436s.

67. Aubier M, Duval X, Knight H, et al. Indacaterol, a novel once-daily β_2-agonist is effective and well tolerated on multiple dosing in patients with mild-to-moderate COPD [abstract]. Eur Respir J 2005;26 (Suppl. 49):287s.

68. Bauwens O, Ninane V, Van de Maele B, et al. 24-hour bronchodilator efficacy of single doses of indacaterol in subjects with COPD: comparison with placebo and formoterol. Curr Med Res Opin 2009;25:463–70.

69. Rennard S, Bantje T, Centanni S, et al. A dose-ranging study of indacaterol in obstructive airways disease, with a tiotropium comparison. Respir Med 2008;102:1033–44.

70. Donohue JF, Fogarty C, Lötvall J, et al. Once-daily bronchodilators for chronic obstructive pulmonary disease: indacaterol versus tiotropium. Am J Respir Crit Care Med 2010;182: 155–62.

71. Beier J, Chanez P, Martinot JB, et al. Safety, tolerability and efficacy of indacaterol, a novel once-daily β_2-agonist, in patients with COPD: a 28-day randomised, placebo controlled clinical trial. Pulm Pharmacol Ther 2007;20:740–9.

72. Kikkawa H, Naito K, Ikezawa K. Tracheal relaxing effects and β_2-selectivity of TA-2005, a newly developed bronchodilating agent, in isolated guinea-pig tissues. Jpn J Pharmacol 1991;57:175–85.

73. Voss H-P, Donnell D, Bast A. Atypical molecular pharmacology of a new long-acting β_2-adrenoceptor agonist, TA-2005. Eur J Pharmacol 1992;227:403–9.

74. Standifer KM, Pitha J, Baker SP. Carbostyril-based β-adrenergic agonists: evidence for long lasting or apparent irreversible receptor binding and activation of adenylate cyclase activity in vitro. Naunyn–Schmiedeberg's Arch Pharmacol 1989;339:129–37.

75. Kikkawa H, Isogaya M, Nagao T, Kurose H. The role of the seventh transmembrane region in high affinity binding of a β_2-selective agonist TA-2005. Mol Pharmacol 1998;53:128–34.

76. Kikkawa H, Kanno K, Ikezawa K. TA-2005, a novel, long-acting and selective β_2-adrenocepter agonist: characterization of its in vivo bronchodilating action in guinea pigs and cats in comparison with other β_2-agonists. Biol Pharm Bull 1994;17:1047–52.

77. Voss H-P. Long-acting β_2-adrenoceptor agonists in asthma: molecular pharmacological aspects. Thesis, Vrije Universiteit, Amsterdam, 1994.

78. Chiesi Farmaceutici S.p.A. Investigator's brochure: CHF 4226. June 2004 (Data on file).

79. Haeussermann S, Acerbi A, Brand P, Poli G, Meyer T. Lung deposition of carmoterol in healthy subjects, patients with asthma and patients with COPD [abstract]. Eur Respir J 2006;28:211s.

80. Kottakis I, Nandeuil A, Raptis H, Savu A, Linberg SE, Woodcock AA. Efficacy of the novel very long-acting β2-agonist carmoterol following 7 days once daily dosing: comparison with twice daily formoterol in patient with persistent asthma [abstract]. Eur Respir J 2006; 28:665s.

81. Nandeuil A, Kottakis I, Raptis H, Roslan H, Ivanov Y, Woodcock A. Safety and tolerability of the novel very long acting β2-agonist carmoterol given as a 2μg qd dose; 8 days comparison with formoterol and placebo in patients with persistent asthma [abstract]. Eur Respir J 2006; 28:665s.

82. Kanniess F, Make BJ, Petruzzelli S. Acute effect of carmoterol, a long-acting beta2-agonist, in patients with COPD [abstract]. Proc Am Thorac Soc 2008;5:A655.

83. Make BJ, Kanniess F, Bateman ED, Linberg SE. Efficacy of 3 different doses of carmoterol, a long-acting beta2-agonist in patients with COPD [abstract]. Proc Am Thorac Soc 2008;5:A961.

84. Bateman ED, Make BJ, Nandeuil MA. Carmoterol – safety and tolerability of a long-acting beta-2 agonist in patients with COPD [abstract]. Proc Am Thorac Soc 2008;5:A653.

85. Rossing TH, Make BJ, Heyman ER. Carmoterol does not induce tolerance in COPD [abstract]. Proc Am Thorac Soc 2008;5:A962.

86. Anonymous. Theravance, Inc. (THRX) announces positive results of clinical program in beyond Advair collaboration. http://www.biospace.com/news_story.aspx?NewsEntityId=51071. Date last accessed 18 January 2009.

87. Lötvall J, Bateman ED, Bleecker ER, et al. Dose-related efficacy of vilanterol trifenatate (VI), a long-acting beta2 agonist (LABA) with inherent 24-hour activity, in patients with persistent asthma. www.ersnet.org ERS2010 (abstract) Session 497. Bronchodilators in airways disease.

88. Spears MATS 2008 – The International Conference of the American Thoracic Society (Part II), Toronto, Canada. IDDB MEETING REPORT http://utility.reference?i_reference_id=913869. Date last accessed 18 January 2009. EXCHANGE TO:

89. Bouyssou T, Casarosa P, Naline E, Pestel S, Konetzki I, Devillier P, Schnapp A. Pharmacological characterization of olodaterol, a novel inhaled beta2-adrenoceptor agonist exerting a 24-hour-long duration of action in preclinical models. J Pharmacol Exp Ther 2010;334(1):53–62. Epub 2010 Apr 6.

90. O'Byrne PM, van der Linde J, Cockcroft DW, Gauvreau GM, Brannan JD, Fitzgerald M, Watson RM, Milot J, Davis B, O'Connor M, Hart L, Korducki L, Hamilton AL, Boulet LP. Prolonged bronchoprotection against inhaled methacholine by inhaled BI 1744, a long-acting beta(2)-agonist, in patients with mild asthma. J Allergy Clin Immunol. 2009 Dec;124(6): 1217–21.

91. van Noord JA, Smeets JJ, Drenth BM, Pivovarova A, Hamilton AL, Cornelissen PJG. Single doses of BI 1744 CL, a novel long-acting β_2-agonist, are effective for up to 24 hrs in COPD patients [abstract]. Proc Am Thorac Soc 2008;5:A961.

92. Brown AD, Bunnage ME, Glossop PA, et al. The discovery of long acting β_2-adrenoreceptor agonists. Bioorg Med Chem Lett 2007;17:4012–15.

93. Brown AD, Bunnage ME, Glossop PA, et al. The discovery of indole-derived long acting β_2-adrenoceptor agonists for the treatment of asthma and COPD. Bioorg Med Chem Lett 2007;17:6188–91.

94. Brown AD, Bunnage ME, Glossop PA, et al. The discovery of adamantyl-derived, inhaled, long acting β_2-adrenoreceptor agonists. Bioorg Med Chem Lett 2008;18:1280–3.

95. Bunnage ME, Glossop PA, James K, et al. The discovery of inhaled, long-acting beta-2 adrenoceptor agonists for the treatment of asthma and COPD [abstract]. 31st National Medicinal Chemistry Symposium. Program and Abstracts June 2008;81.

96. Coghlan M, Shepherd C, Summerhill S, et al. The in vitro biology of UK-503,590 – a novel beta2 adrenoceptor agonist with a long duration of action [abstract]. Proc Am Thorac Soc 2008;5:A488.

97. Wright KN, Holbrook M, Yeadon M, Perros-Huguet C. An inhaled beta2 agonist with greater potency/duration of action (DoA) and superior therapeutic index (TI) to salmeterol in the anaesthetised dog model of bronchoconstriction [abstract]. Proc Am Thorac Soc 2008; 5:A945.

 98. Coghlan M, Shepherd C, Summerhill S, Patel S. The in vitro biology of Compound X – a novel $\beta2$ adrenoceptor agonist with a long duration of action [abstract]. Eur Respir J 2008;32:475s.
 99. Wright K, Yeadon M, Perros-Huguet C. Compound X – an inhaled β_2 agonist with equivalent potency and superior duration of action (DOA)/therapeutic index (TI) to salmeterol in the anaesthetised dog model of bronchoconstriction [abstract]. Eur Respir J 2008;32:476s.
100. Anonymous. Almirall announces promising results with a new compound for asthma and COPD. http://investors.almirall.es/phoenix.zhtml?c=209345&p=irol–newsArticle&ID=1133005& highlight=. Date last accessed 18 January 2009.
101. Hanania NA, Sharafkhaneh A, Barber R, et al. β-Agonist intrinsic efficacy: measurement and clinical significance. Am J Respir Crit Care Med 2002;165:1353–8.

6

The safety of long-acting beta-agonists and the development of combination therapies for asthma and COPD

Victor E. Ortega and Eugene R. Bleecker

Center for Human Genomics and Personalized Medicine, Wake Forest University Health Sciences, USA

6.1 Introduction

β_2-Adrenergic receptor agonists (i.e. beta-agonists) are the most commonly prescribed therapeutic agents for the management of asthma and other obstructive pulmonary diseases, specifically chronic obstructive pulmonary disease (COPD). Two classes of inhaled β_2-adrenergic receptor agonists include the long-acting beta-agonists (LABA: salmeterol, formoterol and arformoterol) and the short-acting beta-agonists (SABA: albuterol, salbutamol, terbutaline, etc.). LABA therapy should be used only in conjunction with inhaled corticosteroids (ICS) for asthma management, while in COPD LABA therapy can be used alone or in combination with an ICS as long-term maintenance therapy.[1] However, SABA therapy is used for acute, as-needed symptom relief or to prevent exercise-induced asthma.[1]

Currently, salmeterol (Serevent®) and formoterol (Foradil® and Performist®) are approved for the treatment of both asthma and COPD; however, a recent advisory panel on the safety of these agents by the United States Food and Drug Administration (FDA) has been conducted (www.fda.gov) and the results of this panel have been reviewed in two recent publications.[2–4] Before the early 1990s, SABAs were the only effective bronchodilator therapies available for the management of asthma and COPD. The short duration of SABA therapy, ranging from 4 to 6 hours, required that patients used several doses to maintain continuous symptom relief, particularly for individuals whose symptoms remained uncontrolled on ICS therapy alone. In contrast, LABAs such as salmeterol and formoterol improve lung function

Advances in Combination Therapy for Asthma and COPD, First Edition. Edited by Jan Lötvall.
© 2012 John Wiley & Sons, Ltd. Published 2012 by John Wiley & Sons, Ltd.

and provide symptom control for at least 12 hours.[5–8] In addition, formoterol has a more rapid onset of action than salmeterol, with an onset of action similar to that of the SABA albuterol.[6,9]

Concern regarding the safety of LABA therapy was raised after these agents were introduced into the market. When salmeterol was introduced in the UK in 1990, a large study called the Serevent Nationwide Surveillance Study showed a statistically insignificant increase in asthma-related deaths related to the use of this agent.[8,9] These potential safety issues were supported by results of the Salmeterol Multicenter Asthma Research Trial (SMART), a surveillance study requested by the FDA at time of the US registration of salmeterol, and a subsequent meta-analysis.[10, 11]

With respect to COPD, adverse cardiovascular events such as supraventricular and premature ventricular beats have been observed with the use of higher doses of formoterol; however, these findings have been limited to those individuals with pre-existing cardiac arrhythmias or severe hypoxaemia.[12] Salmeterol and formoterol may show some β_1-adrenergic receptor activity that might affect heart rate, cardiac rhythm, corrected QT interval, blood pressure and serum potassium concentrations, particularly when these agents are used at higher-than-recommended doses.[13, 14] A meta-analysis performed by Salpeter et al. showed an association of LABA and SABA use with tachycardia and hypokalaemia.[15] Despite these concerns, prospective clinical trials have not shown an increased risk of clinically relevant or fatal adverse cardiovascular events with the use of LABA therapy at appropriate doses when used in the management of COPD.[16–19]

Although there are studies that report data regarding the potential for adverse events related to the use of LABA therapy in the treatment of asthma and COPD, some of these studies have significant design limitations further complicated by the exceedingly low mortality associated with asthma; therefore, definitive conclusions are difficult to make from these studies. Multiple prospective clinical trials have demonstrated that LABA therapy is a very effective therapy for the management of asthma when used in conjunction with ICS therapy. Furthermore, prospective clinical trials have also demonstrated the safety and efficacy of LABA therapy as a monotherapy or combined with ICS therapy in the management of COPD.[20, 21] Thus, the overall therapeutic value of these approaches has led to the development of combination therapies in a single device ensuring the concomitant administration of a LABA and an ICS while improving overall adherence.[22, 23]

6.2 Asthma-related mortality and beta-agonist exposure

Therapeutic use of beta-agonists and asthma-related mortality was first observed in the 1960s; a finding that was primarily related to the dosing regimens and potency of the SABA available at that time. In the UK and other countries a higher dose isoproterenol inhaler (a potent non-specific beta short-acting beta-agonist) was marketed and there was an increase in asthma mortality that disappeared with the withdrawal of this preparation (Figure 6.1).[24] In addition, between 1976 and 1989, fenoterol (a potent less

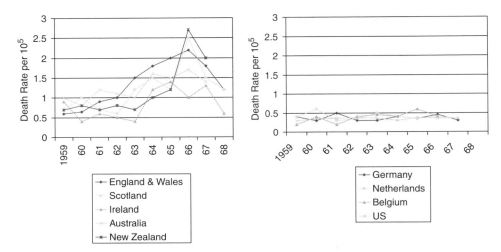

Figure 6.1 Asthma mortality based on National Vital Statistics and the trend of increased asthma mortality observed in the countries that marketed a higher concentration of the nebulized bronchodilator, isoproterenol, during the 1960s. Reproduced from Stolley (1972),[24] with permission.

specific SABA) was marketed in New Zealand as high-dose and regular-dose inhalers. Asthma mortality increased when this agent was released and declined when it was removed from the market (Figure 6.2).[25–29] Additional data, particularly from epidemiological studies such as the Saskatchewan Asthma Epidemiology Project, reported a correlation between the number of prescriptions of fenoterol and other SABAs with

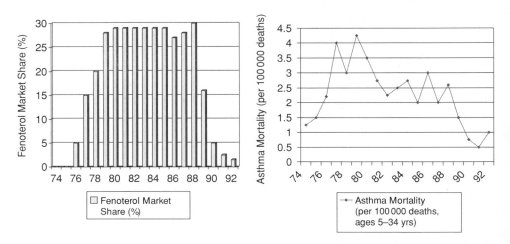

Figure 6.2 The time-trend of increased asthma mortality during the New Zealand asthma mortality epidemic from 1976 to 1989. The increase in mortality was observed in 1976 after the introduction of a potent short-acting beta-agonist (SABA), fenoterol, in New Zealand. The mortality decreased in 1989 after a safety warning was released from the New Zealand Department of Health that resulted in a sudden drop of sales and the eventual removal of fenoterol from the market. Reproduced from Pearce et al. (1995),[27] with permission.

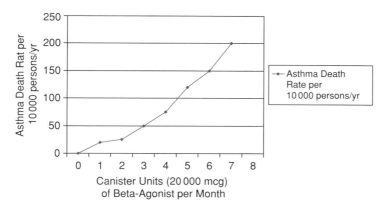

Figure 6.3   Dose–response curve illustrating the relationship between total short-acting beta-agonist (SABA) use and asthma death rates from the Saskatchewan Asthma Epidemiology Project: a retrospective cohort analysis of 12 301 patients with asthma and 46 asthma-related deaths. The observed trend likely reflects increased disease severity rather than a cause and effect relationship. Reproduced from Suissa et al. (1994),[31] with permission.

an increased risk of mortality, which may suggest a cause and effect relationship but may also reflect the fact that an increased frequency of SABA use represents an index of poor asthma control (Figure 6.3).[30,31] In addition, Sears and colleagues, using a prospective clinical trial design, showed that asthma control was worse with the regular use of fenoterol than with as-needed SABA therapy for asthma symptom relief.[32] The National Institutes of Health (NIH) Asthma Clinical Research Network (ACRN) beta-agonist study, BAGS, demonstrated the safety of regular SABA therapy with albuterol but also showed that regular SABA therapy with albuterol therapy did not improve asthma control when compared to as-needed symptomatic use of albuterol.[33] A subsequent sub-analysis of the data from the BAGS trial reported a pharmacogenetic interaction with β_2-adrenergic receptor gene variation, when it was reported that $Arg^{16}Arg$ homozygotes on regular SABA therapy had progressive worsening of lung function during this treatment.[34] This important study supports the concept that pharmacogenetic mechanisms may be important in beta-agonist drug responses and related toxicity.

6.3   Long-acting beta-agonists and increased asthma-related mortality

The first large-scale study to address concerns regarding the safety of LABA therapy and its impact on asthma-related mortality was the Serevent Nationwide Surveillance Study.[8] This study was a prospective, randomized, double-blind, parallel-group study performed in the UK in response to potential concerns regarding the worsening of asthma control with regular fenoterol therapy and other epidemiological studies reporting a correlation of increased beta-agonist use with asthma-related death.[9,25–32] The study enrolled 25 180 participants with asthma of varying severity and compared regular salmeterol therapy with albuterol therapy for a duration of 16 weeks. The study was designed to examine adverse therapeutic events and serious events resulting in study withdrawal. The investigators reported a three-fold increase in the risk of asthma-related deaths in those subjects using salmeterol when compared to those using placebo: a finding that was not statistically significant ($P = 0.105$). Asthma-related death was a rare event in both groups, 12 of 16 787 (0.07%) in the salmeterol group compared to 2 of 8393 (0.02%) in the regular albuterol group, therefore not providing the investigators sufficient power to detect a significant association with asthma-related mortality. Complicating the interpretation of this finding, a significantly larger proportion of asthma and respiratory-related withdrawals were reported in the albuterol group when compared to the salmeterol group ($P = 0.0002$). An important limiting factor of this study was that 31% of the participants in both groups were not receiving ICS therapy at baseline and that adherence to ICS therapy in both groups was not assessed during this study.[9]

The statistically insignificant relationship between the use of salmeterol and asthma-related mortality reported in the Serevent Nationwide Surveillance Study caused the FDA to initiate a larger prospective study to address the effects of salmeterol on respiratory and asthma-related deaths or life-threatening episodes in asthma. The FDA asked GlaxoSmithKline, the manufacturer of salmeterol, to obtain these data in a 'real-world setting'. This resulted in the Salmeterol Multicenter Asthma Research Trial (SMART); a multicentre, placebo-controlled, double-blind, parallel-group, observational surveillance study comparing the addition of salmeterol or placebo to 'usual asthma therapy' for a duration of 28 weeks in a planned initial sample of 60 000 participants. The study was terminated early after a planned interim analysis revealed that the risk for asthma-related death was higher in the salmeterol group compared to the placebo group, especially in African Americans, and due to difficulties in enrolling the larger, proposed population sample. At the time the study was terminated, 26 355 participants had been randomized to study treatment, approximately half of the target number of participants.[10]

A post hoc analysis of the smaller African-American subgroup indicated that the risk of combined asthma-related death or a life-threatening experience was 4.9 times higher in the salmeterol group compared to the placebo group, while the risk was not significant for Caucasians. The results in the African-American subgroup should be interpreted with careful consideration of the following issues related to this ethnic subset: concomitant therapy with ICS was lower in the African-American subgroup, a subgroup that also appeared to have more severe asthma. In addition, the study design included adding salmeterol to current medical therapy, including background regular SABA use. Finally, each participant was given seven canisters of salmeterol at the start of the study, an approach that might result in overuse of the LABA during asthma exacerbations. Unfortunately, only 49% of Caucasians and 38% of African Amercians reported that they were receiving baseline therapy with ICS in this surveillance trial. A further limitation of the SMART trial was in its design as a 'real-world setting' in that participants were not seen in person after the initial clinic visit. Thus, the participants were given a 28-week supply of the study medication and subsequent follow-up was performed by telephone contact every 4 weeks to assess for life-threatening events, changes in asthma therapies, and compliance with the study drug. At no time during the study were objective measures characterized including pulmonary function, symptom assessment or adherence measures. The absence of appropriate monitoring and the lack of consideration for the appropriate use of salmeterol in combination with ICS therapy represent important factors that limit any conclusions drawn from this trial.[10]

A meta-analysis performed by Salpeter and associates compiled data from 19 randomized, placebo-controlled trials with a total of 33 826 subjects, of which more than half were from the SMART trial cohort. The purpose of the meta-analysis was to calculate the risk for severe, life-threatening or fatal asthma exacerbation events related to LABA therapy. The pooled results from the meta-analysis showed an increased risk of exacerbations requiring hospitalization – odds ratio (OR), 2.6; confidence interval (CI), 1.6–4.3, excluding SMART – life-threatening exacerbations (OR, 1.8; CI, 1.1–2.9), and asthma-related deaths in those receiving LABAs compared to placebo (OR, 3.5; CI, 1.3–9.3). This study is limited by the fact that the primary database for this analysis was the life-threatening events assessed in the SMART trial. Specifically, the data regarding asthma-related deaths were obtained solely from the SMART trial. The meta-analysis was further limited by the fact that asthma-related deaths were infrequent, which limits the power of the meta-analysis to calculate a significant association.[11]

A limitation of all these studies is that none of them assessed the impact of the appropriate use of LABA, which is recommended only in combination with ICS for the management of asthma.[10, 11] Salpeter proposed that the rise in asthma mortality since the 1960s was due to the introduction of LABA therapy and the asthma mortality epidemics related to the high dosing and potency of specific SABAs such as isoproterenol and fenoterol, respectively.[24,26–31,35,36] Unfortunately, this statement does not reflect asthma mortality statistics. As outlined in a letter written by Nelson and Dorinsky to the *Annals of Internal Medicine*, asthma mortality has been steadily declining in the USA since the introduction of LABAs in 1994.[37]

In 2005, the FDA held an advisory panel to examine the impact of the SMART study and issued a public health advisory to health-care providers stating that, 'these medicines may increase the chance of severe asthma episodes, and death when those episodes occur'.[38] Thus, in the USA, both salmeterol and formoterol currently carry a boxed warning from the FDA regarding increased risk for serious asthma exacerbations or asthma-related deaths. The FDA has recently held a second advisory meeting and specific recommendations from this meeting are currently pending.[2, 3]

6.4   Safety and efficacy of LABA therapy in asthma: retrospective analyses

Despite the concerns raised by the SMART trial, international asthma guidelines continue to recommend the use of LABA in conjunction with ICS therapy in patients with asthma who remain symptomatic on ICS therapy alone. These guidelines reflect the extensive peer-reviewed literature supporting the benefit of LABA therapy as an adjunct to ICS therapy in the management of asthma, a benefit that outweighs any observed risk to date. Case-control analyses of asthma deaths as well as multiple meta-analyses have failed to show consistently an association between LABA use and risk for asthma-related mortality or severe exacerbations when these agents have been used in conjunction with inhaled corticosteroid therapy.

Anderson and colleagues performed a large case-controlled retrospective analysis evaluating asthma mortality in 532 asthma-related deaths that were ascertained from registry data in the UK that listed asthma as the primary cause of death, and these in-vestigators evaluated medical records of all asthma therapies from up to 5 years prior to death. The investigators did not find a significant association between the use of LABA therapy and risk for asthma-related death when compared to other anti-asthma thera-pies. Implications of the study may be limited due to the fact that the median age of the subjects (53 years) was higher than the participants in the SMART trial, thereby perhaps increasing the probability of a misdiagnosis of asthma as the primary cause of death in the setting of undiagnosed COPD or cardiovascular disease in the older participants.[39]

The Cochrane Airways Group has published several meta-analyses that have sup-ported the safety and efficacy of LABA therapy in combination with ICS therapy.[40,41] The Cochrane Airways Group initially published a meta-analysis using 30 trials that had randomized 9509 participants in order to compare the efficacy and safety of LABA and ICS combination therapy with higher-dose ICS therapy. The authors demonstrated that there was no increase in exacerbation rates requiring systemic corticosteroids or ad-verse events with LABA and ICS combination therapy when compared to higher-dose ICS therapy. In addition, combination therapy with LABA and ICS therapy provided a greater improvement in forced expiratory volume in 1 second (FEV_1), symptom-free days and rescue inhaler use when compared to the higher-dose ICS group.[40] In a large meta-analysis from the Cochrane Airways Group, a total of 42 333 participants from 67 studies where ICS therapy was not a uniformly controlled treatment were included for analysis. The analysis reported that LABA treatment with or without concomi-tant ICS therapy significantly improved symptoms, rescue inhaler use, and quality of life scores when compared to placebo. In addition, there were significant improve-ments in AM peak expiratory flow rate (PEFR), PM PEFR and FEV_1 when compared to placebo.[41]

Another large meta-analysis addressing the safety of LABA therapy when used in conjunction with ICS therapy was performed by Bateman and colleagues, and con-sisted of data from 66 GlaxoSmithKline trials randomizing 20 966 participants. The meta-analysis included 66 randomized, placebo-controlled trials comparing salmeterol plus ICS combination therapy with ICS monotherapy. The authors demonstrated that there was no difference in asthma-related hospitalizations between those treated with combined salmeterol and ICS combination therapy compared to ICS therapy alone. Fur-thermore, a subgroup analysis consisting of 24 trials with treatment duration greater than 12 weeks in which severe exacerbations were reported demonstrated a decreased risk of severe exacerbations with salmeterol and ICS combination therapy when com-pared to ICS therapy alone. One asthma-related intubation and one asthma-related death was reported among those subjects receiving salmeterol plus ICS combination therapy while none were reported among those receiving ICS monotherapy. Asthma-related intubation and death were very rare events in these trials and their infrequency limits the ability of the meta-analysis to calculate risks for these outcomes; however, the analysis did show that salmeterol and ICS combination therapy decreased the risk for severe asthma exacerbations when compared to ICS monotherapy.[42] A larger meta-analysis consisting of over 29 000 participants from 62 studies also demonstrated that LABA therapy when used in conjunction with ICS therapy did not result in a statistically significant difference in asthma-related hospitalizations or serious adverse events.[43]

As the number of clinical trials involving the use of LABAs in the management of asthma has increased, a growing number of meta-analyses addressing the safety of LABA therapy have focused on the safety of specific LABAs. The most recent meta-analyses addressing the safety of LABA therapy in the management of chronic asthma have focused on the safety of individual beta-agonists and have demonstrated somewhat conflicting findings. In two Cochrane Collaboration studies, Cates and colleagues investigated the safety of salmeterol or formoterol therapy by analysing trials that did not randomize participants to concomitant ICS. Cates and colleagues reviewed 22 trials randomizing 8032 participants to regular formoterol therapy or placebo, and 26 trials randomizing 62 630 participants to salmeterol therapy or placebo. The investigators reported that there was an increase in non-fatal serious adverse events with the use of regular formoterol and salmeterol when compared to placebo, with odds ratios of 1.57 (95% CI, 1.06 to 2.31) and 1.15 (95% CI, 1.02 to 1.29), respectively, for the individual LABA investigated in each individual meta-analysis. Neither of the meta-analyses demonstrated a significant increase in asthma-related deaths; however, the number of deaths was too small to draw any definitive conclusions.[44, 45] The results support therapeutic guideline recommendations that LABA therapy should not be used in asthma without concomitant ICS therapy.

In contrast, two additional meta-analyses from Cates and colleagues analysed trials randomizing patients to formoterol and salmeterol with concomitant ICS therapy, and these analyses did not demonstrate an increase in non-fatal serious adverse events with regular LABA therapy with concomitant ICS therapy. These two meta-analyses consisted of 21 trials randomizing 10 816 participants to regular formoterol with ICS therapy, and 33 trials randomizing 12 046 participants to salmeterol with ICS therapy.[46, 47] Finally, a meta-analysis performed by Sears and colleagues analysing data from clinical trials randomizing 68 004 patients reported that among those randomized to formoterol therapy, with or without concomitant ICS therapy, there was a significant decrease in asthma-related serious adverse events when compared to placebo. Among the 68 004 patients in the meta-analysis, there were eight asthma-related deaths among those randomized to formoterol (92% of whom were using ICS therapy) and two asthma-related deaths among those randomized to placebo, a non-significant difference.[48] Although none of these meta-analyses have demonstrated a significant increase in asthma-related deaths, the mortality in these meta-analyses remains too small to make definitive conclusions about the aetiology of these very rare events. Thus, the surrogate marker of asthma hospitalization or severe exacerbations has been used to assess LABA safety.

6.5   Efficacy of LABA therapy as a component of combination therapy with ICS for the management of asthma

The critical issue or question in the long-acting beta-agonist debate is that if a very small risk of severe exacerbations or death does indeed exist with the combination of LABA and ICS therapy, then do the overall therapeutic benefits outweigh this risk. This question was discussed in detail at the December 2008 FDA advisory meeting. While several meta-analyses and a case-control analysis of asthma-related deaths have addressed the concerns raised by the SMART trial and the meta-analysis by Salpeter and colleagues, numerous publications of prospective clinical trials consistently demonstrate the efficacy and safety of LABA in combination with ICS therapy for the management of asthma.

Several clinical trials illustrate the efficacy of LABA therapy when used in combination with ICS therapy and the potential for loss of asthma control that can occur with the use of LABA monotherapy. In 1994, Greening and colleagues showed that the addition of salmeterol to low-dose ICS therapy with beclometasone (400 µg twice daily) resulted in a greater increase in mean a.m. PEFR when compared to increasing the ICS dose by greater than two-fold (500 µg twice daily) in a group of 429 adult asthmatics suboptimally controlled with beclometasone therapy alone (200 µg twice daily).[5] Subsequently, the Formoterol and Corticosteroids Establishing Therapy (FACET) trial study group studied 852 patients with persistent asthma not well controlled on high-dose ICS therapy alone (budesonide 800 µg twice daily). Participants were randomized to one of four treatment strategies for one year: lower-dose ICS (budesonide 100 µg twice daily) with formoterol; lower-dose ICS with placebo; higher-dose ICS (budesonide 200 µg twice daily) with formoterol; and higher-dose ICS with placebo. The addition of LABA therapy to either higher- or lower-dose ICS therapy resulted in a significant reduction in exacerbations rates when compared to placebo (ICS monotherapy). Furthermore, study withdrawals due to severe asthma exacerbations were significantly lower in the treatment groups receiving formoterol ($P = 0.01$ for the difference among the treatment groups). Participants receiving LABA therapy also demonstrated a significant improvement in asthma symptom scores and measures of lung function (FEV_1 and a.m. PEFR) than with ICS monotherapy. The proportion of participants reporting adverse events was similar for all treatment groups.[49]

Four years after the FACET trial, the Oxis and Pulmicort Turbuhaler In the Management of patients with Asthma (OPTIMA) trial demonstrated the efficacy of adding LABA therapy to low- or high-dose ICS therapy in a larger, multicentre cohort of asthma patients in a large cohort with mild, persistent asthma and symptoms requiring the use of rescue bronchodilator therapy at least twice weekly (Figure 6.4). The study was divided into two groups: 698 patients who were ICS naive for greater than or equal to 3 months; and 1272 patients currently treated with low-dose ICS at an equivalent dose of less than or equal to 400 µg per day (ICS-treated group). Among the ICS-naive, budesonide therapy significantly reduced the time to the first severe asthma

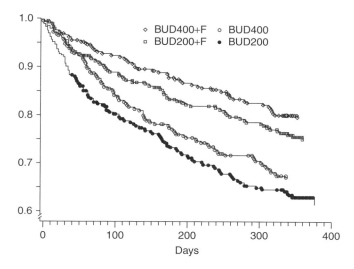

Figure 6.4   Kaplan–Meier survival curve from the Formoterol and Formoterol/Budesonide. In the Management of patients with Asthma (OPTIMA) trial illustrating the time to the first severe asthma exacerbation in the inhaled corticosteroids (ICS)-treated group. Combination therapy resulted in a significantly longer time to the first severe exacerbation when compared to ICS monotherapy (BUD200 and BUD400, budesonide 100 μg and 200 μg twice daily; F, formoterol 4.5 μg twice daily). Reproduced from O'Byrne et al. (2001),[50] with permission.

exacerbation, the number of days with poorly controlled asthma, and exacerbation rates compared to placebo, while the addition of formoterol in these very mild asthma subjects did not affect these outcomes despite significantly improving lung function. In contrast, in those subjects with more persistent asthma, the addition of formoterol to either low- or high-dose budesonide therapy (ICS-treated group) resulted in a significant reduction in the time to the first asthma exacerbation, proportion of days with poorly controlled asthma, and exacerbation rates along with significant improvements in lung function (Figure 6.4). The rate of adverse events was similar in both cohorts and in all treatment groups.[50]

The Salmeterol +/− Inhaled Corticosteroids (SLIC) trial was a randomized, double-blinded, placebo-controlled, double-dummy, parallel-group study performed by the NIH ACRN investigators to evaluate the effect of reducing or eliminating ICS therapy in patients with persistent asthma treated with concomitant LABA therapy. One hundred and seventy-five patients with persistent asthma suboptimally controlled with triamcinolone 400 μg twice daily during a 6-week run-in period were randomized into the SLIC trial. All participants continued the use of triamcinolone therapy and were randomized to receive add-on therapy with salmeterol or placebo during a 2-week 'salmeterol introduction phase'. During this 2-week phase there was an initial improvement in a.m. PEFR, daily asthma symptom scores, daily albuterol rescue inhaler use, FEV_1, and asthma quality of life scores in both the salmeterol-plus and salmeterol-minus groups. Subsequent reduction of the ICS dose by 50% for 8 weeks resulted in treatment failure in 8.3% of those in the salmeterol-minus group compared with 2.8% in the salmeterol-plus group. This difference increased 8 weeks after the elimination of triamcinolone therapy as the percentage of treatment failures increased to 46.3% of those in the salmeterol-minus group compared to 13.7% of those in the salmeterol-plus group. Furthermore, elimination of triamcinolone therapy resulted in a significant deterioration of daily symptom scores, daily albuterol rescue inhaler use, and asthma quality of life scores. The investigators concluded that patients with persistent asthma who are suboptimally controlled with ICS therapy will have an improvement in asthma control with the addition of LABA therapy and that LABAs allow a reduction of the dose of ICS by 50% in over 90% of individuals without a significant loss in asthma control; however, elimination of ICS therapy results in a significant deterioration in asthma control.[51]

The ineffectiveness of LABA therapy as monotherapy for the management of asthma has best been demonstrated by another ACRN study, the Salmeterol or Corticosteroids (SOCS) trial. The SOCS trial was a multicentre, randomized, double-blind, placebo-controlled parallel-group trial comparing the efficacy of salmeterol monotherapy, ICS monotherapy with triamcinolone, or placebo for a duration of 16 weeks followed by a 6-week run-out period during which all participants received placebo.[51,52] One hundred and sixty-four patients with persistent asthma previously controlled on low-dose triamcinolone during the run-in period were randomized to either salmeterol monotherapy, triamcinolone monotherapy or placebo. At the end of the 16-week treatment period, participants in the salmeterol group were significantly more likely to experience treatment failures and asthma exacerbations when compared to triamcinolone. The SOCS trial illustrates that patients with persistent asthma who are well-controlled on low-dose ICS therapy cannot be switched to LABA monotherapy due to the risk of deterioration of asthma control.[52]

The efficacy of LABA therapy in conjunction with ICS therapy using a treatment strategy based on the goal of complete asthma control was investigated by the Gaining Optimal Asthma ControL (GOAL) study. The GOAL study was a randomized, multicentre, placebo-controlled, parallel-group study that compared the efficacy of escalating doses of fluticasone alone and in combination with salmeterol in 3421 patients with uncontrolled asthma for a 1-year period. This study had two phases consisting of a dose escalation phase (phase I) during which the ICS dose was increased in 12-week intervals until asthma control was obtained or the maximum ICS dose was achieved followed by a dose maintenance phase (phase II). Salmeterol and fluticasone combination therapy resulted in a significantly greater number of patients achieving total control of asthma symptoms when compared to escalating doses of fluticasone alone. Participants receiving combination therapy experienced control of asthma more rapidly and at a lower ICS dose when compared to fluticasone alone. In addition, combination therapy resulted in a significant reduction in exacerbation rates when compared to ICS monotherapy.[53]

Why does the addition of a LABA to ICS therapy result in improvements in asthma control, even at lower ICS doses? This fundamental question illustrates an important aspect of combination therapy: the potential for synergy or the enhancement of the effects of LABA and ICS therapies when these agents are combined in the management of asthma.[54] There is *in vitro* evidence that supports the hypothesis that these agents act synergistically. In sputum cells induced from mild to moderate asthmatics, activation of the β_2-adrenergic receptor by a LABA or SABA in combination with ICS therapy results in enhanced translocation of the glucocorticoid receptor into the nucleus, the intracellular location where steroids exert their anti-inflammatory activity.[22,23] The enhanced nuclear translocation associated with combination therapy also results in an increase of steroid-mediated effects such as the suppression of the release of granulocyte-macrophage colony-stimulating factor (GM-CSF), RANTES (regulated upon activation, normal T-cell expressed, or CCL5), and interleukin-8 (IL-8) from induced sputum cells. Furthermore, treatment of these sputum cells with corticosteroids results in a significant increase in β_2-adenergic receptor gene expression.[22] This synergistic interaction causes an enhanced anti-inflammatory effect that represents a potential mechanism explaining why the combination of a LABA and ICS is more effective in improving asthma symptom control with lower ICS doses.

Finally, the STAY trial demonstrated the efficacy of formoterol and budesonide combination therapy as both a maintenance and reliever therapy. The study randomized 2760 participants with moderate to severe persistent asthma to three treatment arms: budesonide 400 μg twice daily with terbutaline reliever therapy; budesonide 100 μg plus formoterol twice daily with terbutaline reliever therapy; and budesonide 100 μg plus formoterol twice daily both as maintenance and reliever therapy. Treatment with budesonide plus formoterol combination therapy as maintenance and reliever therapy resulted in a significant prolongation of the time to first severe asthma exacerbation and a lower risk of experiencing a severe exacerbation. In addition, participants using LABA plus ICS combination therapy as maintenance and reliever experienced statistically significant improvements in severe exacerbation rates, symptoms, nocturnal awakenings and pulmonary function when compared to the other treatment arms.[55]

6.6   Scientific basis of the beneficial and adverse effects of beta-agonist therapy: *in vitro* data and the beta-agonist paradox

Several investigators have demonstrated that LABA therapy does not produce an additional anti-inflammatory effect when added to ICS therapy; however, others have shown that the addition of LABA therapy can allow the reduction of ICS dose without a subsequent rise in airway inflammatory markers.[56,57] Overbeek and colleagues showed that there is no additional anti-inflammatory benefit of formoterol therapy when added to low- or high-dose budesonide therapy when compared to budesonide monotherapy.[58] Subsequently, Jarjour and co-workers demonstrated that asthmatics using fluticasone 250 μg twice daily who were previously uncontrolled with lower doses of fluticasone can tolerate a reduction in ICS dose to 100 μg twice daily with the addition of salmeterol therapy without a worsening of airway inflammation as determined by bronchial biopsy and bronchoalveolar lavage specimens.[59,60] These results support the scientific basis for the use of combination LABA and ICS therapy in treating the inflammatory process of asthma and preventing the clinical 'masking' of inflammation that seems to occur with LABA monotherapy after the withdrawal of ICS therapy.

Over the years, the *in vitro* evidence has suggested that although beta-agonists have beneficial effects, such as smooth muscle relaxation, they may also have potentially counterproductive proinflammatory properties. *In vitro*, albuterol appears to inhibit the production of IL-12 by human monocytes in response to lipopolysaccharide, inhibiting the T helper-1 (Th1) inflammatory pathway favouring the development of T helper-2 cell (Th2) differentiation.[61] Furthermore, increasing concentrations of terbutaline appear to promote the production of IL-4 and IL-5 by monocytes while inhibiting the production of interferon-gamma (IFN-γ), an effect favouring Th2 inflammation.[62] In an ACRN trial, Lazarus and colleagues demonstrated that sputum eosinophils and sputum tryptase concentrations were significantly greater ($P < 0.001$) among those randomized to salmeterol monotherapy when compared to those treated with triamcinolone alone.[52] The proinflammatory nature of beta-agonists as indicated by these *in vitro* findings raises a paradoxical effect with respect to LABA therapy in asthma in which beneficial and adverse effects are simultaneously observed in the same disease process *in vitro*, raising the concern as to whether there is worsening of inflammation in some individuals under specific clinical circumstances with beta-agonist therapy.[4] Unfortunately, such adverse effects are likely to be undetectable *in vivo* making such effects difficult to substantiate or quantify. Thus, alterations in specific aspects of asthmatic inflammation remain a possible contributing factor to the rare adverse events observed when these agents have been used at inappropriate doses or without concomitant ICS therapy in the management of asthma.

6.7   Conclusions regarding the safety of LABA therapy as a component of combination therapy with ICS for the management of asthma

A large number of prospective studies and meta-analyses have established the safety of LABA therapy and its role as an adjunct to ICS therapy in the chronic management of asthma, particularly among those whose symptoms are not optimally controlled with low-dose ICS therapy. In addition, clinical evidence indicates that when used according to these indications LABA therapy does not diminish asthma control but improves it, and reduces asthma exacerbation rates.[5,40,50–53,63] These benefits may be further enhanced with the rapid onset of a LABA such as formoterol and an ICS when they are used as a maintenance and as-needed rescue therapy, but such benefits can be lost when ICS therapy is withdrawn.[52,55] The concerns regarding respiratory-related deaths and loss of asthma control are based primarily on data from trials that used LABAs as a monotherapy and employed suboptimal trial designs.[10,11] It remains uncertain whether these concerns reflect a rare susceptibility to a possible deleterious effect of these medications; however, when these agents have been evaluated in conjunction

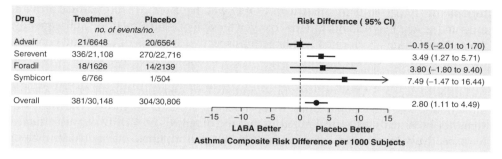

Drug	Treatment	Placebo	Risk Difference (95% CI)
	no. of events/no.		
Advair	21/6648	20/6564	−0.15 (−2.01 to 1.70)
Serevent	336/21,108	270/22,716	3.49 (1.27 to 5.71)
Foradil	18/1626	14/2139	3.80 (−1.80 to 9.40)
Symbicort	6/766	1/504	7.49 (−1.47 to 16.44)
Overall	381/30,148	304/30,806	2.80 (1.11 to 4.49)

LABA Better   Placebo Better
Asthma Composite Risk Difference per 1000 Subjects

Figure 6.5   Differences in the risk of asthma-related death, intubation, or hospitalization and medication use. LABA, long-acting beta-agonist. Reproduced from Kramer (2009),[3] with permission.

with ICS therapy in fixed-dose preparations there is no evidence of any loss of asthma control, increase in severe exacerbations, or increase in respiratory-related deaths. The scientific evidence for the use of concomitant LABA and ICS therapy suggests that these agents act synergistically; however, the absence or withdrawal of ICS therapy may result in the clinical 'masking' of airway inflammation and could contribute to potential deleterious effects of LABA monotherapy (Figure 6.5). This finding was observed in a meta-analysis reported at a FDA advisory meeting on LABA safety. In this meta-analysis, strategies that used fixed LABA and ICS combination therapies were safer, with reduced severe asthma exacerbations compared to LABA alone or LABA added to pre-existing ICS therapy. This finding suggests that there is the potential for differential overuse of LABA and underuse of ICS when these agents are prescribed separately.

6.8   Beta-agonist therapy and adverse events in COPD

The primary safety issue with regular beta-agonist exposure in the management of COPD is related primarily to its potential role for increasing the risk of adverse cardiovascular events such as cardiac arrhythmias. Salmeterol and formoterol are not devoid of β_1-adrenergic receptor activity and may acutely affect heart rate, cardiac rhythm, the corrected QT interval, blood pressure and serum potassium concentrations, particularly when these agents are used at higher-than-recommended doses.[13, 14] Independent of beta-agonist exposure, individuals with COPD are known to have an increased risk of cardiac arrhythmias and prolongation of QT intervals.[64, 65] Large, retrospective cohort analyses from the Saskatchewan health database have shown that there is a higher frequency of smoking in COPD, and cigarette smokers have an increased risk for cardiovascular disease.[66, 67]

Some investigators have postulated that beta-agonist therapy may contribute to an increased risk of cardiac arrhythmias and adverse cardiovascular events in those with COPD, particularly when used at higher doses. Cazzola and co-workers showed that higher-dose formoterol (24 μg), may increase the frequency of supraventricular and ventricular beats when compared to regular-dose salmeterol (50 μg) and lower-dose formoterol (12 µg) in individuals with COPD who have pre-existing cardiac arrhythmias and severe hypoxaemia (arterial oxygen tension of <60 mmHg).[12] Subsequently, Au and co-workers performed two large retrospective analyses of cases and controls: the first from the Group Health Cooperative of Puget Sound and the second from Veterans Administration Medical Centers (VA). The investigators described an association between SABA canister prescriptions and unstable angina or myocardial infarction in two large populations, independent of a COPD diagnosis. The study designs for both analyses were limited in that the diagnosis of COPD was ascertained retrospectively by a history of prior ipratropium prescriptions, questionnaire data or symptom data from the medical record, and that the diagnosis of COPD or asthma was not considered as an inclusion criterion of either analysis.[68, 69] More importantly, SABA use may reflect persistent dyspnoea from either pulmonary disease or cardiovascular disease, particularly since the prevalence of cardiovascular disease was higher among cases in the cohort from the VA medical centres.[69]

A meta-analysis performed by Salpeter and co-workers showed an increased risk of adverse cardiovascular events in those with asthma and COPD who used SABA and LABA therapy. The conclusions of the meta-analysis were limited in that the observed significant association with adverse cardiovascular events was primarily due to an association with tachycardia and hypokalaemia, which may be of questionable clinical relevance. In addition, there was no statistically significant association between beta-agonist use and fatal adverse cardiovascular events.[15]

Although higher doses of LABA therapy have been associated with cardiac arrhythmias, these findings do not necessarily translate into an increase in fatal or serious adverse cardiovascular events, particularly among those without severe hypoxaemia or pre-existing cardiac arrythmias.[12, 15, 68, 69] Subsequent studies using LABA therapy at recommended doses have consistently shown that these agents improve airflow obstruction with an acceptable cardiovascular safety profile.[16–19] Furthermore, the addition of ICS therapy has also been shown to further reduce exacerbation rates and quality of life as well as lung function.[20, 70–72] Thus, the literature showing efficacy and safety of LABA therapy has led to recommendations endorsing LABA monotherapy as an initial therapy for milder COPD and the use of LABA therapy in combination with ICS therapy for the management of moderate to very severe COPD.[73]

6.9   Safety and efficacy of LABA therapy in the management of COPD: the clinical evidence

The cardiovascular safety profile of LABA therapy in the management of COPD has been demonstrated by several clinical trials and meta-analyses. Campbell and co-workers specifically investigated the safety of formoterol 12 µg twice daily for a duration of 8 weeks in 204 patients with COPD using a randomized, double-blind, placebo-controlled study design to assess the cardiovascular safety profile of LABA therapy with 24-hour Holter monitoring. The trial showed that there was no difference in the corrected QT intervals, heart rate or rate of premature ventricular beats between those receiving formoterol and those receiving placebo. Furthermore, there were no episodes of sustained ventricular tachycardia, symptomatic ectopic ventricular beats, or ventricular fibrillation described throughout the duration of therapy, and adverse cardiac events were rare.[16]

Nelson and co-workers also assessed the cardiovascular safety profile of the LABA-formulated therapy in the management of COPD. The cardiovascular effects of therapy were assessed using 24-hour Holter monitoring at baseline and after 12 weeks of therapy. Three hundred and fifty-one patients with COPD were randomized into the study, and Holter monitoring did not detect a significant difference in mean of maximum heart rate, premature ventricular beats, incidence of cardiac arrythmias or the frequency of QT interval prolongation by greater than or equal to 60 ms in those using formoterol when compared to placebo.[17]

A meta-analysis performed by Rodrigo and colleagues further illustrates the safety profile of LABA therapy with respect to respiratory-related outcomes in COPD, utilizing 20 257 randomized patients from 27 randomized controlled trials. The analysis consisted of trials that had included all-cause and respiratory-related deaths as outcomes and demonstrated no significant difference in these outcomes between those who had been treated with a LABA compared to placebo therapy. Furthermore, the group of patients receiving LABA therapy experienced a significant reduction in severe exacerbation rates of 3.3% when compared to placebo therapy. A secondary analysis also showed that among those on LABA therapy, there was a significant improvement in airflow limitation, quality of life as measured by the St George's respiratory questionnaire (SGRQ) score, and rescue inhaler use. Interestingly, the meta-analysis also revealed a potential beneficial effect on the risk of a respiratory-related death among the subset treated with a concomitant ICS when compared to those treated with a LABA alone.[74] Similar findings have been observed in other prospective studies and meta-analyses.[19,75]

6.10   Role of LABA therapy as a component of combination therapy with ICS for the management of COPD

The role of LABA therapy as a long-acting bronchodilator in the treatment of stable COPD has been extensively investigated since 2001 when the initial GOLD guidelines recommended bronchodilators for the primary management of mild COPD.[73] Prior to 2001, there had been some studies that had illustrated the efficacy of LABA therapy in the management of early COPD.[76–79] Subsequently, there have been numerous publications examining data from large, double-blind clinical trials that have provided evidence documenting the efficacy of LABAs in the management of COPD. These studies have consistently shown improvements in airflow obstruction with salmeterol and formoterol therapy with or without other concomitant therapies.[18,19,70–72,76–89] A randomized, double-blind, double-dummy, parallel-group, placebo-controlled study by Mahler and co-workers reported that long-term therapy with salmeterol resulted in greater improvements of trough FEV_1 when compared to either placebo or ipratropium.[79] D'Urzo and co-workers also reported that the combination of formoterol and ipratropium appears to improve trough FEV_1 when compared to the combination of salbutamol and ipratropium.[83] In addition, a randomized trial by Cazzola and co-workers provided initial evidence of the efficacy of combination therapy in the management of COPD by demonstrating that combination therapy consisting of salmeterol with fluticasone or theophylline for 3 months augmented the effects of salmeterol on improving trough FEV_1.[77] A number of different studies have replicated these findings.[76–89]

One of the earlier large prospective trials demonstrating the efficacy and safety of LABA and ICS combination therapy in the management of COPD was performed by Calverley and colleagues from the Trial of Inhaled Steroids and Long-Acting β_2-agonists (TRISTAN) study group. The TRISTAN study randomized 1465 patients with COPD and an FEV_1 between 25% and 70% of the predicted value to salmeterol 50 μg with fluticasone 500 μg, salmeterol 50 μg alone, or placebo, for a duration of 12 months. All active treatment groups showed significant improvements in exacerbation frequency; however, salmeterol in combination with fluticasone significantly improved pretreatment FEV_1, dyspnoea severity scores, rescue inhaler use, and quality of life as measured by the SGRQ when compared to either monotherapy or placebo. Adverse events were not significantly different between the treatment groups with the exception of the incidence of oral candidiasis.[70] Two smaller randomized clinical trials further demonstrated the safety and efficacy of combination therapy in patients with COPD.[79,90]

The beneficial effects of LABA and ICS combination therapy on airflow obstruction, dyspnoea severity, quality of life and exacerbation rates in the management of COPD may be partially attributed to the effects of ICS therapy, a monotherapy that has been studied extensively. In addition to the reduction in exacerbations observed with ICS monotherapy, there are data showing that LABA and ICS combination therapy reduces respiratory-related mortality. Soriano and co-workers performed a retrospective cohort analysis showing a significantly increased 3-year survival in those with COPD using salmeterol and fluticasone therapy. The retrospective cohort consisted of 1045 patients with newly diagnosed COPD who were treated with salmeterol and/or fluticasone, and 3620 patients who did not receive these agents. The largest 3-year survival advantage was observed among the patients who were treated with combination therapy when compared to either monotherapy or the reference group.[91]

A meta-analysis by Sin and co-workers showed a mortality benefit with the use of ICS for at least 12 months. The meta-analysis consisted of 5085 patients from seven randomized trials comparing the effects of ICS therapy with placebo over a follow-up period of 26 months. The analysis showed a statistically significant reduction of approximately 25% in all-cause mortality among those treated with ICS therapy.[92] The database for this analysis included several randomized clinical trials.[68–72,93]

The results of these retrospective analyses in combination with the observed beneficial effects of LABA and ICS therapy on various clinical outcomes, particularly all-cause mortality, prompted the design of the Towards a Revolution in COPD Health, or TORCH trial. The TORCH trial was a multicentre trial designed by the TORCH

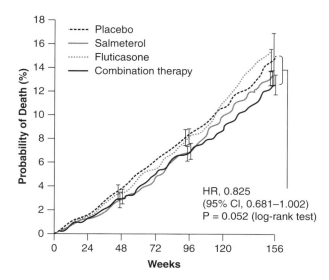

Figure 6.6   Results from the Towards a Revolution in COPD Health (TORCH) trial illustrating the risk of all-cause death with salmeterol and fluticasone combination therapy when compared to placebo over the 3-year study period.

investigators to determine the effects of LABA and ICS therapy on survival among those with COPD and an FEV_1 of less than 65% of the predicted value. Although all-cause mortality was the primary outcome, the study also evaluated, as secondary outcomes, the effects of these agents on the frequency of exacerbations and health status as measured by the SGRQ. At the end of the 3-year treatment period there were 875 deaths, with the proportions of all-cause death being 12.6% in the combination therapy group (LABA and ICS), 13.5% in the salmeterol group, 16% in the fluticasone group, and 15.2% in the placebo group. The absolute risk reduction for death in the combination therapy group when compared to the placebo group was 2.6%, with a hazard ratio of 0.825 corresponding to a total risk reduction of 17.5% for death at any time during the 3-year treatment period. However, these results did not reach statistical significance after an adjustment for an interim analysis ($P = 0.052$) (Figure 6.6). It seems this is a somewhat arbitrary approach since a number of endpoints supported improved disease control in the combination therapy groups. Also of major importance is that the risk of death among those receiving salmeterol monotherapy did not significantly differ from the other groups, indicating that there was no evidence of an increased mortality signal with LABA therapy in COPD. In contrast, the combination therapy group did have a lower likelihood of death when compared to the fluticasone monotherapy group, with a hazard ratio of 0.774 ($P = 0.007$).[20]

With respect to the secondary outcomes in the TORCH study, combination therapy resulted in a statistically significant 25% reduction in annual exacerbation rates and a 17% reduction in annual hospitalization rates when compared to placebo. Patients receiving either monotherapy demonstrated a significant reduction in exacerbation rates when compared to placebo. In addition, quality of life as measured by the SGRQ and

FEV$_1$ was improved throughout the 3-year treatment period in those who received combination therapy when compared to either monotherapy or placebo. Of note, adverse cardiovascular outcomes did not significantly differ in the salmeterol and combination therapy groups when compared to the placebo or fluticasone therapy groups. Finally, those treated with fluticasone or combination therapy did exhibit a statistically significant increased probability of being diagnosed with pneumonia.[20]

6.11   Conclusions regarding the safety of LABA therapy as a component of combination therapy for the management of COPD

Despite a borderline statistically insignificant effect on mortality, combination therapy with a LABA and ICS has been consistently shown to improve airflow obstruction, exacerbation rates and quality of life in the management of moderate to severe COPD in multiple studies including the TORCH trial.[70–72] In addition, LABA therapy, when used as monotherapy or in combination with ICS therapy, has consistently been shown to be safe with respect to adverse cardiovascular outcomes in multiple clinical trials.[70–72,76–78,83,84,86,89] Prior observations have raised concerns regarding the potential for adverse cardiovascular events with the use of LABA therapy; however, no prospective clinical trials have demonstrated an increase in serious or fatal adverse cardiovascular events when salmeterol and formoterol are used at their respective recommended doses.[16,17,74,76] The addition of ICS therapy to LABA therapy appears to provide additional benefits other than just the improvement in airflow obstruction observed with LABA monotherapy, including improvements in exacerbation rates and quality of life.

6.12   Pharmacogenetics of LABAs and combination therapy

Pharmacogenetics is the study of the role of genetic variability in determining individual responses to pharmacological therapies. Hence, pharmacogenetics is an example of gene–environment interactions. A large number of pharmacogenetics studies have evaluated beta-agonist responsiveness to determine the role of genetic variability in predicting the likelihood that an individual will respond favourably or adversely to beta-agonist treatment. Most of pharmacogenetic research with respect to SABA and LABA therapy has involved the clinical response to these agents as it relates to genetic variability within the β_2-adrenergic receptor gene, or *ADRβ2*.

In 1992, Reihaus identified nine genetic variants, or polymorphisms, along the coding region of *ADRβ2*, four of which are single nucleotide changes in the genetic code referred to as single nucleotide polymorphisms (SNPs). SNPs cause coding changes that in turn change the amino acid (AA) product at each codon or amino acid position relative to the start codon. Denoted as $AA_1{}^{codon}AA_2$ (AA_1 and AA_2 referring to the amino acid products of the two differing alleles), two of the most common SNPs include Gly[16]Arg and Gln[27]Glu.[94] Both of these *ADRβ2* polymorphisms have been shown to influence the downregulation of the β_2-adrenergic receptor in *in vitro* studies using Chinese hamster fibroblasts and human airway smooth muscle cells.[95,96] The frequency of Gly[16]Arg and Gln[27]Glu genotypes varies between ethnic groups such as Caucasians and African Americans, independent of asthma disease status, indicating that genetic variation within *ADRβ2* may have a role in determining possible ethnic-specific responses to LABA therapy, particularly the differences in adverse events suggested by the post hoc analysis of the SMART trial.[10,97] Since 1992, nearly 49 different polymorphisms have been identified throughout *ADRβ2*, its promoter region and the 3′ untranslated region, generating multiple, complex *ADRβ2* haplotypes (Figure 6.7).[97–99]

Martinez and co-workers described one of the earliest pharmacogenetic relationships between Gly[16]Arg genotypes and response to a single administration of albuterol in a group of 269 children participating in a longitudinal study of asthma. In this study, Arg[16] homozygotes and Gly[16]Arg heterozygotes were 5.3 times and 2.3 times more likely than Gly[16] homozygotes to show a positive response to albuterol (FEV$_1$ increase greater than 15% predicted), respectively.[100] In 707 asthmatic children from the Childhood Asthma Management Program (CAMP), Silverman and co-workers determined that Gly[16]Arg was associated with post-bronchodilator FEV$_1$, with Arg[16] homozygotes having a higher FEV$_1$ percent of predicted values.[101] Subsequently, Taylor and co-workers retrospectively analysed the genetic effects of Gly[16]Arg during regular LABA and SABA therapy in 115 asthmatics from a placebo-controlled, crossover trial of regular albuterol and salmeterol therapy. Arg[16] homozygotes experienced a higher frequency of exacerbations and a decline in PEFR while using regular albuterol therapy with no adverse effects reported during salmeterol or placebo therapy.[102]

These findings from Taylor and co-workers were replicated in two different Asthma Clinical Research Network (ACRN) trials.[33,103,104] The retrospective analysis of the ACRN BAGS trial analysed Gly[16]Arg genotypes and reported that a.m. PEFR declined among Arg[16] homozygotes using regular beta-agonist therapy when compared to those using as-needed therapy, and the decline was accentuated during the 4-week run-out period. The evening PEFR also declined among Arg[16] homozygotes on regular agonist therapy, with no such effect observed for Gly[16] homozygotes.[103,104]

The Beta Agonist Response by Genotype (BARGE) trial was a prospective, genotype-stratified, placebo-controlled, crossover trial that included 41 Gly[16] homozygotes and 37 Arg[16] homozygotes with mild asthma who were randomized by genotype to regular or as-needed albuterol therapy over a 16-week period then crossed over to the alternative study medication. Exposure to beta-agonist rescue was minimized by using ipratropium bromide as the primary reliever medication. Arg[16] homozygotes showed a significant increase in a.m. PEFR during treatment with placebo, while Gly[16] homozygotes showed a significant increase in a.m. PEFR during regular albuterol therapy. Arg[16] homozygotes experienced significant adverse effects on FEV$_1$, forced vital capacity (FVC), asthma symptom scores and rescue inhaler use during regular albuterol therapy, while Gly[16] homozygotes showed significant improvements in these

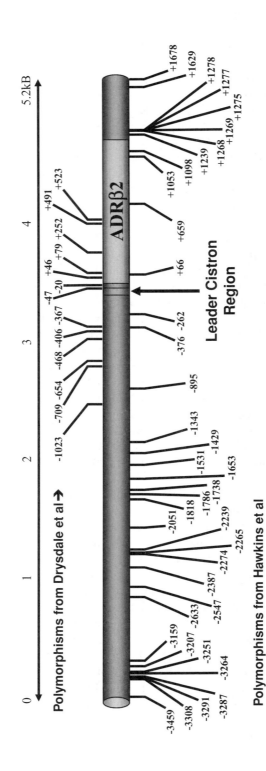

Figure 6.7 Diagram of the β₂-adrenergic receptor gene (*ADRβ2*) with polymorphisms denoted by nucleotide position relative to the start codon. Adapted from Hawkins et al. (2006).[97]

measures during regular beta-agonist therapy. During the run-in period – an interval when albuterol use was minimized since ipratropium was used as the rescue medication – Arg[16] homozygotes experienced a significant increase in a.m. PEFR. Thus, the majority of studies evaluating pharmacogenetic responses to Gly[16]Arg variation in the *ADRβ2* gene showed an effect with regular SABA therapy. However, regular therapy with SABA is not recommended in asthma, and the more important question is whether similar responses are observed with the regular use of LABA in asthma.[34]

Based on the observed *ADRβ2* genotypic effects on therapeutic response demonstrated during regular SABA therapy, subsequent pharmacogenetic studies were designed to evaluate the genotypic effects of *ADRβ2* polymorphisms on response to LABA therapy. In the trial by Taylor described previously, the trial design included a regular SABA treatment arm and a LABA or salmeterol treatment arm. In the salmeterol treatment group, there was no effect of *ADRβ2* Gly[16]Arg genotypes on responses to LABA, with both homozygote and the heterozygote groups showing improved lung function and reduced asthma exacerbations.[102] A second, small retrospective genetic analysis of two randomized, placebo-controlled salmeterol trials designed by the National Heart-Lung and Blood Institute (NHLBI) ACRN, the Salmeterol or Corticosteroids (SOCS) trial and Salmeterol +/− Inhaled Corticosteroid (SLIC) trial, was examined to determine whether there was a *ADRβ2* genotype effect on LABA response. Ninety-six subjects from the SOCS trial and 74 subjects from the SLIC trial were genotyped for genetic variation within *ADRβ2*. The retrospective analysis of both cohorts demonstrated that Arg[16] homozygotes had a lower or decreasing a.m. PEFR when compared to Gly[16] homozygotes during salmeterol therapy, particularly after week 10 of the trial. Within the SLIC cohort, Arg[16] homozygotes on LABA and ICS combination therapy experienced a significantly lower FEV_1, increased rescue inhaler use, and higher asthma symptom scores when compared to Gly[16] homozygotes on similar therapy.[105] The results from this small retrospective study suggested that variation at the Gly[16]Arg locus of *ADRβ2* has a genotypic effect on the response to salmeterol therapy; however, larger subsequent retrospective analyses and a recent prospective, genotype-stratified study have disproved the genotypic effects demonstrated by the analysis of the SOCS and SLIC cohorts.[106]

Bleecker and co-workers initially genotyped five *ADRβ2* SNPs in 183 subjects with persistent asthma who were randomized to regular salmeterol and ICS combination therapy or montelukast for a 12-week period followed by a 2–4-day run-out period. During the 12-week period, all subjects randomized to salmeterol therapy experienced sustained and significant improvements in a.m. PEFR regardless of Gly[16]Arg genotype. During the run-out period, all subjects exhibited a similar and predictable decline in asthma control.[107] Subsequently, Bleecker and co-workers retrospectively analysed two studies consisting of large cohorts of 2250 and 405 asthmatics randomized to combination therapy with formoterol and an ICS as well as salmeterol and fluticasone therapy, both of the currently available LABA combination therapies. These therapies were maintained for 5 to 6 months while evaluating exacerbations and lung function. These cohorts were genotyped for 11 *ADRβ2* SNPs and retrospectively stratified by *ADRβ2* genotype. There was no genotypic effect of Gly[16]Arg genotypes on the percentage of

(a)

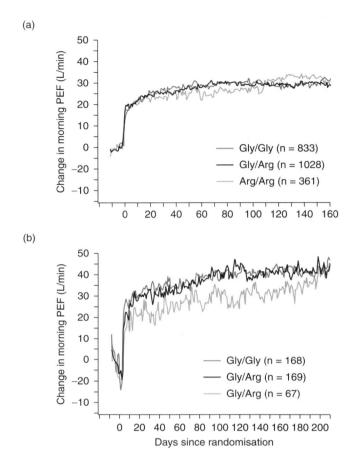

(b)

Figure 6.8   Pharmacogenetic retrospective analysis of two clinical trials (denoted as A and B) using long-acting beta-agonist (LABA) therapy as described by Bleecker et al. These diagrams demonstrate no significant difference in mean daily change from baseline in morning peak expiratory flow (PEF) during the treatment period by $Gly^{16}Arg$ genotype. Reproduced from Bleecker et al. (2007),[108] with permission.

participants with severe exacerbations, with no significant differences observed in time to first asthma exacerbation across all treatment groups. Furthermore, there were no differences in FEV_1, a.m. PEFR, rescue inhaler use or nocturnal awakenings observed between $Gly^{16}Arg$ genotypes (Figure 6.8). In addition, haplotype analysis for this gene revealed no genotype effects on beta-agonist response.[108]

The pharmacogenetic findings reported by Bleecker and co-workers suggest that $Gly^{16}Arg$ genotypes are not a genetic determinant of responses to LABA therapy when administered in the presence of ICS therapy.[107, 108] In addition, a prospective, genotype-stratified, placebo-controlled trial by Bleecker and co-workers did not demonstrate a pharmacogenetic effect among asthmatics receiving LABA therapy with or without concomitant ICS therapy. During the American Thoracic Society International Conference in 2008, the NHLBI ACRN network reported the results of the Long Acting Beta Agonist Response by Genotype (LARGE) study, a genotype-stratified, placebo-controlled, crossover trial investigating the effects of Gly^{16}Arg genotypes on daily peak flow during regular LABA therapy versus placebo with concomitant ICS therapy, in a similar prospective, genotype-stratified design as the BARGE trial. The ACRN investigators demonstrated the lack of a pharmacogenetic effect of Gly^{16}Arg genotypes by showing an identical improvement in lung function between Arg^{16} and Gly^{16} homozygotes after the addition of salmeterol to ICS therapy for 18 weeks. The LARGE trial did demonstrate that Gly^{16} homozygotes had a significant increase in methacholine provocative concentration (PC20), a 'bronchoprotective effect', after the addition of salmeterol to ICS therapy for 18 weeks ($P < 0.0001$) while Arg^{16} homozygotes did not demonstrate any changes ($P = 0.867$). Unfortunately, bronchial responsiveness was only measured 24 hours after the last dose of drug at the end of the study, exceeding the duration of effect for salmeterol. Despite this issue, the findings with respect to bronchial hyperresponsiveness still require further investigation.

Why are there divergent effects observed with respect to Gly^{16}Arg genotype-specific responses to SABA therapy and LABA therapy during the majority of these trials? Specifically, why does genetic variation at the Gly^{16}Arg locus affect the response to regular SABA therapy but does not appear to affect the response to LABA therapy? The absence of a genotype-specific response to LABA therapy with respect to the Gly^{16}Arg locus may reflect the longer duration of activity of LABAs compared to SABAs, which may provide intermittent receptor signalling. Alternatively, the presence of concomitant therapies such as ICS therapy and the variable intrinsic activities of the different beta-agonists may also account for these divergent effects. *In vitro*, corticosteroid therapy upregulates the expression of the β_2-adrenergic receptor while LABAs appear to enhance the anti-inflammatory effects of ICS, thereby generating a drug–drug interaction between beta-agonists and ICS when these agents are used concomitantly.[22, 23] As a result, this interaction has the potential to mask the genotypic effects of *ADRβ2* polymorphisms on the clinical response to LABA therapy when these agents are used in combination with ICS therapy. Other concomitant anti-asthma therapies used during these trials may also mask the genotypic effects of LABA therapy by providing an additional therapeutic effect on asthma control. In addition, beta-agonists with lower intrinsic activities such as the LABA salmeterol, may be less likely to induce receptor downregulation to the extent necessary to generate a genetic effect that can be detected at the clinical level.

Evidence from published studies to date supports the hypothesis that variation in the *ADRβ2* gene at the Gly^{16}Arg locus may affect therapeutic responses during regular SABA therapy.[34, 102, 103, 109] Despite these observations, a similar effect of Gly^{16}Arg genotypes on the response to regular therapy with LABAs has not been demonstrated in larger studies or in genotype-stratified trials.[102, 107, 108]

Our understanding of the genetic effects of the *ADRβ2* gene on individual responses to beta-agonist therapy will improve as pharmacogenetic studies analyse a larger number of *ADRβ2* SNPs, haplotypes and pathway-related genetic variation in larger, more ethnically diverse populations while taking into account interactions with other genes and the environment.[110] Another important approach will be to evaluate rare genetic variants instead of the common variations in the $ADR\beta2$ gene as well as pathway-related genes. Severe adverse events associated with beta-agonist therapy are very rare and it is possible that rare genetic variation may be important. Recently, Ortega and colleagues have performed preliminary studies evaluating the role of rare $ADR\beta2$ genetic variation and asthma exacerbations showing interesting novel associations with asthma phenotypes and exacerbations.[105] In contrast to the genotypic effects studied with respect to LABA therapy in the management of asthma, what we understand about the effect of variation in the $ADR\beta2$ gene on the response to beta-agonist therapy in the management of COPD is very limited with respect to the pharmacogenetics of SABA and LABA therapy. Specifically, there have not been any large or genotype-stratified trials assessing the role of genetic variation of the $ADR\beta2$ gene on the response to LABA therapy with respect to COPD.[111,112]

6.13   Safety and efficacy of LABA therapy and the development of combination therapies for the management of asthma and COPD

Two LABA and ICS combination therapies, salmeterol with fluticasone and formoterol with budesonide, are currently available as fixed-dose LABA and ICS combination preparations – Advair® and Symbicort®, respectively. These preparations offer a convenient means of administering combination therapy that ensures simultaneous, regular therapy with both an ICS and a LABA. A 2-year analysis of prescription refill rates in 3503 patients from a managed care organization demonstrated that adherence with salmeterol and fluticasone combination therapy was better than for other therapies.[113] In addition, the aforementioned analysis by the FDA showed that LABA and ICS fixed-dose combination therapy provides a lower risk of adverse events, including hospitalization.[3] Both of these LABA combination therapies carry the same FDA black box warning regarding the potential for an increased risk of serious asthma exacerbations and asthma-related death as that carried by either salmeterol or formoterol.[38] As the FDA warning implies, there is still concern regarding the potential for adverse effects of LABA therapy even if these events are very rare.

The observed adverse effects of LABA therapy have been found primarily in trials and meta-analyses where these agents have been used in inappropriate clinical settings and at higher-than-recommended doses. Concerns regarding asthma-related deaths and life-threatening exacerbations have been based on data from a trial that used LABA monotherapy within the context of a suboptimal study design and a population size insufficient to assess asthma-related mortality.[10,11] Multiple prospective clinical trials and meta-analyses have shown and replicated the safety and efficacy of LABA therapy in the management of asthma when these agents are used in combination with ICS therapy, while withdrawal of ICS therapy results in a subsequent loss of asthma control.[5,37,40,50–53,63,74] Furthermore, some trials have indicated that the use of the

LABA formoterol, with an ICS on a regular basis and as a rescue inhaler, appears to have further beneficial effects.[55]

Adverse cardiovascular events with the use of LABA therapy in the management of COPD have not been demonstrated in multiple prospective clinical trials and meta-analyses. These studies have shown that LABAs are safe and effective with no significant increases in serious or fatal cardiovascular events when used at their recommended doses.[16,17,74,76] Furthermore, when LABAs are combined with ICS therapy, additional benefits other than improvements in airflow obstruction are observed, such as decreased exacerbation rates and improved quality of life.[70–72]

Large pharmacogenetic trials have not been able to identify a subgroup of patients susceptible to the adverse effects of LABA therapy during the chronic management of asthma,[114,115] although there remains a paucity of data with respect to COPD. However, further studies are indicated to investigate the role of rare gene variations in life-threatening events in asthma.

6.14   Summary and future directions

The issues related to beta-agonist safety and efficacy are complex but extremely important. This class of drugs, including both SABAs and LABAs as well as ultra-long-acting beta-agonists, have therapeutic efficacy in the acute and chronic management of obstructive pulmonary diseases specifically asthma and COPD.[116] The major issue specific to asthma is that therapy with this drug class is associated with very rare but serious adverse events and even death. This is specifically true for the two older preparations of SABA containing higher doses of isoproterenol or fenoterol. However, safety issues are not limited to SABA use since findings from the SMA and SMART studies as well as the FDA analyses show evidence of rare mortality or hospitalizations with LABA therapies when these agents are not administered in fixed dose combinations.

The importance of these rare incidents must be viewed in the context of the major benefits that have been documented using evidence-based, prospective clinical trials as well as retrospective observational or meta-analyses. These issues remain important in the light of continued regulatory reviews, therapeutic recommendations from international treatment guidelines, and the ongoing development of new, longer-acting beta agonists. Interestingly, it does appear that potential risks of LABA are either non-existent or greatly reduced when they are only used in fixed dose combinations with ICS. These fixed dose combination products do not permit regular or excessive use of LABAs in persistent asthma.

What is needed is a specific means to identify higher risk patients with asthma or situations where serious adverse events may occur. What we currently know is that asthma deaths are extremely rare and that in many meta-analyses to date the assumption is made that hospitalization represents a surrogate marker for mortality. How to identify these rare risk-patients, and the biological mechanism of that risk, remains extremely complex. The question remains, how do we predict those who are 'at risk' for these severe beta-agonist-related therapeutic events? Ideally, a pharmacogenetic or molecular biomarker for risk would be extremely useful. The first major problem is that the mortality is so low that obtaining biospecimens is almost impossible unless a national or international network were developed to obtain these biospecimens. Another approach would be to explore the role of rare genetic variants in the *ADRβ2* gene and pathway-related genes in an approach that also requires obtaining relevant biospecimens and DNA. One issue with pharmacogenetic risk is that if genetic variants are the causative mechanisms, they will most probably not represent common gene variation such as Gly[16]Arg but rarer changes that may affect less common therapeutic responses.

Another approach that has been proposed is to perform an adequately designed prospective clinical trial to assess the adverse risk from LABA therapies.[117] Others have responded that such a trial would be prohibitively large because of the statistical power required to detect a rare mortality signal.[115] In conclusion, it remains an extremely important issue to develop mechanisms or clinical approaches for accurate prediction and prevention of serious complications associated with beta-agonist therapy.

Acknowledgement

This is supported by the National Institute of Health grants R01 HL69167 and U01 HL65899.

References

1. Bateman ED, Hurd SS, Barnes PJ et al. Global strategy for asthma management and prevention: GINA executive summary. Eur Respir J 2008;31:143–78.
2. Global Initiative for Chronic Obstructive Pulmonary Disease. Global strategy for diagnosis, management and prevention of Chronic Obstructive Pulmonary Disease. www.goldcopd.com. Accessed on 21 October 2009.
3. Kramer JM. Balancing the benefits and risks of inhaled long-acting beta-agonists – -the influence of values. N Engl J Med 2009;360:1592–5.
4. Taylor DR. The beta-agonist saga and its clinical relevance: on and on it goes. Am J Respir Crit Care Med 2009;179:976–8.
5. Greening AP, Ind PW, Northfield M, Shaw G. Added salmeterol versus higher-dose corticosteroid in asthma patients with symptoms on existing inhaled corticosteroid. Allen & Hanburys Limited UK Study Group. Lancet 1994;344:219–24.
6. Maesen FP, Smeets JJ, Gubbelmans HL, Zweers PG. Bronchodilator effect of inhaled formoterol vs salbutamol over 12 hours. Chest 1990;97:590–4.
7. D'Alonzo GE, Nathan RA, Henochowicz S, Morris RJ, Ratner P, Rennard SI. Salmeterol xinafoate as maintenance therapy compared with albuterol in patients with asthma. JAMA 1994;271:1412–16.
8. Pearlman DS, Chervinsky P, LaForce C et al. A comparison of salmeterol with albuterol in the treatment of mild-to-moderate asthma. N Engl J Med 1992;327:1420–5.
9. Castle W, Fuller R, Hall J, Palmer J. Serevent nationwide surveillance study: comparison of salmeterol with salbutamol in asthmatic patients who require regular bronchodilator treatment. Brit Med J 1993;306:1034–7.

10. Nelson HS, Weiss ST, Bleecker ER, Yancey SW, Dorinsky PM. The Salmeterol Multicenter Asthma Research Trial: a comparison of usual pharmacotherapy for asthma or usual pharmacotherapy plus salmeterol. Chest 2006;129:15–26.

11. Salpeter SR, Buckley NS, Ormiston TM, Salpeter EE. Meta-analysis: effect of long-acting beta-agonists on severe asthma exacerbations and asthma-related deaths. Ann Intern Med 2006;144:904–12.

12. Cazzola M, Imperatore F, Salzillo A, et al. Cardiac effects of formoterol and salmeterol in patients suffering from COPD with preexisting cardiac arrhythmias and hypoxemia. Chest 1998;114:411–15.

13. Bennett JA, Smyth ET, Pavord ID, Wilding PJ, Tattersfield AE. Systemic effects of salbutamol and salmeterol in patients with asthma. Thorax 1994;49:771–4.

14. Guhan AR, Cooper S, Oborne J, Lewis S, Bennett J, Tattersfield AE. Systemic effects of formoterol and salmeterol: a dose-response comparison in healthy subjects. Thorax 2000;55:650–6.

15. Salpeter SR, Ormiston TM, Salpeter EE. Cardiovascular effects of beta-agonists in patients with asthma and COPD: a meta-analysis. Chest 2004;125:2309–21.

16. Campbell SC, Criner GJ, Levine BE, et al. Cardiac safety of formoterol 12 microg twice daily in patients with chronic obstructive pulmonary disease. Pulm Pharmacol Ther 2007;20: 571–9.

17. Nelson HS, Gross NJ, Levine B, et al. Cardiac safety profile of nebulized formoterol in adults with COPD: a 12-week, multicenter, randomized, double- blind, double-dummy, placebo- and active-controlled trial. Clin Ther 2007;29:2167–78.

18. Tashkin DP, Cooper CB. The role of long-acting bronchodilators in the management of stable COPD. Chest 2004;125:249–59.

19. Dahl R, Greefhorst LA, Nowak D, et al. Inhaled formoterol dry powder versus ipratropium bromide in chronic obstructive pulmonary disease. Am J Respir Crit Care Med 2001;164:778–84.

20. Calverley PM, Anderson JA, Celli B, et al. Salmeterol and fluticasone propionate and survival in chronic obstructive pulmonary disease. N Engl J Med 2007;356:775–89.

21. Rossi A, Kristufek P, Levine BE, et al. Comparison of the efficacy, tolerability, and safety of formoterol dry powder and oral, slow-release theophylline in the treatment of COPD. Chest 2002;121:1058–69.

22. Profita M, Gagliardo R, Di GR, et al. Biochemical interaction between effects of beclomethasone dipropionate and salbutamol or formoterol in sputum cells from mild to moderate asthmatics. Allergy 2005;60:323–9.

23. Usmani OS, Ito K, Maneechotesuwan K, et al. Glucocorticoid receptor nuclear translocation in airway cells after inhaled combination therapy. Am J Respir Crit Care Med 2005;172:704–12.

24. Stolley PD. Asthma mortality. Why the United States was spared an epidemic of deaths due to asthma. Am Rev Respir Dis 1972;105:883–90.

25. Grainger J, Woodman K, Pearce N, et al. Prescribed fenoterol and death from asthma in New Zealand, 1981–7: a further case-control study. Thorax 1991;46:105–11.

26. Pearce N, Grainger J, Atkinson M, et al. Case-control study of prescribed fenoterol and death from asthma in New Zealand, 1977–81. Thorax 1990;45:170–5.

27. Pearce N, Beasley R, Crane J, Burgess C, Jackson R. End of the New Zealand asthma mortality epidemic. Lancet 1995;345:41–4.

28. Pearce N, Burgess C, Crane J, Beasley R. Fenoterol, asthma deaths, and asthma severity. Chest 1997;112:1148–50.

29. Crane J, Pearce N, Flatt A, et al. Prescribed fenoterol and death from asthma in New Zealand, 1981–3: case-control study. Lancet 1989;1:917–22.

30. Spitzer WO, Buist AS. Case-control study of prescribed fenoterol and death from asthma in New Zealand, 1977–81. Thorax 1990;45:645–6.
31. Suissa S, Ernst P, Boivin JF, et al. A cohort analysis of excess mortality in asthma and the use of inhaled beta-agonists. Am J Respir Crit Care Med 1994;149:604–10.
32. Sears MR, Taylor DR, Print CG, et al. Regular inhaled beta-agonist treatment in bronchial asthma. Lancet 1990;336:1391–6.
33. Drazen JM, Israel E, Boushey HA, et al. Comparison of regularly scheduled with as-needed use of albuterol in mild asthma. Asthma Clinical Research Network. N Engl J Med 1996;335:841–7.
34. Israel E, Chinchilli VM, Ford JG, et al. Use of regularly scheduled albuterol treatment in asthma: genotype-stratified, randomised, placebo-controlled cross-over trial. Lancet 2004;364:1505–12.
35. Finkelstein FN. Risks of salmeterol? N Engl J Med 1994;331:1314.
36. Speizer FE, Doll R, Heaf P, Strang LB. Investigation into use of drugs preceding death from asthma. Br Med J 1968;1:339–43.
37. Nelson HS, Dorinsky PM. Safety of long-acting beta-agonists. Ann Intern Med 2006;145: 706–10.
38. US Food and Drug Administration. FDA Public Health Advisory: Serevent Diskus (salmeterol xinafoate inhalation powder), Advair Diskus (fluticasone propionate & salmeterol inhalation powder), Foradil Aerolizer (formoterol fumarate inhalation powder). 11-18-2005. 6-29-0008.
39. Anderson HR, Ayres JG, Sturdy PM, et al. Bronchodilator treatment and deaths from asthma: case-control study. Brit Med J 2005;330:117.
40. Greenstone IR, Ni Chroinin MN, Masse V, et al. Combination of inhaled long-acting beta2-agonists and inhaled steroids versus higher dose of inhaled steroids in children and adults with persistent asthma. Cochrane Database Syst Rev 2005;CD005533.
41. Walters EH, Gibson PG, Lasserson TJ, Walters JA. Long-acting beta2-agonists for chronic asthma in adults and children where background therapy contains varied or no inhaled corticosteroid. Cochrane Database Syst Rev 2007;CD001385.
42. Bateman E, Nelson H, Bousquet J, et al. Meta-analysis: effects of adding salmeterol to inhaled corticosteroids on serious asthma-related events. Ann Intern Med 2008;149:33–42.
43. Jaeschke R, O'Byrne PM, Mejza F, et al. The safety of long-acting beta-agonists among patients with asthma using inhaled corticosteroids: systematic review and metaanalysis. Am J Respir Crit Care Med 2008;178:1009–16.
44. Cates CJ, Cates MJ, Lasserson TJ. Regular treatment with formoterol for chronic asthma: serious adverse events. Cochrane Database Syst Rev 2008;CD006923.
45. Cates CJ, Cates MJ. Regular treatment with salmeterol for chronic asthma: serious adverse events. Cochrane Database Syst Rev 2008;CD006363.
46. Cates CJ, Lasserson TJ, Jaeschke R. Regular treatment with salmeterol and inhaled steroids for chronic asthma: serious adverse events. Cochrane Database Syst Rev 2009;CD006922.
47. Cates CJ, Lasserson TJ, Jaeschke R. Regular treatment with formoterol and inhaled steroids for chronic asthma: serious adverse events. Cochrane Database Syst Rev 2009;CD006924.
48. Sears MR, Ottosson A, Radner F, Suissa S. Long-acting beta-agonists: a review of formoterol safety data from asthma clinical trials. Eur Respir J 2009;33:21–32.
49. Pauwels RA, Lofdahl CG, Postma DS, et al. Effect of inhaled formoterol and budesonide on exacerbations of asthma. Formoterol and Corticosteroids Establishing Therapy (FACET) International Study Group. N Engl J Med 1997;337:1405–11.
50. O'Byrne PM, Barnes PJ, Rodriguez-Roisin R, et al. Low dose inhaled budesonide and formoterol in mild persistent asthma: the OPTIMA randomized trial. Am J Respir Crit Care Med 2001;164:1392–7.

51. Lemanske RF Jr, Sorkness CA, Mauger EA, et al. Inhaled corticosteroid reduction and elim-ination in patients with persistent asthma receiving salmeterol: a randomized controlled trial. JAMA 2001;285:2594–603.
52. Lazarus SC, Boushey HA, Fahy JV, et al. Long-acting beta2-agonist monotherapy vs continued therapy with inhaled corticosteroids in patients with persistent asthma: a randomized controlled trial. JAMA 2001;285:2583–93.
53. Bateman ED, Boushey HA, Bousquet J, et al. Can guideline-defined asthma control be achieved? The Gaining Optimal Asthma ControL study. Am J Respir Crit Care Med 2004;170:836–44.
54. Busse W, Koenig SM, Oppenheimer J, et al. Steroid-sparing effects of fluticasone propionate 100 microg and salmeterol 50 microg administered twice daily in a single product in patients previously controlled with fluticasone propionate 250 microg administered twice daily. J Allergy Clin Immunol 2003;111:57–65.
55. O'Byrne PM, Bisgaard H, Godard PP, et al. Budesonide/formoterol combination therapy as both maintenance and reliever medication in asthma. Am J Respir Crit Care Med 2005;171:129–36.
56. Roberts JA, Bradding P, Britten KM, et al. The long-acting beta2-agonist salmeterol xinafoate: effects on airway inflammation in asthma. Eur Respir J 1999;14:275–82.
57. Maneechotesuwan K, Essilfie-Quaye S, Meah S, et al. Formoterol attenuates neutrophilic airway inflammation in asthma. Chest 2005;128:1936–42.
58. Overbeek SE, Mulder PG, Baelemans SM, Hoogsteden HC, Prins JB. Formoterol added to low-dose budesonide has no additional antiinflammatory effect in asthmatic patients. Chest 2005;128:1121–7.
59. Jarjour NN, Wilson SJ, Koenig SM, et al. Control of airway inflammation maintained at a lower steroid dose with 100/50 microg of fluticasone propionate/salmeterol. J Allergy Clin Immunol 2006;118:44–52.
60. McIvor RA, Pizzichini E, Turner MO, Hussack P, Hargreave FE, Sears MR. Potential mask-ing effects of salmeterol on airway inflammation in asthma. Am J Respir Crit Care Med 1998;158:924–30.
61. Panina-Bordignon P, Mazzeo D, Lucia PD, et al. Beta2-agonists prevent Th1 development by selective inhibition of interleukin 12. J Clin Invest 1997;100:1513–19.
62. Agarwal SK, Marshall GD Jr. Beta-adrenergic modulation of human type-1/type-2 cytokine balance. J Allergy Clin Immunol 2000;105:91–8.
63. Nelson HS. Long-acting beta-agonists in adult asthma: Evidence that these drugs are safe. Prim Care Respir J 2006;15:271–7.
64. Shih HT, Webb CR, Conway WA, Peterson E, Tilley B, Goldstein S. Frequency and significance of cardiac arrhythmias in chronic obstructive lung disease. Chest 1988;94:44–8.
65. Stewart AG, Waterhouse JC, Howard P. The QTc interval, autonomic neuropathy and mortality in hypoxaemic COPD. Respir Med 1995;89:79–84.
66. Curkendall SM, DeLuise C, Jones JK, et al. Cardiovascular disease in patients with chronic obstructive pulmonary disease, Saskatchewan Canada cardiovascular disease in COPD patients. Ann Epidemiol 2006;16:63–70.
67. Huiart L, Ernst P, Suissa S. Cardiovascular morbidity and mortality in COPD. Chest 2005;128:2640–6.
68. Au DH, Lemaitre RN, Curtis JR, Smith NL, Psaty BM. The risk of myocardial infarction associated with inhaled beta-adrenoceptor agonists. Am J Respir Crit Care Med 2000;161: 827–30.
69. Au DH, Curtis JR, Every NR, McDonell MB, Fihn SD. Association between inhaled beta-agonists and the risk of unstable angina and myocardial infarction. Chest 2002;121:846–51.

70. Calverley P, Pauwels R, Vestbo J, et al. Combined salmeterol and fluticasone in the treatment of chronic obstructive pulmonary disease: a randomised controlled trial. Lancet 2003;361:449–56.

71. Calverley PM, Boonsawat W, Cseke Z, Zhong N, Peterson S, Olsson H. Maintenance therapy with budesonide and formoterol in chronic obstructive pulmonary disease. Eur Respir J 2003;22:912–19.

72. Szafranski W, Cukier A, Ramirez A, et al. Efficacy and safety of budesonide/formoterol in the management of chronic obstructive pulmonary disease. Eur Respir J 2003;21:74–81.

73. Rabe KF, Hurd S, Anzueto A, et al. Global strategy for the diagnosis, management, and prevention of chronic obstructive pulmonary disease: GOLD executive summary. Am J Respir Crit Care Med 2007;176:532–55.

74. Rodrigo GJ, Nannini LJ, Rodriguez-Roisin R. Safety of long-acting beta-agonists in stable COPD: a systematic review. Chest 2008;133:1079–87.

75. Ferguson GT, Funck-Brentano C, Fischer T, Darken P, Reisner C. Cardiovascular safety of salmeterol in COPD. Chest 2003;123:1817–24.

76. Boyd G, Morice AH, Pounsford JC, Siebert M, Peslis N, Crawford C. An evaluation of salmeterol in the treatment of chronic obstructive pulmonary disease (COPD). Eur Respir J 1997;10:815–21.

77. Cazzola M, Di LG, Di PF, Calderaro F, Testi R, Centanni S. Additive effects of salmeterol and fluticasone or theophylline in COPD. Chest 2000;118:1576–81.

78. Jones PW, Bosh TK. Quality of life changes in COPD patients treated with salmeterol. Am J Respir Crit Care Med 1997;155:1283–9.

79. Mahler DA, Donohue JF, Barbee RA, et al. Efficacy of salmeterol xinafoate in the treatment of COPD. Chest 1999;115:957–65.

80. Aalbers R, Ayres J, Backer V, et al. Formoterol in patients with chronic obstructive pulmonary disease: a randomized, controlled, 3-month trial. Eur Respir J 2002;19:936–43.

81. Brusasco V, Hodder R, Miravitlles M, Korducki L, Towse L, Kesten S. Health outcomes following treatment for 6 months with once daily tiotropium compared with twice daily salmeterol in patients with COPD. Thorax 2006;61:91.

82. Chapman KR, Arvidsson P, Chuchalin AG, et al. The addition of salmeterol 50 microg bid to anticholinergic treatment in patients with COPD: a randomized, placebo controlled trial. Chronic obstructive pulmonary disease. Can Respir J 2002;9:178–85.

83. D'Urzo AD, De Salvo MC, Ramirez-Rivera A, et al. In patients with COPD, treatment with a combination of formoterol and ipratropium is more effective than a combination of salbutamol and ipratropium: a 3-week, randomized, double-blind, within-patient, multicenter study. Chest 2001;119:1347–56.

84. Donohue JF, van Noord JA, Bateman ED, et al. A 6-month, placebo-controlled study comparing lung function and health status changes in COPD patients treated with tiotropium or salmeterol. Chest 2002;122:47–55.

85. Mahler DA, Wire P, Horstman D, et al. Effectiveness of fluticasone propionate and salmeterol combination delivered via the Diskus device in the treatment of chronic obstructive pulmonary disease. Am J Respir Crit Care Med 2002;166:1084–91.

86. Rennard SI, Anderson W, ZuWallack R, et al. Use of a long-acting inhaled beta2-adrenergic agonist, salmeterol xinafoate, in patients with chronic obstructive pulmonary disease. Am J Respir Crit Care Med 2001;163:1087–92.

87. Rutten-van MM, Roos B, van Noord JA. An empirical comparison of the St George's Respiratory Questionnaire (SGRQ) and the Chronic Respiratory Disease Questionnaire (CRQ) in a clinical trial setting. Thorax 1999;54:995–1003.

88. van Noord JA, de Munck DR, Bantje TA, Hop WC, Akveld ML, Bommer AM. Long-term treatment of chronic obstructive pulmonary disease with salmeterol and the additive effect of ipratropium. Eur Respir J 2000;15:878–85.

89. ZuWallack RL, Mahler DA, Reilly D, et al. Salmeterol plus theophylline combination therapy in the treatment of COPD. Chest 2001;119:1661–70.

90. Hanania NA, Darken P, Horstman D, et al. The efficacy and safety of fluticasone propionate (250 microg)/salmeterol (50 microg) combined in the Diskus inhaler for the treatment of COPD. Chest 2003;124:834–43.

91. Soriano JB, Vestbo J, Pride NB, Kiri V, Maden C, Maier WC. Survival in COPD patients after regular use of fluticasone propionate and salmeterol in general practice. Eur Respir J 2002;20:819–25.

92. Sin DD, Wu L, Anderson JA, et al. Inhaled corticosteroids and mortality in chronic obstructive pulmonary disease. Thorax 2005;60:992–7.

93. Burge PS, Calverley PM, Jones PW, Spencer S, Anderson JA, Maslen TK. Randomised, double blind, placebo controlled study of fluticasone propionate in patients with moderate to severe chronic obstructive pulmonary disease: the ISOLDE trial. Brit Med J 2000;320:1297–303.

94. Reihsaus E, Innis M, MacIntyre N, Liggett SB. Mutations in the gene encoding for the beta 2-adrenergic receptor in normal and asthmatic subjects. Am J Respir Cell Mol Biol 1993;8:334–9.

95. Green SA, Turki J, Innis M, Liggett SB. Amino-terminal polymorphisms of the human beta 2-adrenergic receptor impart distinct agonist-promoted regulatory properties. Biochemistry 1994;33:9414–19.

96. Green SA, Turki J, Bejarano P, Hall IP, Liggett SB. Influence of beta 2-adrenergic receptor genotypes on signal transduction in human airway smooth muscle cells. Am J Respir Cell Mol Biol 1995;13:25–33.

97. Hawkins GA, Tantisira K, Meyers DA, et al. Sequence, haplotype, and association analysis of ADRbeta2 in a multiethnic asthma case-control study. Am J Respir Crit Care Med 2006;174:1101–9.

98. Drysdale CM, McGraw DW, Stack CB, et al. Complex promoter and coding region beta 2-adrenergic receptor haplotypes alter receptor expression and predict in vivo responsiveness. Proc Natl Acad Sci U S A 2000;97:10483–8.

99. Ortega VE, Hawkins GA, Peters SP, Bleecker ER. Pharmacogenetics of the beta 2-adrenergic receptor gene. Immunol Allergy Clin North Am 2007;27:665–84.

100. Martinez FD, Graves PE, Baldini M, Solomon S, Erickson R. Association between genetic polymorphisms of the beta2-adrenoceptor and response to albuterol in children with and without a history of wheezing. J Clin Invest 1997;100:3184–8.

101. Silverman EK, Kwiatkowski DJ, Sylvia JS, et al. Family-based association analysis of beta2-adrenergic receptor polymorphisms in the childhood asthma management program. J Allergy Clin Immunol 2003;112:870–6.

102. Taylor DR, Drazen JM, Herbison GP, Yandava CN, Hancox RJ, Town GI. Asthma exacerbations during long term beta agonist use: influence of beta(2) adrenoceptor polymorphism. Thorax 2000;55:762–7.

103. Israel E, Drazen JM, Liggett SB, et al. The effect of polymorphisms of the beta(2)-adrenergic receptor on the response to regular use of albuterol in asthma. Am J Respir Crit Care Med 2000;162:75–80.

104. Israel E, Drazen JM, Liggett SB, et al. Effect of polymorphism of the beta(2)-adrenergic receptor on response to regular use of albuterol in asthma. Int Arch Allergy Immunol 2001;124:183–6.

105. Ortega VE, Hawkins GA, Meyers DA, Bleecker ER. Characterization of asthma cases and controls with rare B2-adrenergic receptor gene polymorphisms in a multi-ethnic population. American Thoracic Society International Conference, May 2009. Poster Discussion Session.

106. Wechsler ME, Lehman E, Lazarus SC, et al. beta-Adrenergic receptor polymorphisms and response to salmeterol. Am J Respir Crit Care Med 2006;173:519–26.

107. Bleecker ER, Yancey SW, Baitinger LA, et al. Salmeterol response is not affected by beta2-adrenergic receptor genotype in subjects with persistent asthma. J Allergy Clin Immunol 2006;118:809–16.

108. Bleecker ER, Postma DS, Lawrance RM, Meyers DA, Ambrose HJ, Goldman M. Effect of ADRB2 polymorphisms on response to longacting beta2-agonist therapy: a pharmacogenetic analysis of two randomised studies. Lancet 2007;370:2118–25.

109. Hancox RJ, Sears MR, Taylor DR. Polymorphism of the beta2-adrenoceptor and the response to long-term beta2-agonist therapy in asthma. Eur Respir J 1998;11:589–93.

110. Hall IP. Pharmacogenetics of asthma. Eur Respir J 2000;15:449–51.

111. Ho LI, Harn HJ, Chen CJ, Tsai NM. Polymorphism of the beta(2)-adrenoceptor in COPD in Chinese subjects. Chest 2001;120:1493–9.

112. Joos L, Weir TD, Connett JE, et al. Polymorphisms in the beta2 adrenergic receptor and bronchodilator response, bronchial hyperresponsiveness, and rate of decline in lung function in smokers. Thorax 2003;58:703–7.

113. Stempel DA, Stoloff SW, Carranza R Jr, Stanford RH, Ryskina KL, Legorreta AP. Adherence to asthma controller medication regimens. Respir Med 2005;99:1263–7.

114. Masoli M, Fabian D, Holt S, Beasley R. The global burden of asthma: executive summary of the GINA Dissemination Committee report. Allergy 2004;59:469–78.

115. Drazen JM, O'Byrne PM. Risks of long-acting beta-agonists in achieving asthma control. N Engl J Med 2009;360:1671–2.

116. Cazzola M, Segreti A, Matera MG. Novel bronchodilators in asthma. Curr Opin Pulm Med 2009 (epub ahead of print).

117. Knobil K. Long-acting beta agonists in asthma. N Engl J Med 2009;361:208–9.

7

Inhaled combination therapy with glucocorticoids and long-acting β_2-agonists in asthma and COPD, current and future perspectives

Jan Lötvall

Krefting Research Centre, University of Gothenburg, Göteborg, Sweden

7.1 Pharmacological management guidelines of asthma and COPD

During the last 25 years we have observed a massive improvement in the management of asthma thanks to guidelines from most countries implementing inhaled glucocorticoid treatments. Since the publication of the Swedish Medical Product agency guidelines in 1986,[1] most if not all guidelines have enforced a baseline therapy using inhaled glucocorticoid therapy if the patient has any regular symptoms of asthma.[2] Since the early 1990s, the recommendation has been to add a long-acting β_2-agonist (LABA) if the asthma symptoms remain uncontrolled despite the baseline glucocorticoid therapy.[3] When the use of inhaled glucocorticoid therapy was implemented in Sweden in the mid-1980s, a marked reduction in hospitalizations due to asthma was observed.[4] Internationally, the Global Initiative for Asthma[5] has taken a strong stance to develop guidelines that are comprehensive for the treatment of adult asthma, and for the treatment of paediatric asthma the European and US Allergy Academies (EAACI and AAAAI) developed a collaborative consensus statement called PRACTALL.[6]

The development of guidelines for the management of chronic obstructive pulmonary disease (COPD) came later, and is internationally represented by the GOLD guidelines (Global Initiative for Chronic Obstructive Lung Disease).[7] The pharmacological management part of these guidelines is based on a series of very large studies showing efficacy of different therapies in COPD, including inhaled glucocorticoids, inhaled antimuscarinics, inhaled LABAs, as well as inhaled combinations of glucocorticoids and LABAs.

Advances in Combination Therapy for Asthma and COPD, First Edition. Edited by Jan Lötvall.
© 2012 John Wiley & Sons, Ltd. Published 2012 by John Wiley & Sons, Ltd.

Both asthma and COPD guidelines currently recommend a stepwise approach to treat patients with these respective diseases, depending on either degree of control (asthma)[5] or severity (COPD – based on measured forced expiratory volume in first second, or FEV_1).[7] Efforts are being made to develop these guidelines to be more closely related to asthma and COPD phenotype characteristics, achieving more individualized therapy. There is no question that guidelines in themselves make a difference for patients, not only because the advice on how to utilize pharmacological treatments is simplified, but also because of the greater efficiency in distributing the recommendations to a wide audience.

A weakness with the current guidelines for both asthma and COPD is that they seldom or never take into account the fact that both diseases are fundamentally different in different individuals, with different treatment responses depending on different expression of disease phenotypes.[8,9] Indeed, it has been proposed that, for example, asthma is a syndrome encompassing several disease entities that are called 'asthma endotypes',[10] and development of novel treatments that are mechanism specific should ideally be focusing on basic processes of each disease endotype. Hopefully the future will provide better evidence of effects of different treatments in different subgroups of patients, as the understanding of the mechanisms of disease phenotypes develops.[10]

The current chapter will primarily focus on the use of combinations of inhaled glucocorticoids and LABAs in the treatment of asthma and COPD, both now and in the future.

7.2   Steroid treatment in asthma

The first inhaled glucocorticoid that was effectively used for asthma was beclometasone, which early showed to be beneficial in reducing the need for oral steroid treatment in those with severe disease.[11–13] This drug became clinically available in the early 1970s, but the widespread use of inhaled glucocorticoids in asthma did not start until the 1980s, when new inhaled glucocorticoids and inhaler devices were registered and marketed.[4,14] Inhaled glucocorticoids have importantly been shown to reduce the risk of asthma deaths,[15,16] and to reduce the frequency and the severity of asthma exacerbations.[4,17,18] Inhaled glucocorticoids are also effective in asthma by improving lung function, reducing the need for bronchodilator therapy, and reducing symptoms of bronchial hyperresponsiveness; they may also maintain lung function over time.[17–19] A crucial property of any inhaled glucocorticoid is that the drug has low oral bioavailability, reducing the proportion of the drug that is absorbed through the gut.[20] The first significant signs of the clinical effects of inhaled glucocorticoids can be observed only a few hours after the first inhalation,[21] but the improvement in the control of asthma can be seen over several days and even months after the initiation of treatment.[22] Since there is massive evidence of the beneficial effects of inhaled glucocorticoids in all severities of asthma, they are recommended in the regular management of the disease if symptoms occur regularly, each week. The three most commonly used inhaled glucocorticoids worldwide are beclometasone, fluticasone propionate and budesonide; also triamcinolone and flunisolide are used clinically in some countries, including the USA.[23,24]

A series of new inhaled glucocorticoids have been developed over the last decade, including ciclesonide, mometasone and fluticasone furoate, which have come into clinical use for different indications.[24–27] These are typically more potent glucocorticoids, exhibiting very low oral bioavailability and, hypothetically at least, increasing the therapeutic ratio of these drugs even further compared to the older drugs.[28,29]

The systemic side effects of inhaled glucocorticoids are limited at the doses usually recommended today, up to approximately 800–1000 μg, but at higher doses systemic effects can be observed. The risk of osteoporosis and subsequent fractures is low, but has been documented with higher doses of the older inhaled glucocorticoids.[30] The clinically more common side effects are oral candidiasis and effects on voice/hoarseness, which in rare cases can be quite difficult to manage.[31]

The concept of inhaled glucocorticoids as a baseline therapy for most patients with asthma will probably prevail for many years to come. However, not all asthma patients are fully or efficiently controlled by inhaled glucocorticoids alone,[32,33] which is why the addition of a LABA or another complementary treatment is often indicated.[32]

7.3 Effects of adding LABA to inhaled glucocorticoids in asthma

By the mid-1990s it was shown that adding a LABA to a baseline treatment of inhaled glucocorticoids produced a clear improvement in symptom control as well as lung function.[34] In the FACET study, it was also shown that a very clear reduction in the frequency of exacerbations of asthma can be observed when inhaled corticosteroids (ICS) and LABAs are given together.[35] This was a very important discovery, since there was an extensive debate going on at the time, suggesting that LABAs may be increasing the risk of severe asthma attacks.[36,37] Eventually, treating asthma with inhaled glucocorticoids complemented with a LABA inhaler was shown to produce additional improvement of asthma symptoms, and several combination inhalers became available in the mid- to late 1990s.[32,38,39] A very large number of studies have shown the efficacy of combination inhalers in different degrees of asthma severity, in different countries and in patients with different genetic backgrounds. Importantly, patients who have been included in these studies have uncontrolled asthma despite baseline inhaled glucocorticosteroid (GCS) therapy, or express clear improvement in FEV_1 when reversibility to salbutamol or another rapid-acting β_2-agonist is tested.[34,35,39,40] Thus, there is very little evidence that combining inhaled GCS and LABAs in patients who are controlled on inhaled GCS alone adds any effect of clinical importance.

Daytime asthma symptoms are clearly improved by adding LABAs to inhaled GCS, a phenomenon that is very closely associated with improvement in lung function measures such as FEV_1 or peak expiratory flow (PEF).[39,40] This improvement is usually observed immediately, after the first inhaled dose, or after a few days of combining these medications.[35] The observed bronchodilation is maintained for weeks, months and years of treatment, and there is no tendency for progressive tolerance to this function of LABAs after the first few doses.[35] Improving lung function and symptoms is of course important in managing asthma, but is only one measure of the success of treating asthma, albeit one that is easy to quantify and statistically assess. This quantifiable aspect of lung function has been retained as a key factor in acceptance of new treatments for distribution to different markets, but other key clinical effects of asthma drugs may be even more important for the patients.[41,42]

Night-time symptoms of asthma are indicative of uncontrolled disease, and are significantly improved in studies where LABAs are added to inhaled GCS.[34,35,40] Awakenings due to asthma are a sign of severe and uncontrolled disease, and probably reflect greater disease activity at that time. Night-time asthma is thus not a separate disease entity, but signs of improvement of this variable suggest that combined inhaled GCS and LABAs help in controlling disease activity.

Overall asthma control tests have been developed over the last decade, and studies show uniformly that the control that these questionnaires define, which includes daytime symptoms, night-time symptoms, ability to perform activities and lung function, is improved by combining inhaled GCS and LABAs[43] (Figure 7.1). Critics have

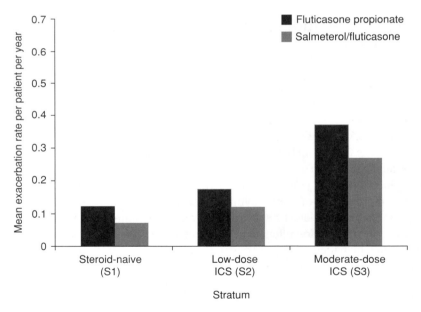

Figure 7.1 Asthma exacerbations per patient per year among patients treated with salmeterol/ fluticasone or fluticasone propionate only in the GOAL study. ICS, inhaled corticosteroid. Reproduced with permission from Bateman ED, Boushey HA, Bousquet J, Busse WW, Clark TJ, Pauwels RA, Pedersen SE; GOAL Investigators Group. Can guideline-defined asthma control be achieved? The Gaining Optimal Asthma Control study. Am J Respir Crit Care Med. 2004 Oct 15;170(8):836–44 © American Thoracic Society.

suggested that these measures themselves bias results towards showing efficacy of adding a LABA to inhaled GCS instead of adding another therapy or intensifying the inhaled anti-inflammatory therapy by itself. However, these tools are simple and straightforward, and when medication is adjusted to improve control, the future risks of asthma, such as exacerbations, are also reduced.[44]

Exacerbations are strong markers of severity of asthma, and their frequency and severity are therefore key endpoints in studies of any asthma medication. It was early shown that inhaled glucocorticoids reduce the frequency of exacerbations of asthma, although some exacerbations occur despite high doses of inhaled glucocorticoids, suggesting that some of these are steroid insensitive.[18] The FACET study in 1997 showed that adding a LABA to a chronic treatment with inhaled glucocorticoids will further reduce the frequency of exacerbations.[35] Specifically, more than 800 patients becoming controlled with a high dose of glucocorticoids during a run-in period, and checked for adherence to taking medication, were randomly assigned to two doses of budesonide (200 or 800 μg daily divided in two doses), plus addition of formoterol 12 μg or placebo given at the same time by a different inhaler. Firstly, budesonide 800 μg reduced exacerbation frequency to a greater extent than 200 μg, but adding formoterol to either dose of budesonide further reduced the frequency of asthma exacerbations.[35] This was a pivotal finding at the time, since there was an extensive debate ongoing suggesting that treatment with inhaled β_2-agonists in general, and perhaps LABAs in particular, increased the risk of asthma exacerbations. However, this suggestion was strongly disproved by the FACET study, and similar studies that followed. Importantly, in the FACET study the inhaled glucocorticoid and the LABA were given in two separate inhalers and in a controlled clinical study environment. In a real-life situation, however, it has been recognized that some patients stop using their controller inhaled GCS but maintain use of the LABA, which clearly increases the risk of the detrimental effects of LABA treatment.[45,46] By contrast, maintaining inhaled GCS therapy totally abolishes any risk with inhaled LABAs, arguing for a positive interaction of these drugs in controlling asthma.[47] Since the groundbreaking FACET study, a large series of additional studies have determined the effects of combinations of inhaled GCS and LABAs on the frequency of asthma exacerbations, including the combinations of fluticasone propionate combined with salmeterol, and budesonide combined with formoterol.[39,40,43] These results are consistent with combined inhaled GCS and LABAs interacting positively in asthma when given concomitantly, resulting in reduced risk of severe events and/or asthma exacerbations.[46]

There is also evidence that giving patients combinations of inhaled GCS and LABAs does not in any way increase the risk for severe asthma events, which have been documented in studies where LABAs have been allowed to be taken without inhaled GCS.[46,47] Indeed, a recent meta-analysis showed no tendency of increased risk of asthma exacerbations if the LABA was given together with the inhaled GCS.[47] However, all clinicians treating asthmatics with inhaled GCS and LABAs in two separate inhalers have experienced patients who stop taking the controller inhaled GCS but maintain the LABA, which in itself can lead to risk. Therefore, it is reasonable to treat patients with asthma with a LABA only if the LABA is given together with an inhaled GCS in the same inhaler.

7.4   Steroid treatment in COPD

Inhaled glucocorticoids are seldom used alone in COPD, as several studies show no or weak evidence of effect on the long-term loss in lung function in COPD. However, in COPD patients with reduced lung function, inhaled glucocorticoids have been shown to reduce the frequency of exacerbations, and in some patients withdrawal of inhaled glucocorticoids can itself lead to an exacerbation. It is possible that only a subgroup of patients with COPD respond well to inhaled glucocorticoids given alone, as the small signals seen in large studies could depend on efficacy attributed to a subgroup of patients. Recent studies argue for some efficacy of inhaled glucocorticoids in all severities of COPD,[48, 49] although one study also showed an increased risk of pneumonia in COPD patients if high doses of inhaled glucocorticoids are given over a long period of time.[50, 51] It has previously been suggested that COPD patients with some degree of eosinophilic inflammation will have more prominent clinical effects with inhaled glucocorticoids, an aspect that should be more carefully evaluated in prospective studies using subgroups of patients with such phenotype expression.

7.5   Effects of LABAs in COPD

Bronchodilators including anticholinergics and LABAs are well established in the management of COPD, both when given alone and, in the case of LABAs, sometimes when given with inhaled glucocorticoids.[7,49–52] Improvement in lung function has been shown in a multitude of studies of LABAs given to patients with COPD of different severity over variable periods of time as maintenance therapy. The induced bronchodilation achieved in COPD patients with the LABAs salmeterol and formoterol given twice daily is usually sustained over the study periods for up to one or several years,[49,50,52] although some loss in FEV_1 can be observed in parallel with progression of the disease. Thus, these studies show no evidence of clinically important tolerance to the direct bronchodilating effects of LABAs in patients with COPD.[50,52] Analysis of data from the TORCH study even argues that salmeterol may have the capacity to slightly reduce the rate of decline in lung function in patients with COPD, although this effect was on average small in patients with COPD.[53] One important clinical effect of LABAs given to patients with COPD is a substantially increased tolerance to strenuous exercise.[54] Not all studies with different LABAs are consistent in their results, but especially in relation to endurance tests, improvements in exercise tolerance can be observed when COPD patients are treated with either formoterol or salmeterol,[54,55] although the effects of these drugs on maximal exercise performance are less convincing.

The effects of LABAs on COPD exacerbations also vary from study to study, perhaps partly dependent on inclusion criteria for the studies and their overall design. However, the TORCH study that was performed over three years in a large cohort of patients showed that salmeterol reduced the annual rate of COPD by 15% compared with placebo ($P < 0.001$), but a slightly numerically greater reduction in exacerbations was observed when salmeterol was given in combination with fluticasone.[50]

7.6   Combination inhalers versus two separate inhalers for inhaled GCS and LABAs

Numerous studies have compared the clinical effects on patients with asthma of giving combinations of LABAs and inhaled GCS in either separate inhalers or combined in one inhaler.[39, 40] These studies have consistently shown that giving either formoterol and budesonide or salmeterol and fluticasone propionate in one inhaler is at least as good as giving the same drugs in two separate inhalers. Indeed, there is a tendency that combination inhalers result in a more rapid onset of effect compared to when the two drugs are given by different inhalers (Figure 7.2). However, in controlled study environments the differences are small.

From both a clinical and commercial perspective, it is clear that the combination of inhaled GCS and LABAs achieves improved asthma control, and this is especially evident when these two drugs are combined in a single inhaler. There has been extensive

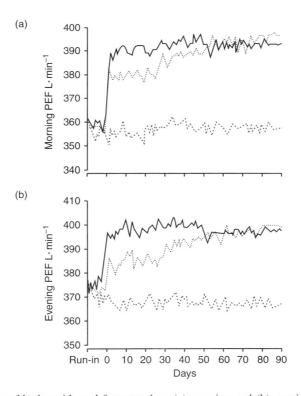

Figure 7.2   Effect of budesonide and formoterol on (a) morning and (b) evening peak expiratory flow (PEF) when given in separate or single inhalers, with a tendency of more rapid effect when the combination is utilized. Reproduced with permission from Zetterström O, Buhl R, Mellem H, Perpiñá M, Hedman J, O'Neill S, Ekström T. Improved asthma control with budesonide/formoterol in a single inhaler, compared with budesonide alone. Eur Respir J. 2001 Aug;18(2):262–8. © European Respiratory Society.

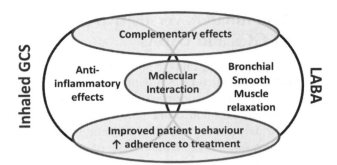

Figure 7.3   Hypothesis for the mechanisms behind the efficacy of combinations of inhaled gluco-corticosteroids (GCS) and long-acting β₂-agonists (LABAs) involves the separate anti-inflammatory and bronchodilating effects complementing each other, molecular interaction increasing the efficacy of the respective drugs, and increased adherence to medication.

scientific discussion concerning why the combination of these drugs is efficient, and I here present four key arguments that have been supported by different degrees of scientific evidence (Figure 7.3).

Firstly, inhaled GCS and LABAs have pharmacologically totally different effects in asthma, with the inhaled GCS having clear anti-inflammatory properties and the LABA primarily being a bronchodilator.[34, 56, 57] Thus, these two types of drugs have complementary effects in the airways, through fundamentally different pharmacological processes affecting different aspects of the asthma disease. The utilization of drugs having complementary effects on disease is found in other fields, such as in the treatment of hypertension. In the case of combination inhalers, the LABA provides bronchodilation of the airways, which is not achieved by the inhaled GCS. Even though GCS are very efficient anti-inflammatory drugs, the elimination or substantial reduction of inflammation is often insufficient to fully eliminate the tendency of the airways to narrow in patients with asthma, which is why bronchodilators add to symptom relief.

Secondly, combining a LABA with an inhaled GCS has been shown to increase the adherence to regular inhaled treatments in asthma, when measured by refills of prescriptions,[58] but also supported by clinical experience. When asthma patients are prescribed the inhaled GCS and the LABA in two separate inhalers, some individuals get confused, and it is not uncommon that they stop using the GCS inhaler but continue with the LABA only, which causes more obvious subjective symptom relief.[59] Such behaviour is potentially dangerous in asthma, as treatment with a LABA alone can hide the symptoms of an emerging asthma exacerbation.[46] Taking only a LABA, and no inhaled GCS, is also related to an increased risk of severe asthma events,[46] and is therefore never recommended. However, no evidence has been published to suggest that LABAs in a combination inhaler with GCS increase the risk of severe asthma attacks.[47] By contrast, it has been repeatedly shown that adding a LABA to a fixed dose of inhaled GCS reduces the frequency of both mild and severe exacerbations.[37]

Thirdly, the positive clinical interaction between inhaled GCS and LABAs to further reduce the frequency of asthma exacerbations is surprising from a molecular perspective. The finding that adding a LABA to an inhaled GCS improves lung function is logical, but when the exacerbation frequency is reduced, a clinical synergistic effect influencing the core process of the disease is implied. Over the last 10–15 years, extensive research has determined that β_2-agonists in general interact with GCS at the molecular level, primarily by enhancing the transport of GCS–receptor from the cytoplasm to the nucleus, resulting in more pronounced anti-inflammatory effects in a vast number of cell culture models[60, 61] and in humans.[62] The clinical consequence of this molecular effect is likely to be the observed reduction in exacerbations when LABAs are added to inhaled GCS.[37] Indeed, it is likely that this clinical effect is synergistic, as LABA treatment alone has no effect on exacerbation frequency, or sometimes even increases the risk of an exacerbation,[46, 63] whereas combining the LABA with an inhaled GCS reduces exacerbations.35,39 It could also be speculated that the interaction between the GCS and LABA is optimized when these two drugs are given by a single inhalation, rather than with two separate breaths from two different inhalers. Thus, during a single inhalation, it is likely that the two medications will deposit to the same regions of the lung, allowing for optimal molecular interaction. Thus, if the drugs are given by two different inhalers, the two drugs may deposit slightly differently, which would not favour the molecular interaction.[60, 61]

Fourthly, it has over recent years become clear that asthma is not one disease, but rather a syndrome encompassing a series of different disease entities, that still are vaguely described but may be present within clusters of phenotypes.[10, 63, 64] Indeed, it has been proposed that the subgroups of asthma should be identified as asthma endotypes, encompassing an endogenous molecular mechanism[10] but with different responses to treatment. It has also been shown that some asthma patients respond well to an inhaled GCS, whereas other patients have weak or no short-term responses to such therapy.[65] One possible advantage of using a combination inhaler in managing the 'undefined' patient with asthma could thus be that any type of asthma will respond to the therapy, and those individuals with an asthma endotype less responsive to inhaled GCS will still have a beneficial clinical effect. The same could be argued for a group seldom studied, which includes those with mixed asthma and COPD, or symptoms that overlap the two disorders. Again, COPD patients respond very weakly to inhaled GCS, but do respond significantly to inhaled LABAs.[52] Therefore, combination inhalers are more likely to show clinical efficacy in a larger proportion of patients, regardless of exact molecular mechanisms driving the disease, and regardless of whether the patients have some degree of mixed asthma and COPD.

7.7   Regular treatment alone versus additional formoterol-containing combinations as reliever therapy

The combination inhalers with inhaled GCS and LABAs have been studied and clinically implemented primarily as regular therapy, in most instances prescribed as one or two inhalations taken twice daily. This approach is well documented to reduce both exacerbations of asthma and COPD in clinical study settings, and to elicit all the other benefits of giving inhaled GCS and LABAs at the same time. It has also been recommended in guidelines.[5]

The two major LABAs that have been used to date, salmeterol and formoterol, both have a long duration of effect, with a majority of effects sustained for up to 16 h after inhalation, and even some measurable bronchodilation still observable at 24 h after a single inhalation.[66,67] However, half of the induced bronchodilation is gone after approximately 14–18 h after inhalation, which is why both of these drugs, from a practical and pharmacodynamic perspective, are useful primarily as twice-daily treatments.

Other pharmacological features of salmeterol and formoterol are, however, fundamentally different. Thus, it is well documented that formoterol has a more rapid onset of effect than salmeterol.[68] Indeed, formoterol has a similarly rapid onset of effect as salbutamol.[69] However, salmeterol has a clearly shorter onset of effect, taking 1–3 hours to achieve full bronchodilation.[68] This is one reason why formoterol has in some instances been approved for use as rescue medication.[70]

Another reason why formoterol can be used as rescue in asthma is because of its high pharmacological efficacy at the β_2-receptor. Thus, during severe bronchial smooth muscle contraction *in vitro*, addition of salmeterol to the tissue will result in some bronchodilation, but adding formoterol will lead to a greater relaxation. This ability to reverse severe bronchoconstriction to a greater extent has been documented also in humans, where formoterol shows a greater protective effect than salmeterol on methacholine responsiveness.[71] This would argue that formoterol could be used as rescue medication in acute asthma, which has been documented in several clinical studies.[72]

The rapid onset and high pharmacological efficacy of formoterol on bronchial smooth muscle would also allow the use of combination inhalers with formoterol and any inhaled GCS for immediate symptom relief. The combination of formoterol and budesonide developed by AstraZeneca in the Turbuhaler has been tested for such use.[73,74] With the designs utilized for clinical testing, the use of this combination both as regular morning and evening therapy, as well as reliever therapy, reduces the frequency of exacerbations of asthma.

From a conceptual viewpoint, the use of a combined rapid-onset LABA (currently formoterol) with an inhaled GCS at a time when a patient with asthma feels the need for reliever therapy, allows for an anti-inflammatory drug to be introduced to the lung at the very time of any insult causing symptoms of asthma. Indeed, some such insults may be proinflammatory, such as exposure to inhaled allergen, and receiving a booster dose of inhaled GCS to arrest the progression of the induced inflammation may give added benefit compared with taking only symptom-relieving bronchodilator therapy. Several studies have taken this approach in large cohorts of patients, and documented a further reduction in asthma exacerbation frequency during regular treatment with combination therapy.[75,76] The key study that has evaluated this approach, compared the frequency of asthma exacerbations with only regular combination therapy and a short-acting β_2-agonist (terbutaline) as reliever, or only formoterol as reliever, or the combination of formoterol and budesonide as reliever medication.[77] The results showed unequivocally that replacing terbutaline with formoterol as reliever reduced the frequency of asthma exacerbation when used during regular combined formoterol and budesonide treatment. The key finding was, however, that replacing the rescue medication with a combination of formoterol and budesonide further reduced the frequency of exacerbations, showing that adding a small dose of an inhaled glucocorticoid in a rescue medication benefits the patient.[75–77] Thus, time to first severe exacerbation was longer when formoterol plus budesonide was given as rescue compared to when formoterol was given. The reported rate of severe exacerbations was 37, 29 and 19 per 100 patients per year when the rescue medication used was terbutaline, formoterol or the combination of formoterol plus budesonide, respectively, and again all patients were treated with regular formoterol and budesonide given in the morning and the evening as baseline therapy. These findings are in line with a study where the combination of salbutamol and beclometasone was used as rescue medication in patients with very mild asthma, resulting in fewer exacerbations and a similar degree of reduction of exacerbations as regular beclometasone treatment, which led to a substantially higher overall dose of inhaled GCS.[78]

The combination of formoterol and budesonide for both maintenance and reliever therapy has been accepted by regulatory authorities in many countries, but not in the USA. However, the evidence is compelling that adding a small dose of glucocorticoid to a rescue β$_2$-agonist reduces the frequency of asthma exacerbations and increases overall control of asthma, and this may become more widely used in the long term. For the future, it is possible that new combinations, with formoterol as the bronchodilating component, and any other inhaled GCS, will also be used as maintenance and reliever therapy. Importantly, scientific evidence so far argues strongly that this therapy should be utilized in those having symptoms despite current therapy with combinations of inhaled GCS and LABAs.

7.8   Currently available combination inhalers

Salmeterol + fluticasone combinations

The combination of salmeterol and fluticasone propionate was the first combination of a LABA and an inhaled GCS for the treatment of asthma, and subsequently was approved also for the treatment of COPD. The market name for this product, developed by GlaxoSmithKline is Seretide (same product as Advair, Adoair and Viani). This combination product is available both as dry powder inhaler (Diskus inhaler) and as a spray inhaler (Evohaler), and the dose is one puff per treatment occasion with the dry powder inhaler, but two puffs per treatment occasion with the spray inhaler.[40] This combination maintains a stable dose of salmeterol (50 µg in Diskus and 25 µg in the Evohaler), but variable doses of fluticasone propionate (with doses of 100, 250 and 500 µg per dosing occasion). The combination of salmeterol and fluticasone is only recommended for twice-daily treatment[43] and cannot be used as rescue medication.

Formoterol + budesonide combinations

The combination of formoterol and budesonide became clinically available in the year 2000 for treating asthma,[39] and has subsequently been approved also for the treatment of COPD.[52] The market name for this product, developed by AstraZeneca, is Symbicort. This combination product is available both as a dry powder inhaler (Turbohaler inhaler) and as a spray inhaler (pMDI; pressurized metered dose inhaler). This combination also has a mixture of available doses, including formoterol/budesonide at 4.5/80 μg and 4.5/160 μg, as well as 9/320 μg respectively. Traditionally, the dose is one puff per treatment occasion with the dry powder inhaler, but two puffs per treatment occasion with the spray inhaler. The most common recommendation is to treat asthma patients with one dose morning and evening. In some markets this combination has also been approved for use as rescue medication in patients taking it regularly (see above), and has been approved in some countries as once-daily treatment for patients with milder asthma.[79]

Formoterol + beclometasone combinations

The combination of formoterol and beclometasone was launched a few years ago, and is marketed in an hydrofluoroalkane (HFA) pMDI, which delivers an extrafine aerosol fraction, known to reach the more distal airways to a greater extent. This combination was developed by Chiesi, and is sold by UCB as well as Chiesi in different markets, under the market name of Innovair or Fostair. This combination has been shown to provide efficacy equivalent to other inhaled GCS/LABA combinations, as measured by most asthma outcomes.[80] It is not clear scientifically whether the extra fine aerosol distribution leads to a greater efficacy in the peripheral airways that is clinically relevant. This combination has not been studied as a reliever therapy, despite its formoterol content, but the onset of action on bronchodilation is documented to be similar to that of formoterol given in combination with budesonide.[81]

Formoterol + mometasone combinations

The combination of mometasone and formoterol has been approved for treatment of asthma in the USA, but is currently not being pursued for registration in Europe.[82, 83] This combination, marketed as Dulera, has similar effects on lung function parameters and asthma exacerbation frequency as other combinations. Even though mometasone is documented to be an effective inhaled GCS when given once daily, the combination has only been documented for twice-daily treatment since formoterol has only a moderate effect persisting 24 h after inhalation of a single dose.[67] Studies show consistently that the combination of mometasone and formoterol is superior to mometasone alone in improving control of asthma symptoms, reducing night-time awakenings due to asthma, and reducing use of short-acting β_2-agonists, which is evident when patients uncontrolled on inhaled GCS alone are recruited.[82, 83]

7.9   Upcoming and alternative combinations of inhaled GCS and LABAs

A large number of new combinations of inhaled GCS and LABAs are in different phases of development, and many of these will surely reach the marketplace. In principle, there are two types of combinations that will be launched in the future, those containing currently available inhaled GCS and LABAs, and those with totally new compounds. Specifically, new LABAs that have bronchodilating efficacy measurable over 24 h are used for novel combinations, and are envisaged to be taken once daily. The new combinations using older compounds will primarily be used as twice-daily therapy.

Vilanterol trifenatate + fluticasone furoate

The new combination that is closest to market is probably the one combining fluticasone furoate (FF) with vilanterol trifenatate (VI). Vilanterol trifenatate is a LABA with a longer than 24-hour activity in humans, and is being developed to be used in combination with FF. According to experimental studies, VI is potent on the β_2-receptor, and in comparison with salmeterol it has a faster onset of action and clinically longer duration of effect.[84] Vilanterol trifenatate is also highly selective for the β_2-receptor, with over 1000-fold greater selectivity compared to β_1-receptors.[85] Fluticasone furoate is a GCS that has been shown in clinical studies also to be active for 24 hours.[86,87] Importantly, FF is not the same drug as fluticasone propionate (FP), even though they share part of the name, because the furoate salt changes the structure of the molecule, allowing extended binding to the GCS receptor.[86] According to reports, the combination of these drugs is being developed for the treatment of COPD as well as asthma, and the planned tradename is Relovair. Very few clinical data are available on the effect of this combination in patients with obstructive lung disease, but one study has reported the effect of regular treatment in patients with COPD. Over 2 weeks it was documented that patients with COPD observed improved lung function when this treatment was given once daily in the morning.[88] In lung function measures, there is no evidence that VI induces tolerance.[84] The combination of VI and FF will most likely be the first clinically available combination of a LABA and an inhaled GCS that can be used in a once-daily regimen.

Indacaterol + mometasone

It has been reported that studies are underway looking at the combination of indacaterol and mometasone – a once-daily LABA and a once-daily inhaled GCS, respectively. However, no data have been presented to suggest that the launch of such a combination for the treatment of asthma or COPD is imminent.

Formoterol + fluticasone propionate combinations

The combination of fluticasone propionate and formoterol (500/20 µg, given twice daily) has been documented to be at least as effective as fluticasone propionate and formoterol given in two separate inhalers with respect to FEV_1 and symptom control, and has been shown to produce greater improvement in lung function than fluticasone propionate alone.[89,90] Thus, adding formoterol to fluticasone propionate results in similar improvement in lung function as with other previously studied and registered combination products, and this combination has a similar safety and tolerability profile to the two separate components given in separate inhalers. The market name of this combination will be Flutiform, and it is administered with an aerosol delivery system. This combination will be given in a twice-daily regimen.

Formoterol + ciclesonide combination

It has been suggested that the potent and once-daily inhaled GCS ciclesonide can be combined with formoterol in one inhaler, and both patents and clinical trials have been filed, but no scientific data are available. Such a combination would likely be used in a twice-daily regimen, since formoterol is given on a twice-daily basis in most patients.

Out-of-patent drug combinations

The lack of patent protection of many potent inhaled GCS and effective LABAs will provide a new environment for asthmatic patients, with a vast portfolio of combination drugs becoming available in the marketplace in future. Copies of the first combinations of salmeterol with fluticasone propionate and formoterol with budesonide are also in the pipeline. Clearly, the inhalation devices may be different, as the patent protection of those technical products is much longer than the pharmaceuticals placed inside them.

7.10   Future of combined inhalation therapy in respiratory disease

The future combination therapies in asthma and COPD will have two diverse profiles. One will comprise combinations of drugs that have been on the market for many years, such as any combination of the inhaled GCS fluticasone propionate, budesonide or ciclesonide, and any of the two LABAs formoterol or salmeterol. Most new combinations are utilizing formoterol as the LABA component, possibly because it has a more rapid onset of effect, which allows for immediate bronchodilation when taken as rescue medication. What will be the added benefits of the complex mixtures of combination products that will be available for the treatment of both asthma and COPD? Clearly, more companies are getting involved in the field, and commercial competition may reduce the costs of these medications. However, the clinical efficacy and side-effect profiles are likely to be very similar to currently available combinations.

The other series of combinations will primarily be based on new drugs, giving the added benefit of once-daily treatment. These combinations, using a once-daily LABA such as indacaterol or vilanterol trifenatate, and once-daily inhaled GCS such as fluticasone furoate or mometasone, may provide different clinical profiles. These regimens may indeed give added clinical benefit for some patients with asthma or COPD, by the use of drugs with improved therapeutic ratio and longer duration of effect.

References

1. Beerman B, Boe J, Boye NP, et al. Farmakoterapi vid astma – rekommendationer från en expertgrupp [Pharmacotherapy in asthma – recommendations from an expert group]. Läkartidningen 1986;83:2385–8 [in Swedish].

2. British Thoracic Society and others. Guidelines for management of asthma in adults: I – chronic persistent asthma. Brit Med J 1990;301:651–3.

3. Andrén L, Beerman B, Benson L, et al. Farmakoterapi vid astma – rekommendationer från en expertgrupp [Pharmacotherapy in asthma – recommendations from an expert group]. Läkartidningen 1992;98:2608–11 [in Swedish].

4. Wennergren G, Kristjánsson S, Strannegård IL. Decrease in hospitalization for treatment of childhood asthma with increased use of antiinflammatory treatment, despite an increase in prevalence of asthma. J Allergy Clin Immunol 1996;97:742–8.

5. Bateman ED, Hurd SS, Barnes PJ, et al. Global strategy for asthma management and prevention: GINA executive summary. Eur Respir J 2008;31:143–78.

6. Bacharier LB, Boner A, Carlsen KH, et al. Diagnosis and treatment of asthma in childhood: a PRACTALL consensus report. Allergy 2008;63:5–34.

7. Rabe KF, Hurd S, Anzueto A, et al. Global strategy for the diagnosis, management, and prevention of chronic obstructive pulmonary disease: GOLD executive summary. Am J Respir Crit Care Med 2007;176:532–55.

8. Wenzel SE. Asthma: defining of the persistent adult phenotypes. Lancet 2006;368:804–13.

9. Han MK, Agusti A, Calverley PM, et al. Chronic obstructive pulmonary disease phenotypes: the future of COPD. Am J Respir Crit Care Med 2010;182:598–604.

10. Lötvall J, Akdis CA, Bacharier LB, et al. Asthma endotypes: A new approach to classification of disease entities within the asthma syndrome. J Allergy Clin Immunol 2011;127: 355–60.

11. Brown HM, Storey G, George WH. Beclomethasone dipropionate: a new steroid aerosol for the treatment of allergic asthma. Br Med J 1972;1:585–90.

12. Lal S, Harris DM, Bhalla KK, Singhal SN, Butler AG. Comparison of beclomethasone dipropionate aerosol and prednisolone in reversible airways obstruction. Br Med J 1972;3: 314–7.

13. Godfrey S, König P. Beclomethasone aerosol in childhood asthma. Arch Dis Child 1973;48:665–70.

14. Toogood JH, Baskerville JC, Jennings B, Lefcoe NM, Johansson SA. Influence of dosing frequency and schedule on the response of chronic asthmatics to the aerosol steroid, budesonide. J Allergy Clin Immunol 1982;70:288–98.

15. Ernst P, Spitzer WO, Suissa S, et al. Risk of fatal and near-fatal asthma in relation to inhaled corticosteroid use. JAMA 1992;268:3462–4.

16. Ishihara K, Hasegawa T, Okazaki M, et al. Long-term follow-up of patients with a history of near fatal episodes; can inhaled corticosteroids reduce the risk of death from asthma? Intern Med 1995;34:77–80.

17. Dahl R, Lundback B, Malo JL, et al. A dose-ranging study of fluticasone propionate in adult patients with moderate asthma. International Study Group. Chest 1993;104:1352–8.

18. Busse WW, Chervinsky P, Condemi J, et al. Budesonide delivered by Turbuhaler is effective in a dose-dependent fashion when used in the treatment of adult patients with chronic asthma. J Allergy Clin Immunol 1998;101:457–63.

19. O'Byrne PM, Pedersen S. Measuring efficacy and safety of different inhaled corticosteroid preparations. J Allergy Clin Immunol 1998;102:879–86.

20. Grove A, Allam C, McFarlane LC, McPhate G, Jackson CM, Lipworth BJ. A comparison of the systemic bioactivity of inhaled budesonide and fluticasone propionate in normal subjects. Br J Clin Pharmacol 1994;38:527–32.
21. Engel T, Dirksen A, Heinig JH, Nielsen NH, Weeke B, Johansson SA. Single-dose inhaled budesonide in subjects with chronic asthma. Allergy 1991;46:547–53.
22. Juniper EF, Kline PA, Vanzieleghem MA, Ramsdale EH, O'Byrne PM, Hargreave FE. Long-term effects of budesonide on airway responsiveness and clinical asthma severity in inhaled steroid-dependent asthmatics. Eur Respir J 1990;3:1122–7.
23. Kelly HW. Comparison of inhaled corticosteroids. Ann Pharmacother 1998;32:220–32.
24. Postma DS, Sevette C, Martinat Y, Schlösser N, Aumann J, Kafé H. Treatment of asthma by the inhaled corticosteroid ciclesonide given either in the morning or evening. Eur Respir J 2001;17:1083–8.
25. Larsen BB, Nielsen LP, Engelstätter R, Steinijans V, Dahl R. Effect of ciclesonide on allergen challenge in subjects with bronchial asthma. Allergy 2003;58:207–12.
26. Bernstein DI, Berkowitz RB, Chervinsky P, et al. Dose-ranging study of a new steroid for asthma: mometasone furoate dry powder inhaler. Respir Med 1999;93:603–12.
27. Kaiser HB, Naclerio RM, Given J, Toler TN, Ellsworth A, Philpot EE. Fluticasone furoate nasal spray: a single treatment option for the symptoms of seasonal allergic rhinitis. J Allergy Clin Immunol 2007;119:1430–7.
28. Tayab ZR, Fardon TC, Lee DK, et al. Pharmacokinetic/pharmacodynamic evaluation of urinary cortisol suppression after inhalation of fluticasone propionate and mometasone furoate. Br J Clin Pharmacol 2007;64:698–705.
29. Lee DK, Fardon TC, Bates CE, Haggart K, McFarlane LC, Lipworth BJ. Airway and systemic effects of hydrofluoroalkane formulations of high-dose ciclesonide and fluticasone in moderate persistent asthma. Chest 2005;127:851–60.
30. Weatherall M, James K, Clay J, et al. Dose-response relationship for risk of non-vertebral fracture with inhaled corticosteroids. Clin Exp Allergy 2008;38:1451–8.
31. Ishizuka T, Hisada T, Aoki H, et al. Gender and age risks for hoarseness and dysphonia with use of a dry powder fluticasone propionate inhaler in asthma. Allergy Asthma Proc 2007;28:550–6.
32. O'Connor RD, Stanford R, Crim C, et al. Effect of fluticasone propionate and salmeterol in a single device, fluticasone propionate, and montelukast on overall asthma control, exacerbations, and costs. Ann Allergy Asthma Immunol 2004;93:581–8.
33. Zeiger RS, Bird SR, Kaplan MS, et al. Short-term and long-term asthma control in patients with mild persistent asthma receiving montelukast or fluticasone: a randomized controlled trial. Am J Med 2005;118:649–57.
34. Greening AP, Ind PW, Northfield M, Shaw G, Allen & Hanburys Limited UK Study Group. Added salmeterol versus higher-dose corticosteroid in asthma patients with symptoms on existing inhaled corticosteroid. Lancet 1994;344:219–24.
35. Pauwels RA, Löfdahl CG, Postma DS, et al. Effect of inhaled formoterol and budesonide on exacerbations of asthma. Formoterol and Corticosteroids Establishing Therapy (FACET) International Study Group. N Engl J Med 1997;337:1405–11.
36. Taylor DR, Sears MR, Herbison GP, et al. Regular inhaled beta agonist in asthma: effects on exacerbations and lung function. Thorax 1993;48:134–8.
37. Sears MR, Taylor DR. Bronchodilator treatment in asthma. Increase in deaths during salmeterol treatment unexplained. Brit Med J 1993;306:1610–11.
38. Palmqvist M, Arvidsson P, Beckman O, Peterson S, Lötvall J. Onset of bronchodilation of budesonide/formoterol vs. salmeterol/fluticasone in single inhalers. Pulm Pharmacol Ther 2001;14:29–34.

39. Zetterström O, Buhl R, Mellem H, et al. Improved asthma control with budesonide/formoterol in a single inhaler, compared with budesonide alone. Eur Respir J 2001;18:262–8.

40. Chapman KR, Ringdal N, Backer V, Palmqvist M, Saarelainen S, Briggs M. Salmeterol and fluticasone propionate (50/250 microg) administered via combination Diskus inhaler: as effective as when given via separate Diskus inhalers. Can Respir J 1999;6:45–51.

41. Reddel HK, Taylor DR, Bateman ED, et al. An official American Thoracic Society/European Respiratory Society statement: asthma control and exacerbations: standardizing endpoints for clinical asthma trials and clinical practice. Am J Respir Crit Care Med 2009;180:59–9.

42. Juniper EF, Guyatt GH, Epstein RS, Ferrie PJ, Jaeschke R, Hiller TK. Evaluation of impairment of health related quality of life in asthma: development of a questionnaire for use in clinical trials. Thorax 1992;47:76–83.

43. Bateman ED, Boushey HA, Bousquet J, et al. Can guideline-defined asthma control be achieved? The Gaining Optimal Asthma ControL study. Am J Respir Crit Care Med 2004;170:836–44.

44. Meltzer EO, Busse WW, Wenzel SE, et al. Use of the Asthma Control Questionnaire to predict future risk of asthma exacerbation. J Allergy Clin Immunol 2011;127:167–72.

45. Mcivor RA, Pizzichini E, Turner MO, Hussack P, Hargreave FE, Sears MR. Potential masking effects of salmeterol on airway inflammation in asthma. Am J Respir Crit Care Med 1998;158:924–30.

46. Nelson HS, Weiss ST, Bleecker ER, Yancey SW, Dorinsky PM; SMART Study Group. The Salmeterol Multicenter Asthma Research Trial: a comparison of usual pharmacotherapy for asthma or usual pharmacotherapy plus salmeterol. Chest 2006;129:15–26.

47. Weatherall M, Wijesinghe M, Perrin K, Harwood M, Beasley R. Meta-analysis of the risk of mortality with salmeterol and the effect of concomitant inhaled corticosteroid therapy. Thorax 2010;65:39–43.

48. Boorsma M, Lutter R, van de Pol MA, Out TA, Jansen HM, Jonkers RE. Long-term effects of budesonide on inflammatory status in COPD. COPD 2008;5:97–104.

49. Jenkins CR, Jones PW, Calverley PM, et al. Efficacy of salmeterol/fluticasone propionate by GOLD stage of chronic obstructive pulmonary disease: analysis from the randomised, placebo-controlled TORCH study. Respir Res 2009;10:59.

50. Calverley PM, Anderson JA, Celli B, et al. Salmeterol and fluticasone propionate and survival in chronic obstructive pulmonary disease. N Engl J Med 2007;356:775–89.

51. Crim C, Calverley PM, Anderson JA, et al. Pneumonia risk in COPD patients receiving inhaled corticosteroids alone or in combination: TORCH study results. Eur Respir J 2009;34:641–7.

52. Calverley PM, Boonsawat W, Cseke Z, Zhong N, Peterson S, Olsson H. Maintenance therapy with budesonide and formoterol in chronic obstructive pulmonary disease. Eur Respir J 2003; 22:912.

53. Celli BR, Thomas NE, Anderson JA, et al. Effect of pharmacotherapy on rate of decline of lung function in chronic obstructive pulmonary disease: results from the TORCH study. Am J Respir Crit Care Med 2008;178:332.

54. Brouillard C, Pepin V, Milot J, Lacasse Y, Maltais F. Endurance shuttle walking test: responsiveness to salmeterol in COPD. Eur Respir J 2008;31:579–84.

55. Berton DC, Reis M, Siqueira AC, et al. Effects of tiotropium and formoterol on dynamic hyperinflation and exercise endurance in COPD. Respir Med 2010;104:1288–9.

56. Ullman A, Svedmyr N. Salmeterol, a new long acting inhaled beta 2 adrenoceptor agonist: comparison with salbutamol in adult asthmatic patients. Thorax 1988;43:674–8.

57. Gauvreau GM, Doctor J, Watson RM, Jordana M, O'Byrne PM. Effects of inhaled budesonide on allergen-induced airway responses and airway inflammation. Am J Respir Crit Care Med 1996;154:1267–71.

58. Stoloff SW, Stempel DA, Meyer J, Stanford RH, Carranza Rosenzweig JR. Improved refill persistence with fluticasone propionate and salmeterol in a single inhaler compared with other controller therapies. J Allergy Clin Immunol 2004;113:245–51.

59. Jonkers RE, Bantje TA, Aalbers R. Onset of relief of dyspnoea with budesonide/formoterol or salbutamol following methacholine-induced severe bronchoconstriction in adults with asthma: a double-blind, placebo-controlled study. Respir Res 2006;7:141.

60. Eickelberg O, Roth M, Lörx R, et al. Ligand-independent activation of the glucocorticoid receptor by beta2-adrenergic receptor agonists in primary human lung fibroblasts and vascular smooth muscle cells. J Biol Chem 1999;274:1005–10.

61. Nie M, Corbett L, Knox AJ, Pang L. Differential regulation of chemokine expression by peroxisome proliferator-activated receptor gamma agonists: interactions with glucocorticoids and beta2-agonists. J Biol Chem 2005;280:2550–61.

62. Usmani OS, Ito K, Maneechotesuwan K, et al. Glucocorticoid receptor nuclear translocation in airway cells after inhaled combination therapy. Am J Respir Crit Care Med 2005;172:704–12.

63. Lazarus SC, Boushey HA, Fahy JV, et al. Long-acting beta2-agonist monotherapy vs continued therapy with inhaled corticosteroids in patients with persistent asthma: a randomized controlled trial. JAMA 2001;285:2583–93.

64. Haldar P, Pavord ID, Shaw DE, et al. Cluster analysis and clinical asthma phenotypes. Am J Respir Crit Care Med 2008;178:218–24.

65. Berry M, Morgan A, Shaw DE, et al. Pathological features and inhaled corticosteroid response of eosinophilic and non-eosinophilic asthma. Thorax 2007;62:1043–9.

66. Rabe KF, Jörres R, Nowak D, Behr N, Magnussen H. Comparison of the effects of salmeterol and formoterol on airway tone and responsiveness over 24 hours in bronchial asthma. Am Rev Respir Dis 1993;147:1436–41.

67. Lötvall J, Langley S, Woodcock A. Inhaled steroid/long-acting beta 2 agonist combination products provide 24 hours improvement in lung function in adult asthmatic patients. Respir Res 2006;7:110.

68. Palmqvist M, Persson G, Lazer L, Rosenborg J, Larsson P, Lötvall J. Inhaled dry-powder formoterol and salmeterol in asthmatic patients: onset of action, duration of effect and potency. Eur Respir J 1997;10:2484–9.

69. Seberová E, Andersson A. Oxis (formoterol given by Turbuhaler) showed as rapid an onset of action as salbutamol given by a pMDI. Respir Med 2000;94:607–11.

70. Pauwels RA, Sears MR, Campbell M, et al. Formoterol as relief medication in asthma: a worldwide safety and effectiveness trial. Eur Respir J 2003;22:787–94.

71. Palmqvist M, Ibsen T, Mellén A, Lötvall J. Comparison of the relative efficacy of formoterol and salmeterol in asthmatic patients. Am J Respir Crit Care Med 1999;160:244–9.

72. Najafizadeh K, Sohrab Pour H, Ghadyanee M, Shiehmorteza M, Jamali M, Majdzadeh S. A randomised, double-blind, placebo-controlled study to evaluate the role of formoterol in the management of acute asthma. Emerg Med J 2007;24:317–21.

73. O'Byrne PM, Bisgaard H, Godard PP, et al. Budesonide/formoterol combination therapy as both maintenance and reliever medication in asthma. Am J Respir Crit Care Med 2005;171:129–36.

74. Barnes PJ. Scientific rationale for using a single inhaler for asthma control. Eur Respir J 2007;29:587–95.

75. Kuna P, Peters MJ, Manjra AI, et al. Effect of budesonide/formoterol maintenance and reliever therapy on asthma exacerbations. Int J Clin Pract 2007;61:725–36.

76. Aubier M, Buhl R, Ekström T, et al. Comparison of two twice-daily doses of budesonide/formoterol maintenance and reliever therapy. Eur Respir J 2010;36:524–30.

77. Rabe KF, Atienza T, Magyar P, Larsson P, Jorup C, Lalloo UG. Effect of budesonide in com-
    bination with formoterol for reliever therapy in asthma exacerbations: a randomised controlled,
    double-blind study. Lancet 2006;368:744–53.
78. Papi A, Canonica GW, Maestrelli P, et al. Rescue use of beclomethasone and albuterol in a single
    inhaler for mild asthma. N Engl J Med 2007;356:2040–52.
79. Kuna P, Creemers JP, Vondra V, et al. Once-daily dosing with budesonide/formoterol com-
    pared with twice-daily budesonide/formoterol and once-daily budesonide in adults with mild to
    moderate asthma. Respir Med 2006;100:2151–9.
80. Papi A, Paggiaro PL, Nicolini G, Vignola AM, Fabbri LM; Inhaled Combination Asthma Treat-
    ment versus SYmbicort (ICAT SY) Study Group. Beclomethasone/formoterol versus budes-
    onide/formoterol combination therapy in asthma. Eur Respir J 2007;29:682–9.
81. Cazzola M, Pasqua F, Ferri L, Biscione G, Cardaci V, Matera MG. Rapid onset of bronchodilation
    with formoterol/beclomethasone Modulite and formoterol/budesonide Turbuhaler as compared
    to formoterol alone in patients with COPD. Pulm Pharmacol Ther 2011;24:118–22.
82. Nathan RA, Nolte H, Pearlman DS; P04334 Study Investigators. Twenty-six-week efficacy and
    safety study of mometasone furoate/formoterol 200/10 microg combination treatment in pa-
    tients with persistent asthma previously receiving medium-dose inhaled corticosteroids. Allergy
    Asthma Proc 2010;31:269–79.
83. Weinstein SF, Corren J, Murphy K, Nolte H, White M; Study Investigators of P04431. Twelve-
    week efficacy and safety study of mometasone furoate/formoterol 200/10 microg and 400/10
    microg combination treatments in patients with persistent asthma previously receiving high-dose
    inhaled corticosteroids. Allergy Asthma Proc 2010;31:280–9.
84. Lötvall J, Bateman ED, Bleecker ER, et al. Dose-related efficacy of vilanterol trifenatate (VI),
    a long-acting beta2 agonist (LABA) with inherent 24-hour activity, in patients with persistent
    asthma. *ERS Congress 2010 Barcelona*, 5554, online http://dev.ersnet.org/uploads/Document/
    29/WEB_CHEMIN_5358_1258548454.pdf.
85. Procopiou PA, Barrett VJ, Bevan NJ, et al. Synthesis and structure-activity relationships of
    long-acting beta2 adrenergic receptor agonists incorporating metabolic inactivation: an antedrug
    approach. J Med Chem 2010;53:4522–30.
86. To Y, Adcock I, Johnson M, Barnes PJ. Fluticasone furoate (FF): Prolonged duration of ac-
    tion compared with other ICS. *ERS Congress 2010 Barcelona, P1242*, online http://dev.ersnet.
    org/uploads/Document/29/WEB_CHEMIN_5358_1258548454.pdf.
87. Busse WW, Bleecker E, Bateman E, et al. Fluticasone furoate (FF), an inhaled corticosteroid
    (ICS), demonstrates efficacy in asthma patients symptomatic on moderate doses of ICS ther-
    apy. *ERS Congress 2010 Barcelona, P1168*, online http://dev.ersnet.org/uploads/Document/
    29/WEB_CHEMIN_5358_1258548454.pdf.
88. Lötvall J, Bakke P, Bjermer L, et al. Safety and efficacy of fluticasone furoate/vilanterol trifenatate
    (FFVI) in COPD patients. *ERS Congress 2010 Barcelona*, 5556, online http://dev.ersnet.org/
    uploads/Document/29/WEB_CHEMIN_5358_1258548454.pdf.
89. Bodzenta-Lukaszyk A, Pulka G, Dymek A, Mansikka H. Fluticasone propionate/formoterol
    fumarate combination therapy has an efficacy and safety profile similar to that of its individ-
    ual components administered concurrently in the treatment of asthma. *ERS Congress 2010
    Barcelona, P1207*, online http://dev.ersnet.org/uploads/Document/29/WEB_CHEMIN_5358_
    1258548454.pdf.
90. Bumbacea D, Pulka G, Dymek A, Mansikka H. Fluticasone propionate/formoterol fumarate
    combination therapy is more effective than fluticasone propionate alone in the treatment of
    asthma. *ERS Congress 2010 Barcelona, P1208*, online http://dev.ersnet.org/uploads/Document/
    29/WEB_CHEMIN_5358_1258548454.pdf.

8

Novel anti-inflammatory treatments for asthma and COPD

Paul A. Kirkham[*], **Gaetano Caramori**[†],
K. Fan Chung[*] **and Ian M. Adcock**[*]

[*]*Airways Disease Section, National Heart and Lung Institute, Imperial College London; and MRC-Asthma UK Centre for Allergic Mechanisms in Asthma, UK*
[†]*Section of Respiratory Diseases, University of Ferrara, Ferrara, Italy*

8.1   Introduction

Asthma is one of the most common chronic inflammatory diseases, with a worldwide incidence of $\sim$300 million; this is predicted to rise by an additional 100 million, mainly in children, over the next 15–20 years.[1] Chronic obstructive pulmonary disease (COPD) is the fourth commonest cause of death worldwide,[2] and presents a major but neglected global healthcare problem,[3,4] which is associated predominantly with lower socioeconomic groups.[5] Asthma and COPD have profound direct healthcare costs in terms of emergency room visits and hospitalizations and also have enormous indirect costs, and together are one of the leading causes of work and school absenteeism.[6] Most patients with asthma respond well to current therapies; however, a small percentage (5–10%) have severe disease that often fails to respond to conventional therapy, and these patients account for more than 50% of the total asthma healthcare costs.[7] The limited efficacy of current therapies for COPD indicates a pressing need to develop new treatments to prevent the progression of the disease, which results in a large consumption of healthcare resources.[4]

Asthma and COPD are chronic inflammatory diseases of the lower airways

Asthma is a chronic inflammatory disorder of the airways in which many cells and elements play a role. The chronic inflammation is associated with increased airway hyperresponsiveness leading to recurrent episodes of wheezing, breathlessness, chest tightness and coughing, particularly at night or in the early morning. These episodes are usually associated with widespread but variable airflow obstruction that is often

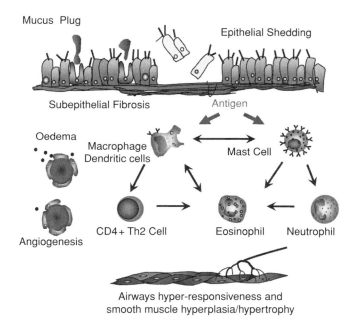

Figure 8.1 Even before asthma becomes symptomatic, exposure to an allergen produces structural changes to the airways, including subepithelial fibrosis and epithelial denudation. Inhaled allergens encounter antigen-presenting cells (dendritic cells, macrophages) that line the airways, and mast cells, which release mediators such as histamine. The antigen-presenting cells migrate to the lymph nodes, where they induce the proliferation and activation of CD4[+] T-lymphocytes (Th2 cells). These express a variety of cytokines and chemokines, under the control of intracellular kinases and down-stream transcription factors, which lead to the differentiation, migration and pathobiological effects of eosinophils. These inflammatory processes lead to pathological effects, such as airway hyper-responsiveness and airway remodelling including vasodilation and angiogenesis. Neutrophils are increasingly important in severe asthma.

reversible either spontaneously or with treatment.[8] The chronic airway inflammation of asthma is unique in that the airway wall is infiltrated by T-lymphocytes of the T-helper type 2 phenotype (Th2), eosinophils, macrophages/monocytes and mast cells[9, 10] (Figure 8.1). In addition, an 'acute-on-chronic' inflammation may be observed during exacerbations, with an increase in eosinophils and sometimes neutrophils.[9, 10]

Chronic obstructive pulmonary disease is a preventable and treatable disease with some significant extrapulmonary effects that may contribute to the severity in individual patients. Its pulmonary component is characterized by airflow limitation that is not fully reversible. The airflow limitation is usually progressive and associated with an abnormal inflammatory response of the lung to noxious particles or gases.[11] The main cause of COPD is cigarette smoking.[4] The pathological hallmarks of COPD are destruction of the lung parenchyma, which characterizes pulmonary emphysema, inflammation of the peripheral airways, which characterizes respiratory bronchiolitis, and inflammation of the central airways.[12] Airflow obstruction in COPD is caused by small (peripheral) airway lesions.[13] Most patients with COPD have all three pathological conditions (chronic obstructive bronchiolitis, emphysema and mucus plugging), but the relative extent of emphysema and obstructive bronchitis within individual patients can vary widely. Pathological studies show that inflammation in COPD occurs in the central and peripheral airways (bronchioles) and lung parenchyma.[14]

There is a marked increase in macrophages and neutrophils in bronchoalveolar lavage (BAL) and induced sputum. Patients with COPD have infiltration of T-cells (with an increased proportion of CD8+ relative to CD4+ T-cells) and macrophages and an increased number of neutrophils within the bronchial mucosa and lung parenchyma.[12, 14] The bronchioles are obstructed by fibrosis and mucus plugging and infiltrated predominantly by macrophages and T-lymphocytes.[13] In contrast to the situation with asthma, eosinophils are not prominent except in patients with concomitant asthma or in some patients during viral-induced exacerbations.[13, 15]

The pattern of pulmonary inflammation in COPD is specific, predominantly affects the small airways and lung parenchyma, and increases in intensity with the disease severity[13] (Figure 8.2). For example, alveolar macrophages are increased 25-fold in

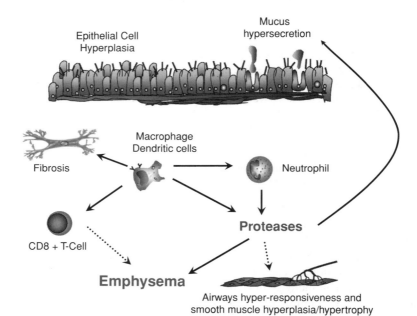

Figure 8.2 COPD is mainly related to cigarette smoking. The cigarette smoke activates macrophages and airway epithelial cells. Dendritic cells also play an important role in the pulmonary response to toxic particles in the smoke. Once activated, these cells release mediators that recruit and activate CD8+ T-lymphocytes (CD8+ T-cells) and neutrophils. The inflammatory process also mediates fibrosis through the proliferation of fibroblasts, an effect that eventually leads to obstructive bronchiolitis. Macrophages and neutrophils release proteases that break down connective tissue, producing emphysema and stimulating mucus hypersecretion. Although the role of CD8+ T-cells in the pathophysiology of COPD is not yet clear, it is thought that they contribute to the development of emphysema.

COPD patients compared to smokers with normal lung function,[16] are localized to sites of alveolar destruction and are activated. It is proposed that the inflammatory response in the small airways and lung parenchyma may underlie the accelerated loss of lung function that is characteristic of COPD.[17]

Thus, the specific characteristics of the inflammatory response and the site of inflammation differ between asthma and COPD but both involve the recruitment and activation of inflammatory cells and changes in the structural cells of the lung. Asthma and COPD are characterized by an increased expression of components of the inflammatory cascade including cytokines, chemokines, growth factors, enzymes, receptors and adhesion molecules. The increased expression of these proteins seen in asthma and COPD is the result of enhanced gene transcription since many of the genes are not expressed in normal cells but are induced in a cell-specific manner during the inflammatory process.

By understanding the different types of airway inflammation in various subtypes of asthma and COPD it should be possible to address some of the important questions in the area, such as:

1. What triggers/factors underlie airway smooth muscle hyperresponsiveness?
2. What are the processes (genetic/environmental) underlying different subtypes of asthma and COPD?
3. Which aspects of airway remodelling are important in disease subtypes?
4. What are the best biomarkers of disease progression and/or treatment response?
5. Why are some patients less responsive to conventional therapies?

For example, it is now recognized that there are distinct asthma phenotypes,[18] and that distinct therapeutic approaches may only impinge upon some aspects of the disease process, or at least outcome measures, within each subgroup. Thus, treatments may affect exacerbation rates without altering day-to-day symptoms or lung function. This reflects the fact that distinct cells/mediators in the lung could drive airway hyperresponsiveness and/or specific inflammatory components and that treatments directed at a single cell/mediator may only affect a single aspect of disease.[19] Although the diagnosis, the assessment of severity, and the monitoring of COPD still rely on lung function tests, there is an increasing interest in characterizing the type and intensity of lower airways inflammation, and to investigate whether this provides useful information for the management of this disease. For example, what were considered in the 1990s as COPD patients with a significant reversibility after a course of glucocorticoids and having the pathological characteristics of asthma, with an increased number of eosinophil granulocytes in their bronchial mucosa,[20] would not be considered as having COPD under present guidelines. The current reductionist approach to understanding the disease has led to the development of drugs targeting specific pathways or mediators. In future, we may need to target and assess several outcome measures and biomarkers simultaneously, and perform subgroup analyses of the responses obtained when evaluating combinations of new drugs.

8.2   Current asthma and COPD therapies

Asthma

Initial approaches to treating asthma emphasized the relief of bronchoconstriction with bronchodilators, particularly β_2-adrenergic agonists, but the discovery of airway inflammation as an important pathophysiological component of asthma has led to the use of inhaled corticosteroids (ICS) as the mainstay of asthma therapy.[21] Asthmatic inflammation is characterized by eosinophilia, mast cell infiltration and activation of T-helper 2 (Th2)-cells that express interleukin-4 (IL-4), IL-5 and IL-13, which are exquisitely sensitive to ICS. Structural changes such as goblet cell hyperplasia, airway smooth muscle hypertrophy and hyperplasia along with subepithelial fibrosis are also present, even in mild disease, although these features may be more prominent in severe disease (Figure 8.1). The functional effects of these structural changes are unclear, but they may contribute to chronic airflow obstruction and reduced airway responses to bronchodilators and/or ICS.[22]

Long-term treatment with ICS reverses airflow obstruction, reduces exacerbations and the need for hospitalization, and improves quality of life. ICS may have also contributed to the reduction in asthma deaths over recent years.[23] Concerns about the long-term detrimental effects of high-dose ICS therapy include cataracts, osteoporosis in elderly patients and stunting of growth in children,[24] but for the majority of patients on low/moderate doses of ICS, there is a high safety margin. However, ICS may not modify the progression of asthma and are not curative since asthma symptoms and inflammation recur on discontinuation of treatment.[25]

There is now evidence that long-acting β_2-agonists, in contrast with glucocorticoids, inhibit neutrophilic inflammation in the airways. In a study of patients with mild asthma, salmeterol for 6 weeks significantly reduced neutrophils in the airway mucosa and in BAL, whereas an inhaled glucocorticoid, fluticasone, was ineffective.[26] In this study, salmeterol, but not placebo or fluticasone, was associated with a reduction in symptom-free days and nights and a reduction in airway hyperresponsiveness, but it is unknown whether this is a result of the bronchodilator action of the long-acting β_2-agonist or the reduction in airway neutrophils. In patients with mild asthma who had an elevated induced sputum neutrophil count in, treatment with inhaled formoterol (24 μg twice a day) for 4 weeks caused a significant reduction in neutrophilia without any effect on eosinophil counts, whereas a high dose of inhaled glucocorticoids (budesonide 400 μg twice a day) had the reverse effect with a reduction in eosinophils but no effect on neutrophils.[27] The reduction in neutrophils by formoterol was associated with a reduction of sputum CXCL8 (IL-8) concentrations, a major neutrophilic chemoattractant, which were unaffected by the inhaled glucocorticoid.

The effectiveness of ICS, particularly at low/moderate doses, in controlling asthma and reducing exacerbations is improved by combination with long-acting β_2-agonists (LABAs) and is better than that shown by higher doses of ICS alone.[28] This has led to the use of ICS and LABA combination therapies in the treatment of moderate-to-severe asthma,[28] and has now become established as the most efficacious treatment.[1] Due to the rapid action of formoterol compared to salmeterol it is also possible to use the combination of formoterol/budesonide or formoterol/beclometasone as both maintenance and reliever medication. An alternative approach to asthma control has been taken with the salmeterol/fluticasone combination where the GOAL study showed that comprehensive asthma control could be achieved in the majority of patients.[29] It must be emphasized that LABAs are not recommended as a monotherapy maintenance treatment of asthma.

COPD

In contrast to asthma, long-acting inhaled β_2-agonists are minimally useful in the regular treatment of stable COPD.[30] In addition to prolonged bronchodilation, long-acting inhaled β_2-agonists exert other effects *in vitro* that may be of clinical relevance. These include inhibition of airway smooth muscle cell proliferation and inflammatory mediator release, as well as non-smooth-muscle effects, such as stimulation of mucociliary transport, reduction of the bronchial epithelial damage caused by bacterial products, and attenuation of neutrophil recruitment and activation.[31] Airway biopsy studies are required to evaluate whether long-acting inhaled β_2-agonists have a significant *in vivo* anti-inflammatory activity in COPD patients in addition to their known bronchodilator properties. Several clinical trials showed that long-acting inhaled β_2-agonists are indeed effective as symptomatic treatment in COPD, with significant decreases in dyspnoea and improved quality of life.[30,32–34] Most of these trials have been conducted with salmeterol and only a few with formoterol.[35,36] More recently, the TORCH (TOwards a Revolution in COPD Health) study[37] has shown that 3 years' treatment with salmeterol compared to placebo improved lung function – post-bronchodilator forced expiratory volume in one second (FEV_1) – symptoms and exacerbation rate but had no significant effect on quality of life and mortality.

Several large controlled clinical trials of combination therapy in stable COPD have shown that combination therapy is well tolerated and produces a modest, but statistically significant, improvement in number of severe exacerbations, FEV_1, quality of life and respiratory symptoms in stable COPD patients, with no greater risk of side effects (bruising or clinically significant falls in serum cortisol) than that with use of either component alone.[38–40]

The TORCH study showed a 17% relative reduction in mortality over 3 years for patients receiving salmeterol/fluticasone although this just failed to reach significance.[37] In addition, the patients on combination therapy had a significant improvement in exacerbation rate (but not on the number of hospitalizations), lung function and health status compared to either monotherapy. Importantly, this long-term study in elderly COPD patients did not show any effect of salmeterol on heart disease mortality, which has been a concern in asthmatics.[41,42] It is likely, therefore, that this effect of the salmeterol/fluticasone combination is a class effect rather than a specific drug combination effect, although this needs to be confirmed.

Treatment with salmeterol/fluticasone also has anti-inflammatory effects on sputum and bronchial biopsies from both current and former smokers with COPD, and this may contribute to its clinical efficacy. Thus, salmeterol/fluticasone reduces sputum differential (but not total) cell counts; sputum neutrophils and eosinophils; bronchial $CD45^+$, $CD8^+$ and $CD4^+$ cells; and cells expressing the mRNA for tumor necrosis factor-α (TNF-α) and interferon-γ (IFN-γ). These anti-inflammatory effects were accompanied by improvements in pre-bronchodilator FEV_1.[43]

Anticholinergics and COPD

Bronchodilators are the mainstay of current drug therapy for COPD.[4] Bronchodilators only give a small increase in FEV_1 in patients with COPD, but these drugs may improve symptoms by reducing hyperinflation and thus dyspnoea, and they may improve exercise tolerance.[4, 44] COPD appears to be more effectively treated by anticholinergic drugs than by β_2-agonists as monotherapies. This is in sharp contrast to asthma, for which β_2-agonists are more effective.[44] Tiotropium has prolonged and selective antagonism at the muscarinic receptor subtype 3 (M_3). Importantly, tiotropium decreases the number of hospital admissions for severe COPD exacerbations, suggesting the presence of non-bronchodilating effects.[45, 46] Recent studies have demonstrated that acetylcholine is produced both in cholinergic nerves and non-neuronal cells in the lower airways. These cells include bronchial epithelial cells, endothelial cells, smooth muscle, lymphocytes and macrophages, configuring a true extraneuronal airway cholinergic system.[47] This suggests the possibility that anticholinergic drugs might have inhibitory effects on inflammatory cells and that this may account for the 25% reduction in exacerbations of COPD seen in long-term studies with tiotropium.[48]

There is clear evidence for the additive effects of inhaled short-acting anticholinergics with inhaled short-acting β_2-agonists, leading to the introduction of combination inhalers. There is also emerging evidence that LABAs and tiotropium may also have additive effects. Thus, Tashkin and colleagues reported the preliminary results of a large controlled clinical trial (Understanding Potential Long-term Impacts on Function with Tiotropium: UPLIFT) investigating the long-term (4 years) effect of tiotropium on COPD mortality and FEV_1 decline. The majority of patients with moderate-to-very-severe disease demonstrate meaningful increases in lung function following administration of tiotropium when used in combination with formoterol.[49] A once-daily inhaler with a once-daily LABA and anticholinergic would, therefore, be ideal. The potential steroid-sparing activity of tiotropium alone or in combination (with LABAs and/or low-dose theophylline) in asthma and COPD deserves to be investigated in controlled clinical trials, some of which are already underway.

8.3   The need for new therapies

Asthma

In most ($\sim$90%), but not all, asthmatics ICS/LABA combination therapy is effective.[50] However, even existing patients who are apparently 'well controlled' by existing therapies may benefit from more efficacious therapies to which such patients are more compliant.[25] Telephone surveys of asthmatics have surprisingly reported a high degree of morbidity among asthmatics who reported that their asthma was well controlled.[25] This may reflect either a lack of compliance or that existing medications are not as efficacious in day-to-day practice as in controlled trial situations. Improved compliance in the mild-to-moderate asthmatic may be achieved by developing safe oral versions of conventional treatments or of new, more efficacious treatments than those currently available, particularly if these agents alter the course of the disease or point towards a 'cure'. The drive to find new drugs has led to a widening of the targets for asthma treatments, which now include inflammatory and immune cytokines and chemokines, transcription factors, enzymes and immune cells.[18]

Poorly controlled severe asthmatics who do not respond well to combination therapy are another major unmet need. One characteristic of this group is relative corticosteroid insensitivity.[22] These patients may have corticosteroid-dependent, or more rarely, corticosteroid-resistant (CSR) asthma.[22] It is important to highlight that these CSR patients are a subset of those patients with severe asthma, and the terms are not interchangeable since some CSR patients do not have severe disease and some patients with severe asthma are not treatment-insensitive.[51] The Severe Asthma Research Program (SARP)[51] and ENFUMOSA[52] have highlighted the need to understand the molecular and cellular mechanisms present in severe asthma to enable the identification of novel targets for asthma and to speed the drug development process.[53] Clarifying the mechanisms relating to disease subtypes in CSR may not only indicate selective responsiveness to novel therapies in severe asthma but also point to similar subtypes and treatment responsiveness in patients with mild/moderate asthma.

Some pathological characteristics of patients with severe asthma have recently been observed. The thickness of the airway epithelium, of sub-basement membrane and of the airway smooth muscle in the airways of patients with severe asthma is greater than in non-severe asthma,[54,55] and is associated with altered expression of markers of epithelial proliferation.[55] Simultaneously, a number of unbiased techniques such as hierarchical clustering of BAL cytokine expression,[56] cluster analysis of inflammation and responses to treatment,[57] the analysis of volatile organic components of exhaled breath using an electronic nose,[58] and the analysis of bronchial biopsies[59] have supported the possibility of several distinct phenotypes of patients with severe asthma. Targeting nodal points in these clusters may highlight potential novel sites for drug intervention.

COPD

With few exceptions, COPD is caused by tobacco smoking, and smoking cessation is the only truly effective treatment of COPD. Once smoking has caused COPD, the disease is still largely irreversible and progressive. Current pharmacological treatment of COPD is unsatisfactory, as it does not significantly influence the severity of the disease or its natural course.[4] Bronchodilators (including long-acting inhaled β_2-agonists and long-acting inhaled antimuscarinics) are the only pharmacological treatment that improves symptoms, quality of life and lung function in COPD patients, but they do not significantly influence the natural course of the disease. Apart from the treatment and prevention of exacerbations, systemic and inhaled glucocorticoids have not been shown to be consistently effective in COPD, either in reducing symptoms or for improving lung function and the course of the disease.

One clear difference between COPD and other chronic inflammatory diseases of the lower airways such as asthma, is the clinical responsiveness to glucocorticoids,[60,61] this is despite the fact that combination therapy of inhaled glucocorticoids and long-acting inhaled β_2-agonists in the same inhaler is slightly more effective than monotherapy in the treatment of patients with stable COPD.

Even high doses of inhaled or oral glucocorticoids are virtually ineffective in patients with COPD compared to the marked responses seen in asthma, suggesting that the inflammation in COPD is essentially steroid insensitive.[60,61] In COPD there is a marked increase in oxidative stress, which may contribute to glucocorticoid-insensitivity.[61,62] Understanding the molecular mechanisms involved may lead to the development of an effective therapeutic strategy for COPD.[63]

8.4   Improving current therapies

New longer-acting bronchodilators for asthma and COPD

The LABAs, salmeterol and formoterol, have a 12-hour bronchodilator effect, and in conjunction with ICS improve asthma and COPD control and reduce exacerbation rates compared with short-acting β_2-agonists.[64] Several 'ultra-long-acting' β_2-agonists under development, including indacaterol, carmoterol and vilanterol, act for more than 24 hours, are fast acting and suitable for once-daily dosing.[65] It is also possible to increase the duration of ICS action, which in combination with the once-a-day fast-onset LABAs, will result in a combination therapy with prolonged action that, although possibly no more efficacious than current drugs, will improve compliance.[65] Although other classes of bronchodilators exist, such as vasoactive intestinal peptide (VIP), other neuropeptide (such as calcitonin gene-related peptide, or CGRP) analogues and K^+-channel openers, they have proved difficult to develop due to their potent systemic vasodilator effects.[12]

New glucocorticoids with reduced systemic side effects

Glucocorticoids are still the most effective anti-inflammatory treatments for asthma. Moreover, asthma severity is sometimes defined according to corticosteroid responsiveness.[22] Lung absorption of ICS contributes to systemic side effects, which are seen particularly with higher doses. To circumvent this, various ways of reducing systemic side effects have been developed (Figure 8.3) including systemic or local inactivation, administration of an inactive prodrug that is only converted to active drug in the airways (e.g. ciclesonide[66]), or targeted airway deposition using monodispersed particles.[67] Another approach has been to develop dissociated glucocorticoids that cannot activate mechanisms that lead to side effects while preserving therapeutic anti-inflammatory effects. Many of the detrimental side effects of glucocorticoids

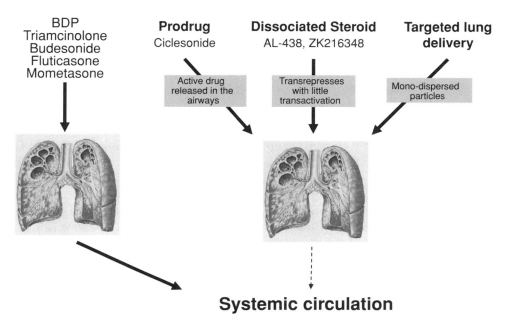

BDP
Triamcinolone
Budesonide
Fluticasone
Mometasone

Prodrug
Ciclesonide

Dissociated Steroid
AL-438, ZK216348

**Targeted lung
delivery**

Active drug
released in the
airways

Transrepresses
with little
transactivation

Mono-dispersed
particles

Systemic circulation

Figure 8.3   Current inhaled corticosteroids are absorbed through the lung into the systemic circulation and cause the detrimental side effects associated with high-dose inhaled corticosteroid usage. Several approaches are being taken to reduce systemic absorption including the use of prodrugs such as ciclesonide, which is activated to release the active form des-ciclesonide only in the lungs, and the use of corticosteroids that are able to repress inflammatory gene expression without affecting the induction of corticosteroid-inducible genes, many of which are responsible for the side effects. Alternatively, using new delivery devices it may be possible to deliver monodispersed corticosteroid particles to specific parts of the airway thereby dramatically reducing the dose of inhaled drug required to obtain the equivalent clinical benefit.

have been linked to transactivation (i.e. activation of gene transcription through DNA-binding of the activated glucocorticoid receptor) whereas most beneficial effects are associated with transrepression (i.e. activated glucocorticoid receptor binding to other transcription factors rather than to DNA sites), although this requires confirmation in humans.[24,68,69] These dissociated glucocorticoids may be just as effective as conventional ICS, have a better safety profile and might even lead to safer oral glucocorticoids.[69] Linking the development of dissociated glucocorticoids to drugs with a non-steroidal backbone, such as AL-438 and ZK 216348, may further improve the therapeutic index as these drugs will also lack activity at other nuclear hormone receptors that also cause side effects.[70] Finally, addition of a nitric oxide (NO)-donating group to prednisolone (NCX1015) and budesonide (NCX1020) has resulted in improved glucocorticoid efficacy against lipopolysaccharide (LPS)-induced inflammatory responses and prevented LPS-induced airway hyperresponsiveness, eosinophilia and neutrophilia in animals. In contrast, only a small effect on eosinophilia was seen with the parent compounds.[71,72] In a similar manner, NO groups have been tagged to β_2-agonists.[73] This probably results from donation of the NO moiety to specific residues within the respective ligand-binding domains thereby affecting receptor function. New combinations of these drugs are likely to be more effective alone but more so as combinations in both asthma and COPD.

Lipid mediator blockade

Many inflammatory mediators have been implicated in asthma and COPD, with specific inhibitors and antagonists against many of these having been developed (Table 8.1). However, the only mediator antagonists that are currently used are antileukotrienes, which block cysteinyl-leukotriene (CysLT) receptors or block LT synthesis.[74] CysLT$_1$ receptor antagonists such as montelukast, improve lung function and asthma symptoms in some patients with mild-to-moderate asthma, but their efficacy is reduced compared to low-dose ICS. Moreover, they are less effective in severe asthma,[75] although a study has suggested that they may also be beneficial in smoking asthmatics.[76] Zileuton, a 5-lipoxygenase (5-LO) inhibitor that blocks cysLT and LTB$_4$ synthesis, also provided similar efficacy to montelukast in asthma.[77]

The expression of LTB$_4$, which can recruit and activate neutrophils in the lungs, is increased in patients with COPD,[78, 79] and further increased during COPD exacerbations,[80] and this may account for the greatly increased numbers of neutrophils in the sputum and airway lumen of COPD patients.[81] Interestingly, preliminary clinical observations suggest that 5-lipoxygenase inhibitors (such as zileuton) significantly

Table 8.1   Summary of some of the compounds in preclinical and initial clinical development for asthma and COPD.

Drug class	Target	Example
Ultra-long-acting β_2-agonist	β_2-Adrenergic receptor	Indacaterol, carmoterol, vilanterol
Dissociated steroid	Glucocorticoid receptor	AL-438, ZK 216348
CCL11 antagonist/blocking Ab	CCR5	CAT-213
CCR3 antagonist	CCR3	Met ionine CCL5
Th2 blocker	IL-4/IL-13 receptor	Pitrakinra, CAT-354, IMI-358
CXCR1/2 antagonists	CXCL8/IL-8, CXCL1	GSK-656933, repertaxin
E-selectin inhibitor	E-selectin	Bimosiamose
PGD2/CRTh2 inhibitors	CRTh2 receptor	ODC9101, ramatroban
Sphingosine receptor blocker	Sphingosine-1 phosphate receptor	FTY720
PDE4 inhibitor	PDE4	Roflumilast
NF-κB inhibitor	IKK-2	MIN425
p38 MAP kinase inhibitor	p38 MAP kinase-α	SCIO-469
PI3Kγ inhibitor	PI3Kγ	None known
Antioxidants	Oxidative stress	SOD analogues

CCL, CC chemokine ligand; CCR, CC chemokine receptor; CXCR, CXC chemokine receptor; GROα, ; IKK-2, inhibitor of κB kinase-2; IL, interleukin; MAP kinase, mitogen-activated protein kinase; PDE, phosphodiesterase; PGD, prostaglandin D; PI3Kγ, phosphoinositide 3-kinase-γ; SOD, superoxide dismutase; Th2, T-helper cell type 2. CXCL, CXC chemokine ligand.

improve lung function in COPD patients, in contrast to cysteinyl leukotriene receptor antagonists.[82] However, potent 5-LO inhibitors have been difficult to develop; zileuton is a relatively weak 5-LO inhibitor that has a short duration of action. Its effect in asthma is greater than leukotriene receptor antagonists, particularly in severe asthma, indicating a possible role of LTB_4 in asthma. A pilot study with BAYx1005 in patients with COPD showed only a modest reduction in sputum LTB_4 concentrations but no effect on neutrophil activation markers.[83]

Antagonizing the receptors for LTB_4 – BLT_1 and peroxisome proliferator-activated receptor-α (PPAR-α) – may be an alternative approach for suppressing LTB_4 actions. Proinflammatory LTB_4 activities are mediated by BLT_1, while the inactivation of LTB_4 is promoted by PPAR-α.[84] The number of $BLT_1{}^+$ T-cells is increased in the asthmatic airways,[85] and those of $BLT_1{}^+$ macrophages, neutrophils and $CD8^+$ T-cells in COPD peripheral lung.[86] Importantly, in animal models BLT_1 antagonists prevent airway inflammation and airway hyperresponsiveness,[85] and also inhibit neutrophil chemotaxis in response to sputum from patients with COPD.[86] However, the LTB_4 receptor antagonist, LY293111, had no effect on allergen challenge in a small group of asthmatic patients,[87] and the BLT_1 antagonist LTB019 did not decrease sputum neutrophil number in patients with COPD.[88]

Recently, the 5-lipoxygenase-activating protein (FLAP, ALOX5AP) gene has been linked to risk for myocardial infarction, stroke and coronary restenosis. The early FLAP inhibitors showed some efficacy in clinical trials in asthma but were not developed commercially. However, new safer FLAP inhibitors such as DG031 may be particularly useful in patients with distinct genetic/phenotypic backgrounds and particularly as a steroid add-on therapy in the treatment of asthma exacerbations and in COPD.[89]

Prostaglandin PGD_2, produced by mast cells, acts predominantly through the G-protein-coupled receptor DP_2 (also known as CRTh2, chemoattractant receptor-homologous molecule expressed on Th2 lymphocytes) to mediate Th2 recruitment and activation.[90] Ramatroban, a thromboxane receptor (TP) antagonist and a partial DP_2 antagonist, is used to treat perennial rhinitis in Japan,[90] and more selective and potent DP_2 antagonists are being developed for asthma. For example, TM30089 is effective in animal models of asthma, and a once-day oral molecule, ODC9101, is now in phase IIa clinical trials in asthma.[90] Other prostanoids and isoprostanes have been reported to be involved in the inflammatory process seen in COPD.[91] The novel chemical analogue RESPIR 4-95 is able to relax human small airways where contraction was induced by many bronchoconstrictor stimuli (such as LTD_4, histamine, acetylcholine and PGD_2 exposure). This was independent of both transient receptor potential cation channel subfamily V number 1 (TRPV1) antagonism and current bronchodilator drug mechanisms.[92]

The endogenous anti-inflammatory eicosanoid lipoxin A_4 (LXA_4) is reduced in severe asthma[93] and in COPD compared to subjects with mild asthma,[94] and LXA_4 therapy may be considered as an anti-inflammatory agent for these patients.[93] Despite initial promise, inhibitors of other lipid mediators, including prostaglandins and platelet-activating factor (PAF), have proved ineffective in the treatment of asthma and COPD.[95]

8.5 Targeting chemokines and their receptors in asthma and COPD

Recruitment of inflammatory cells into the airway by chemokines is a crucial process in the development of asthma and COPD. Chemokines are classified into four families based on a conserved cysteine motif as follows: C, CC, CXC and CX3C, and act through specific receptors according to the ligand class.[85]

Chemokines, their receptors and cell adhesion molecules regulate migration of immune cells into inflamed tissue. Each inflammatory cell type is activated and recruited by a specific pattern of chemokines. For example Th1 cells express a distinct repertoire of chemokine receptors such as CCR5 and CXCR3. In contrast, Th2 cells mainly express CCR3, CCR4, CCR8 and CRTh2.[96]

The major focus of interest in asthma has been initially on CCR3 and its ligands (CCL11, CCL24 and CCL26), which are increased in asthma[97] and mediate eosinophil recruitment[85] (Figure 8.4). CCR3 is also expressed on mast cells and some Th2 cells. CCL11 is increased temporally prior to induction of CCL24 and CCL26 following allergen challenge.[98] Targeting of CCR3 would therefore be more reasonable than targeting its ligands, as is the case with most chemokine receptors. Antisense oligonucleotides that inhibit CCR3 and IL-5R led to a reduction in sputum eosinophilia following allergen challenge associated with an inhibition of the early response but only a trend for a reduced late response.[99] Furthermore, inhibitors of CCR3 have been effective in inhibiting eosinophilic inflammation, airway hyperresponsiveness and goblet cell hyperplasia in mouse models,[100, 101] and are currently undergoing clinical trials for asthma. Increased numbers of eosinophils have also been reported in COPD sputum, BAL and bronchial mucosa particularly during exacerbations or in patients with concomitant asthma.[102] This is also reflected in elevated levels of CCL11 and CCL5 in

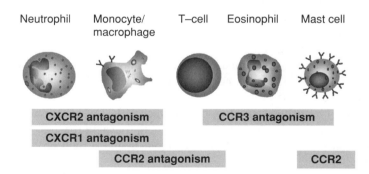

Figure 8.4 Chemokine receptor modulation in asthma. Prevention of inflammatory cell migration into the airways might be achieved by modulation of chemokine receptors. CCR3 antagonists would be predicted to prevent T-cell, eosinophil and mast cell recruitment and activation in the airways, whereas CXCR2 antagonism would target monocytes/macrophage and neutrophil infiltration. Antagonism of the CCR2 receptor or biologicals against its ligands would prevent mast cell, monocytes/macrophage and T-cell effects in asthma.

COPD, particularly during exacerbations,[103] and in increased IL-4 and IL-5 expression in plasma cells associated with submucosal glands.[104] Inhibitors of eosinophil recruitment may also therefore be effective in subgroups of COPD patients.[102]

Other chemokines may be important in the pathogenesis of asthma. For example, the expression of CCL17 and CCL22[105] and the number of CCR4+ Th2-cells are increased in asthmatic airways after allergen challenge,[106] and antibodies directed against CCL17 and CCL22 are effective in animal models of asthma.[85] CCR2, which is expressed on monocytes and T-cells, and CCR4 and CCR8, which are expressed on Th2 cells, are also targets for asthma therapy[85] (Figure 8.4).

In contrast, CXCL8, acting through CXCR1, is important for neutrophil chemotaxis.[107] CXCL8 levels are markedly elevated in the sputum of patients with COPD, and are correlated with disease severity[108, 109] and increase during exacerbations.[110] Blocking antibodies to CXCL8 and related chemokines inhibit certain types of neutrophilic inflammation in experimental animals[111] and significantly reduce the neutrophil chemotactic activity of sputum from patients with COPD.[86] This reduction, however, is only of the order of around 30%, indicating that other neutrophil chemotactic factors such as LTB_4 and the activated complement factor C5a are important. A human monoclonal antibody (mAb) to CXCL8 showed minimal clinical benefit in a clinical study in COPD apart from a small reduction in dyspnoea,[112] although a larger study is currently being undertaken. Significantly, other CXC chemokines are also involved in COPD and would not be inhibited by this specific blocking antibody. Furthermore the antibody blocked only free CXCL8, and the effect of bound CXCL8 cannot be excluded.[107]

CXCL8 activates neutrophils via a specific low-affinity receptor (CXCR1) and a high-affinity receptor (CXCR2).[107] CXCL1 and CXCL5 may also be involved in neutrophilic inflammation acting via CXCR2. There is an increase in CXCL1 and CXCL5 expression in the lungs of patients with COPD in both stable COPD and during exacerbations,[113–115] and of CXCL1 in COPD sputum BAL.[115] This may result from the increased basal and TNF-α- and IL-17-induced enhanced CXCL1 secretion by COPD alveolar macrophages and airway epithelial cells.[116–118]

CXCL5 is derived predominantly from bronchial epithelial cells and also activates CXCR2.[119] CXCL5 levels are increased in the BAL of COPD patients[120] and in bronchial epithelial cells during exacerbations of COPD.[113] Because concentrations of CXCL1, CXCL5 and CXCL8 seem to be increased in COPD airways and because these chemokines signal through CXCR2, blocking this common receptor could reduce the chemotaxis of neutrophils. Small molecule inhibitors of CXCR2 have been developed and are entering clinical trials. It is possible that dual blockers of CXCR1 and CXCR2 would be more effective than selective CXCR2 antagonists in the treatment of COPD and for patients with severe asthma or asthma exacerbations with evidence of neutrophilia.[107]

CCL5 is also a CCR1 ligand, and levels of CCL5 are significantly increased in COPD sputum, where they correlated with the number of sputum neutrophils,[121] and during COPD exacerbations.[122] Interestingly, CCR5-knockout mice have reduced BAL neutrophilia in an animal model of cigarette-smoking-induced pulmonary inflammation.[123]

In one study wild-type and CCR5-knockout mice were subjected to subacute and chronic cigarette smoke exposure. In the CCR5-knockout mice, cigarette smoke induced increases in CCR5 ligands, yet BAL inflammatory cells and peribronchial lymphoid follicles were all significantly attenuated compared with wild-type animals.[123] Importantly, chronic cigarette smoke exposure induced airspace enlargement in wild-type mice, while CCR5-knockout mice were partially protected against the development of emphysema. However, CCR5 deficiency did not affect cigarette smoke-induced airway remodelling, which was similar to that of wild-type mice.[123]

Most chemokine receptors bind several ligands, and small molecules that block the binding site for one specific chemokine may be unable to inhibit binding of other ligands. Targeting the receptor transmembrane helices has proved to be an effective strategy in the case of CCR5.[124] The first successful small molecule against a chemokine receptor is TAK-799 (Takeda), which binds near the extracellular part of CCR5. It has been used to block CCR5, which also functions as a coreceptor of HIV-1.[125] Other CCR5 antagonists have been studied for the treatment of HIV infection, but no reports are currently available on COPD. Another interesting strategy to inhibit chemokine receptor activation is the truncation of the N-terminus of their ligands, so as to abrogate the signalling activity but not the binding proprieties. Similarly the extension of the N-terminus has the same antagonist effect. Several N-terminal modified CCR5 antagonists have been used, including Met-RANTES (methionine-CCL5),[126] AOP-RANTES[127] and PSC-RANTES. They have all been successfully used to prevent vaginal SHIV transmission in primates.[128] To the best of our knowledge there are no clinical trials with CCR5 antagonists underway in patients with COPD.

Yet another CC chemokine receptor, CCR6, and its corresponding ligand CCL20, have been implicated in the pathogenesis of COPD, in particular that associated with lung destruction.[129] In COPD patients with emphysema there is a significant increase in the number of CCR6$^+$ dendritic cells and B-cells, along with CCL20 expression within the lung. Furthermore, CCR6-deficient mice exhibited less emphysema compared to wild-type mice when exposed to cigarette smoke.[130] Unfortunately, there are no good CCR6 antagonists available as yet.

The T-cells in the bronchial mucosa of patients with stable COPD express high levels of CXCR3 in some[105] but not all[131] studies. CXCL9 (monokine-induced by IFN-γ, or MIG), CXCL10 (interferon-inducible protein-10, or IP-10) and CXCL11 (interferon-inducible T-cell alpha chemoattractant, or I-TAC) are three known ligands for CXCR3 produced by bronchial epithelial cells and T-cells and are required for homing of Th1 cells.[96] The number of CXCR3$^+$ cells is increased in the small airways of patients with stable COPD.[132] In the peripheral lung of patients with COPD and emphysema there is an increased number of CD4$^+$ and CD8$^+$ T-lymphocytes that express CXCR3 and secrete more CXCL9 and CXCL10.[133] CCR5 was also detected in a high percentage of CD4$^+$ and CD8$^+$ T-lymphocytes from the lung removed from the same patients. CD8$^+$ T-cells and dendritic cells in the peripheral lung of patients with stable COPD showed an increased expression of CXCR3 and CXCL9 that correlated with the severity of COPD.[134] Collectively these results suggest the presence of a Th1 response in the lungs of people with COPD.

The compound T0906487 (originally from Tularik), a CXCR3 antagonist, has been developed further by Amgen and Chemocentryx. The compound was evaluated in a phase II clinical trial in patients with moderate to severe psoriasis, a Th1-like disease, but the treatment had no effect on psoriasis.[135] High-affinity selective CXCR3 antagonists, including aryl-1 and -4 diazepane ureas and 3-phenyl-3H-quinazolin-4-ones, have been identified using cell-based assays and are effective at ~100 nM. Other antagonists such as NBI74330 have been developed from the T487 series. NBI74330 is selective for CXCR3, and has differential potency against the three CXCR3 ligands with the rank order CXCL11 ≫ CXC10 > CXCL9. However, there are currently no CXCR3 antagonists in clinical trials for COPD.[107] Because it is thought that T-cells expressing both CXCR3 and CCR5 are actively recruited to sites of lung inflammation in COPD, double antagonists such as the compound TAK779, which acts on both receptors, might be more effective.[136]

Finally, the glycosaminoglycan heparin is coreleased with histamine from mast cells and can, in addition to its well-described anticoagulant properties, combine with chemokines to prevent their action and thereby prevent exercise-induced bronchoconstriction.[137] A phase II study of IVX-0142, a novel heparin-derived oligosaccharide, in mild asthma has been completed (http://clinicaltrials.gov/ct2/show/NCT00232999?term=ivx+0142+asthma&rank=1).

8.6 Targeting T-cell-derived and proinflammatory cytokines in asthma and COPD

Cytokines are major targets for new asthma therapies because of their key role in chronic inflammation and in remodelling of the airway.[95] The concept of asthma as a Th2-driven disease and the demonstration that inhibition of Th2-derived cytokines in many animal models of asthma prevented all aspects of disease drove the development of antagonists and antibodies directed against these cytokines (Figure 8.1). However, this has not been replicated in asthma, illustrating the limitations of the animal models used, and this problem needs to be urgently addressed. Activated CD4/CD8 T-cells are also increased in the small airway wall of smokers with severe COPD,[138] particularly of the Th1/Tc1 type[139] with expression of the chemokine CXCL10, which may control the release of elastolytic matrix metalloproteinases (MMPs)[132] and of the transcription factor signal transducer and activator of transcription (STAT4).[140] In severe emphysema, T-cells isolated from lung tissues showed oligoclonal expansion following conventional antigenic stimuli.[141] An autoantigen, antielastin antibody, has been reported in COPD patients and may underlie the autoimmune response.[142]

IL-4 and IL-13

Both IL-4 and IL-13 are important in B-cell IgE isotype switching, and IL-4 is also important in maintaining the Th2 phenotype. IL-13 also modulates eosinophilic inflammation, airway smooth muscle hyperplasia, induction of goblet-cell hyperplasia, monocyte and T-cell recruitment, and induction of a corticosteroid-insensitive airway inflammation.[143] Early studies with a soluble recombinant human IL-4 receptor (altrakincept) in mild-to-moderate asthma showed some efficacy in maintaining asthma control when inhaled corticosteroids were being withdrawn,[144] but this effect was not subsequently confirmed in a phase III trial. Humanized IL-4-specific and IL-4Rα-blocking antibodies together with peptide-based vaccines against IL-4 are now being tested.[145] A study has showed that IL-4 muteins (pitrakinra), which can inhibit the binding of IL-4 and IL-13 to IL-4Ra complexes, reduced the allergen-induced late-phase response in asthmatic subjects.[146] Several monoclonal antibodies against IL-13, including CAT-354 and IMA-638, are currently undergoing clinical trials for asthma and these may have a better therapeutic index than small molecule inhibitors due to the large size of the binding pocket preventing selectivity.[145]

An increase in IL-4-positive cells in mucus-secreting cells and associated plasma cells of the airway mucosa of chronic bronchitis patients has been reported.[103] Although IL-18 expression appears to be increased in pulmonary macrophages of COPD patients, IL-13 gene expression appears to be decreased in emphysematous lung.[147] However, an increase in IL-4- and IL-13-positive cells in the bronchial submucosa in chronic bronchitis has been reported.[148] Much evidence for a role of IL-13 in COPD comes from work in mice. Overexpression of the Th2 cytokine IL-13 in lungs of adult mice induces emphysema, mucus goblet-cell hyperplasia, and airway inflammation with macrophages, lymphocytes and eosinophils, and increased matrix metalloproteinases, which are many of the features associated with COPD.[149] The induction of emphysema was related to the release of metallo- and cysteine-proteases.[149] Interestingly, the proinflammatory cytokine IL-18 can induce lung inflammation and emphysema through the production of IL-13 but not through IFN-γ,[150] despite IFN-γ also being capable of inducing emphysema in this model.[151]

IL-5

Interleukin-5 is critical for terminal differentiation of eosinophils and for eosinophilic inflammation; however, a blocking antibody to IL-5 had no effect on airway hyper-responsiveness, lung function or exacerbation frequency in asthmatic patients despite depletion of blood and sputum eosinophilia.[152, 153] In a subsequent study, an IL-5 antibody failed to prevent eosinophilia within the airway submucosa and resulted in some beneficial effects on aspects of airway remodelling.[154] It is possible that anti-IL-5 therapy may be more effective in patients with high levels of circulating and sputum eosinophils, as it has been shown to be effective in the treatment of hypereosinophilic syndrome.[155] Recent evidence suggests that anti-IL-5 treatment may improve exacerbation rates in patients with severe asthma and high sputum eosinophils.[156]

Suplatast tosilate selectively inhibits IL-4 and IL-5 from T-cells *in vitro* and attenuates allergen-induced goblet-cell metaplasia, reduces blood and sputum eosinophilia and airway hyperresponsiveness in mild-to-moderate asthmatics.[145] In small clinical trials, suplatast was as effective as budesonide in decreasing blood and sputum eosinophils, blood and sputum eosinophil cationic protein, sputum mast cell tryptase, exhaled nitric oxide and airway responsiveness in patients with mild-to-moderate asthma or cough-variant asthma without causing significant side effects.[157] Interestingly, *in vitro* suplatast may inhibit monocyte-mediated IL-8 production and the release of oxidants from neutrophils, suggesting that it could also have some efficacy in COPD patients.[158]

Thymic stromal lymphopoietin (TSLP)

This is highly expressed in airway epithelial cells of asthmatic patients and can either activate dendritic cells to orchestrate an allergic pattern of inflammation through the activation of Th2 cells or directly stimulate Th2 cytokine expression from T-cells.[159, 160] Additionally, *Tslp* knockout mice fail to develop an antigen-specific Th2-mediated inflammatory response in the airways. Clinical studies are now needed in patients with all types of asthma. TSLP is also expressed in increased levels in airway smooth muscle (ASM) and bronchial mucosa of patients with COPD.[131, 161]

IL-10 and IL-12

Some cytokines are intrinsically anti-inflammatory and are therefore potential therapeutic agents. IL-10 and IL-12 expression is reduced in patients with severe asthma,[162, 163] and restoration of levels has been proposed to re-establish asthma control. However, repeated IL-12 injections had no effect on airway hyperresponsiveness despite marked effects on blood eosinophilia.[164]

The potent immunosuppressive and anti-inflammatory action of IL-10 has suggested that it may be useful therapeutically in the treatment of asthma and COPD.[165, 166] IL-10 administration has proved effective in animal models of asthma but no studies have been reported in asthma or COPD despite IL-10 being approved for Crohn's disease and psoriasis.[167] In addition, both IL-12 and IL-10 have unacceptable side effects, and an alternative strategy to enhance endogenous IL-10 expression through immunomodulatory pathways (see below) is preferable.

TNF-α

Tumor necrosis factor-α (TNF-α), a multifunctional cytokine, is released in the airways from mast cells, alveolar macrophages and CD8 T-lymphocytes,[168] and elevated levels of TNF-α have been demonstrated in the bronchial biopsies and sputum from asthmatic and COPD patients.[108, 169] TNF-α levels in BAL increase after allergen challenge in atopic asthmatics.[170] In addition, TNF-α is an important chemotactic protein for neutrophils. In fact the inhalation of TNF-α induces sputum neutrophilia and airway hyperresponsiveness in patients with mild asthma.[166] Humanized monoclonal anti-TNF-α antibodies (infliximab) and soluble TNF receptors (etanercept) are already on the market for the treatment of inflammatory bowel disease, rheumatoid arthritis and psoriasis.[171]

In a small study in symptomatic moderate asthmatics,[172] and in two studies in severe corticosteroid-insensitive asthmatics who failed to respond to conventional therapy,[173, 174] anti-TNF-α therapy resulted in improved lung function. This was particularly the case with etanercept, a soluble TNF-α receptor blocker, in patients who had high levels of surface TNF-α on peripheral blood cells.[173] These results promised a new treatment regime for these patients; however, a subsequent larger study failed to show clinically significant improvements in lung function or exacerbation rates in refractory severe asthmatics.[175]

In addition, a multicentre, randomized, double-blind, placebo-controlled, parallel-group study of moderate to severe COPD patients who received infliximab demonstrated no treatment benefit as measured by quality of life scores, prebronchodilator FEV_1, 6-min walk distance or exacerbation rates.[176] Worryingly, more cases of cancer and pneumonia were observed in the infliximab-treated subjects. In contrast, Suissa and colleagues reported an observational study in a cohort of 15 771 patients diagnosed with both rheumatoid arthritis (RA) and COPD.[177] There was a 50% reduction in rate ratios of COPD hospitalization in subjects treated with etanercept but not infliximab. Anti-TNF-α therapies therefore demonstrate different efficacies in asthma and COPD, and further supportive clinical data are needed. This is particularly so for those subsets of patients who could benefit the most from these therapies. However, extreme care must be given in weighing up these risks due to their potentially lethal side effects.

8.7   Targeting adhesion molecules in asthma and COPD

There has been considerable effort to exploit the importance of adhesion molecules in several important facets of asthma, such as leukocyte migration, exocytosis, cytokine production and respiratory burst, by developing drugs targeting these molecules[85] (Figure 8.1). Much interest has revolved around the very late antigen-4 (VLA-4, $\alpha_4\beta$ integrin), which is involved in the recruitment of eosinophils and T-cells.[85] However, the clinical outcome of trials for these agents in asthma has been disappointing and, indeed, the development of some classes of these drugs (e.g. $\alpha_4\beta$ integrin antagonists) was placed on hold by the US Food and Drug Administration (FDA) due to reports of progressive multifocal leukoencephalopathy in patients taking natalizumab (Tysabri, Biogen and Elan Pharmaceuticals). Although now lifted, the ban delayed approval causing widespread implications for the development of adhesion molecule antagonists for the treatment of asthma.[85]

The leucocyte $\alpha M\beta_2$ integrin, also known as Mac-1 or CD11b/CD18, functions as an adhesion molecule facilitating neutrophil diapedesis. Overexpression of CD11b has been reported in blood neutrophils[178, 179] and sputum[180] of COPD patients compared to control subjects. CD62E (E-selectin), the major ligand of CD11b, is critical for converting the initial cell tethering into a steady slow rolling of neutrophils in the vessel lumen.[181] CD62E expression is also increased in bronchial biopsies of patients with stable COPD,[182] but the expression of CD11b on neutrophils in the bronchial mucosa of patients with stable COPD is still unknown. Despite elevated blood neutrophil CD11b expression, these cells show an impaired chemotaxis and migration in response to IL-8 and formyl-Met-Leu-Phe (FMLP).[183] Targeting CD11b may prove effective in COPD, however.

CD44 is a ubiquitous multistructural and multifunctional cell surface adhesion molecule involved in cell–cell and cell–matrix interactions. CD44 belongs to the family of hyaluronan-binding type I transmembrane glycoprotein receptors. Hyaluronan, an extracellular matrix component, is the main ligand for CD44[184] and, interestingly, CD44 knock-out animals have an increased influx of neutrophils into their lungs.[185] This suggests a negative regulatory role for CD44 in neutrophil migration.

8.8 Growth factor blockers in asthma and COPD

Central airway squamous metaplasia as measured by expression of involucrin expressed in stratified epithelium increases with severity of COPD;[186] recently, increased IL-1β expression by squamous cells has been postulated to lead to integrin-mediated activation of transforming growth factor-β1 (TGF-β1) to amplify pathological epithelial-mesenchymal interactions in COPD.[102] A small increase in the proliferative rate of the epithelium of small airways of COPD patients has been reported,[187] possibly due to the increased expression of growth factors such as TGF-β1,[188–191] fibroblast growth factors (FGFs)[192] and oxidant responsive genes.[193]

Microarray analysis of lung tissue from GOLD stage 2 patients has found an increased expression of the growth factors TGF-β1 and connective tissue growth factor (CTGF), with a reduction in the expression of collagen type 1.[194] Increased TGF-β1 with possible activation of MMP-12 could lead to elastolytic effects with fibrotic effects, depending on its localization in the airway or in the parenchyma.

In animal models cigarette smoke can result in the activation of latent TGF-β1, with stimulation of lower airway fibrosis.[195] There are several mechanisms by which latent TGF-β1 can be activated in COPD; these include mediation by thrombospondin-1,[196] by integrins,[197,198] by serine proteases such as neutrophil elastase[199] and by oxidants.[200]

Activation of the epithelial growth factor receptor (EGFR) cascade is also increased in bronchial epithelium from smokers with or without COPD compared to non-smokers,[201,202] and smoking cessation does not lead to a reduction in EGFR expression.[203] This indicates that chronic cigarette exposure may lead to permanent changes in the bronchial epithelium that are linked to preneoplastic lesions of this epithelium and development of lung cancer, emphasizing the importance of targeting these factors. Many compounds preventing growth factor activity are either in development or in clinical use for cancer, but their efficacy and safety for the long-term treatment of COPD have not yet been established.[204]

8.9 Mucous cells, submucosal glands and mucus production in asthma and COPD

Increased goblet cell hyperplasia and mucus production are characteristic of both asthma and smokers with COPD.[9] While an earlier study indicated no predictive value of mucus hypersecretion to mortality in COPD,[205] other studies have associated chronic sputum production with the risk of hospitalization, an excessive yearly decline in FEV_1 and the development of COPD.[206] Antimucolytics have proved ineffective in asthma but have shown some efficacy in preventing COPD exacerbations.[207,208] Increased expression of the major secreted mucins of the airways, MUC5B and MUC5AC, has been reported in the central and small airways of COPD patients,[202,209] and in the bronchial mucosa of asthmatics.[210] The synthesis of these mucin glycoproteins in the airways is most likely regulated by inflammation and respiratory pathogens that activate mitogen-activated protein kinase (MAPK) pathways, and in turn through RAS activate nuclear factor-κB (NF-κB), Sp1 (specificity factor 1) or AP-1 (activator protein 1) transcription factors.[211]

8.10   Infections in asthma and COPD

Some small uncontrolled serological studies suggest that *Chlamydia pneumoniae* infection may amplify the inflammation that occurs in severe persistent asthma and that asthma will subsequently improve with antibiotic therapy.[212–214] However, that is not the case in all asthmatics.[215–218] Similar reports have also associated the onset of persistent asthma with *Mycoplasma pneumoniae* infection.[215,219] In addition to treating the infection present, macrolide antibiotics have been show to have some direct anti-inflammatory effects. For example, clarithromycin treatment in asthmatic patients could reduce the oedematous area as identified by α_2-macroglobulin staining, which may lead to airway tissue shrinkage and cause an artificial increase in the number of blood vessels.[220]

Respiratory viral and/or bacterial infections are a major cause of asthma exacerbations.[1] Therefore, antiviral treatments may be beneficial for asthma exacerbations. Telithromycin, a macrolide antibiotic, caused a small but significant reduction in asthma symptoms without changes in lung function compared to placebo when administered to patients with acute exacerbations of asthma.[221] In addition, clarithromycin can reduce CXCL8 levels and sputum neutrophilia and improve asthma quality of life in patients with refractory non-eosinophilic asthma.[222] It is unclear whether these macrolide antibiotics act by directly inhibiting infections or by inhibiting neutrophil-based inflammation. Despite the increasing evidence that persistent infection with *Chlamydia pneumoniae* is linked to chronic diseases including atherosclerosis and myocardial infarction, the role of *Chlamydia pneumoniae* infection in the onset of COPD remains controversial. The majority (54–77%) of patients with COPD show serological evidence of past infection with *Chlamydia* pneumoniae,[223–225] but the incidence is similar to that seen in age-matched healthy subjects.[223,226,227] There is some evidence that persistent *Chlamydia pneumoniae* infection may amplify the inflammation that occurs in COPD,[228,229] but a prospective serological study suggests that chronic *Chlamydia pneumoniae* infection is not a major risk factor for progressive airflow obstruction.[230] Clearly, further studies are necessary to determine whether chronic infection with *Chlamydia pneumoniae* is important in the pathogenesis of COPD or whether the organism is simply a 'bystander'.

Therapeutic interventions aimed at treating viral or bacterial infections by inhibition of Toll-like receptors (TLRs) are also under investigation, although evidence in animal models is inconclusive.[231]

Furthermore, rhinovirus infection can reduce glucocortico receptor (GR) nuclear translocation and corticosteroid function,[232] and, conversely, inhibition of the GR-associated heat-shock protein-90 (hsp-90) by geldanomycin or its analogues can attenuate rhinovirus replication without the formation of drug-resistant strains,[233] implying mutual antagonism between viral infection and corticosteroids.

8.11   Intracellular signalling pathways

Phosphodiesterase-4 inhibitors in asthma and COPD

Phosphodiesterase-4 (PDE4) inhibitors such as roflumilast and cilomilast prevent eosinophilic inflammation in ovalbumin-sensitized (OVA) Brown Norway rats with an efficacy similar to budesonide.[234] Moreover, PDE4 inhibitors are able to suppress neutrophilic inflammation and exert distinct anti-inflammatory effects compared to those seen with corticosteroids,[235] suggesting that PDE4 inhibitors may be potentially useful in the treatment of severe asthma[235] (Figure 8.4). Both cilomilast and roflumilast show dose-dependent inhibition of early- and late-phase responses to allergen and exercise challenges.[235] In a parallel-group trial, cilomilast caused small improvements in FEV_1 at 6 weeks but this was lost by 12 months.[235] In contrast, roflumilast (500 μg daily) produced greater effects and caused improvements in FEV_1, morning and evening peak flow, and asthma symptoms over 12 weeks similar to those seen with 400 μg beclometasone dipropionate.[236]

Roflumilast and cilomilast are able to suppress neutrophilic inflammation in response to smoking and exert distinct anti-inflammatory effects compared to the response seen with corticosteroids. *In vitro* work comparing several PDE4 inhibitors shows that these agents reduce the activity of neutrophils, macrophages and $CD8^+$ T-lymphocytes and the expression of many inflammatory mediators. This suggests that PDE4 inhibitors may be potentially useful in the treatment of asthmatics who smoke,[237] particularly those who are at risk from developing COPD.[238] In animal models of COPD, PDE4 inhibitors are effective anti-inflammatory agents, in contrast to the lack of effect seen with dexamethasone.[239] More importantly, in COPD patients, cilomilast (15 mg b.i.d. for 12 weeks) was able to reduce airway tissue $CD4^+$ and $CD8^+$ T-lymphocyte subsets by 42% and 48%, respectively, and neutrophil accumulation by 37%.[240] In particular, cilomilast was able to reduce the expression of $CD68^+$ macrophages in bronchial biopsies of COPD patients by 47%. This is in contrast to the lack of effect seen with combination (corticosteroid/LABA) therapy as demonstrated in a similar biopsy study by the same group.[43] The problem of nausea and vomiting that occurs at the top of the dose–effect curve has not been overcome despite improved isoform selectivity. Therefore administration of these compounds by inhalation is being considered in order to try and overcome these side effects when taken orally.

Kinase inhibitors in asthma and COPD

Kinases play a critical role in the expression and activation of inflammatory mediators in the airway, in both resident and infiltrating cells, as well as in airway

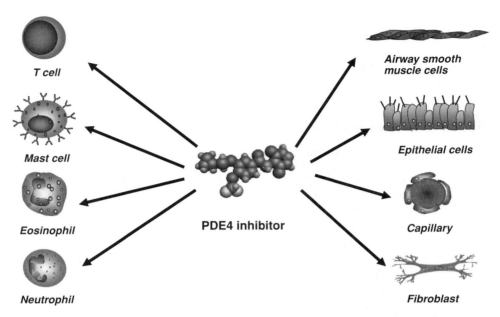

T cell

Mast cell

Eosinophil

Neutrophil

PDE4 inhibitor

Airway smooth muscle cells

Epithelial cells

Capillary

Fibroblast

Figure 8.5 Phosphodiesterase-4 (PDE4) inhibitors target the key inflammatory cells in asthma: CD4$^+$ T-lymphocytes (Th2 cells), mast cells and eosinophils. They also modify airway hyperresponsiveness and remodelling by reducing smooth muscle cell proliferation and migration, the proinflammatory activity of epithelial cells and plasma exudation leading to oedema (as a result of increased permeability of the microvasculature). The suppressive activity of PDE4 inhibitors on inflammatory cells in asthma involves the inhibition of the generation of cytokines, chemokines, oxidants, proinflammatory mediators, the reduction or inhibition of eosinophilic migration and the attenuation of degranulation.

remodelling.[241,242] (Figure 8.5). Although different kinase pathways can activate specific downstream transcription factors there is considerable cross-talk between the pathways.[241,242] Changes in kinase activation status have been reported in COPD and in all asthmatics, but particularly in severe asthma where an association with reduced glucocorticoid responsiveness has been proposed.[243] Thus, enhanced activation of ERK, c-Jun N-terminal kinase (JNK) and p38 MAPKs, and JAK/STATs have all been proposed to play a role in steroid-insensitive asthma in a stimulus-dependent manner.[22,244,245]

MAPK inhibitors

The kinase p38 MAPK is involved in many inflammatory processes in the lower airways and in tissue remodelling. Selective second-generation p38 MAPK inhibitors such as SB2439063 and ISIS 101757[241] reduce the release of inflammatory mediators and lessen some characteristics of allergic inflammation in animal models[241] with no hepatic or neurological toxicity.[241] Interestingly, the corticosteroid insensitivity seen in peripheral blood cells and BAL macrophages of patients with severe asthma can be overcome by the combination of a p38 MAPK inhibitor and dexamethasone.[22,246]

The activity of p38 MAPK is elevated in COPD,[247] and selective inhibitors such as SB239063[248] and SD-282[249] can reduce neutrophil infiltration and the concentrations of IL-6 and matrix metalloproteinase 9 in BAL fluid of rats after inhaled endotoxin. Moreover, it can also suppress tobacco-smoke induced inflammatory cell infiltration, IL-6 and cyclo-oxygenase-2 (COX-2) expression, indicating its potential as an anti-inflammatory agent in COPD. It is likely that such a broad-spectrum anti-inflammatory drug will have some toxicity during long-term use, but again, inhalation may be a feasible therapeutic approach. An alternative approach is to target downstream substrates such as MAPKAPK2 since, in contrast to p38 MAPK knockout mice, MAPKAPK2 knockouts are viable and exhibit an anti-inflammatory phenotype.[250]

JNK activity is increased in CSR asthma,[251] and SP600125, a JNK inhibitor, reduces BAL accumulation of eosinophils and lymphocytes, cytokine release, serum IgE production and smooth muscle proliferation after repeated allergen exposure in acute and chronic animal models of asthma.[252,253] and COPD.[254]

Syk inhibitors

Spleen tyrosine kinase (Syk, p72^{Syk}) plays a pivotal role in triggering mast cell degranulation through the high-affinity IgE receptor (FcεRI).[255] Syk is also involved in B- and T-lymphocyte antigen receptor signalling and in eosinophil survival, suggesting that this might be an important potential target for the development of new anti-asthma drugs.[256] BAY 61-3606, a potent and selective inhibitor of Syk kinase-inhibited lipid mediator release, cytokine synthesis and mast cell degranulation, had inhibitory effects on human basophils, eosinophils and monocytes,[257] and attenuated ovalbumin-induced airway inflammation in rats.[257] The Syk inhibitor, R112, given topically rapidly reduced symptoms of allergic rhinitis,[258] and its follow-up, R343, began phase I studies in asthma in late 2007.

PI3K inhibition

Phosphoinositide 3-kinases (PI3Ks) catalyse the phosphorylation of phosphoinositides and regulate a number of distinct cellular responses including cell growth/division, cell apoptosis/survival and activation in response to cytokines, antigens and costimulatory molecules.[242,259] PI3Ks may also contribute to the pathogenesis of asthma by affecting airway smooth muscle proliferation and eosinophil recruitment.[242,259] PI3Kγ is involved in neutrophil recruitment and activation. Knockout of the PI3Kγ gene results in inhibition of neutrophil migration and activation.[260] Intriguingly, knockout models of PI3Kγ failed to restore corticosteroid sensitivity after cigarette smoke exposure. In contrast, PI3Kδ-deficient mice were able to maintain corticosteroid efficacy after cigarette smoke exposure.[261] This suggests that a combination of a PI3Kγ and a PI3Kδ inhibitor could be of therapeutic benefit for COPD, as it would be both anti-inflammatory and restorative of corticosteroid function. The broad specificity profile and associated toxicity of existing PI3K inhibitors limits their current use in asthma and COPD.[262] However, isoform-specific small molecule inhibitors of PI3Kγ and PI3Kδ are in development. Moreover, a combined PI3Kγ/PI3Kδ inhibitor may prove the most effective in COPD given the evidence above.

8.12   Inhibition of transcription factors in asthma and COPD

NF-κB

NF-κB is induced by many factors involved in asthmatic inflammation including allergen challenge, cytokines, chemokines, and bacterial and viral infections, and induces the expression of many mediators, growth factors, receptors and enzymes important in the inflammatory cascade, leading to a feed-forward enhancement of inflammation.[241] NF-κB activation is enhanced in mild asthma and further increased in severe asthma,[263, 264] and genetic studies also implicate the NF-κB pathway in CSR asthma.[265] NF-κB expression and activity are also enhanced in COPD lung particularly during exacerbations.[266–268] Small molecule inhibitors targeting the stimulating kinase (inhibitor of IκB kinase-2, or IKK2) completely suppressed inflammatory responses in animal models of asthma and in BAL macrophages from asthmatics[269,270] (Figure 8.6). Targeting IKK2 may also have additional benefits as it appears that current IKK2 inhibitors can also modulate the corticosteroid-insensitive IP10 release induced by IFN-γ[271,272] and directly modulate mast cell degranulation.[273] There are concerns, however, that inhibition of NF-κB may cause side effects, such as increased susceptibility to infections.[241] Delivery by inhalation may decrease the risk of serious side effects, and these drugs may be particularly effective for exacerbations.

NF-κB is a major target for corticosteroids, and downstream coactivators or corepressors may also be potential therapeutic targets as steroid-sparing agents. Histone deacetylase 2 (HDAC2) recruitment is involved in GR-mediated suppression of NF-κB, and its expression and activity are reduced in some corticosteroid-insensitive diseases.[274, 275] Importantly, overexpression of HDAC2 in corticosteroid-insensitive cells can restore corticosteroid responsiveness.[276] The suppression of HDAC2 activity may be due to tyrosine nitration,[276] further implicating a potential therapeutic role for antioxidants or nitric oxide synthase 2 (NOS2) inhibitors in restoring corticosteroid responsiveness. Theophylline and curcumin both enhance HDAC2 activity under conditions of oxidative stress leading to a restoration of corticosteroid responsiveness.[267,277] This may explain why adding a low, sub-bronchodilator dose of theophylline is more effective than increasing the dose of inhaled corticosteroids in patients with poorly controlled disease and why theophylline withdrawal worsens control of patients with severe asthma.[278]

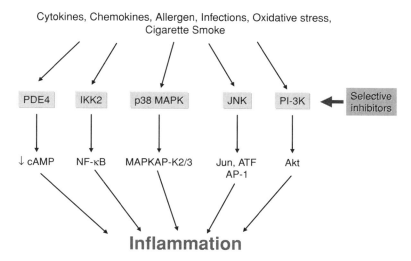

Figure 8.6   Many stimuli including cytokines, allergens, chemokines and infectious agents known to be important in asthma and asthma exacerbations can activate key intracellular signalling pathways in a cell- and stimulus-dependent manner. Activation of these pathways results in enhanced recruitment and activation of infiltrating and resident cell types and increases the expression of inflammatory mediators including other cytokines and chemokines that can act, in turn, in either an autocrine and/or paracrine manner to further drive the inflammatory response in asthma. Selective inhibitors of these pathways are under development with the intention of dampening the inflammatory response. Some of these pathways (e.g. IKK2 and MAPK) are also implicated in corticosteroid function, and suppression of these may be corticosteroid-sparing. In addition, inhibitors of Syk kinase are able to prevent mast cell degranulation. Abbreviations: Akt, v-akt murine thymoma viral oncogene homolog; AP-1, activator protein-1; ATF, activating transcription factor; cAMP, cyclic adenosine monophosphate; IKK, inhibitor of κB kinase; JNK, c-Jun N-terminal kinase; MAPK, mitogen-activated protein kinase; MAPKAP-K, MAPK-activated protein kinase; NF-κB, nuclear factor κB; PDE, phosphodiesterase; PI3K, phosphoinositide-3 kinase; Syk, spleen tyrosine kinase.

GATA-3

GATA-3 expression is markedly increased in T-cells and bronchial biopsies from asthmatics,[279,280] and in BAL cells after allergen challenge.[281] GATA-3 also regulates early T-cell development in the thymus, the differentiation of invariant natural killer T-cells (iNKT cells),[282] and participates in the control of regulatory T-cells (T_{reg}).[283] GATA-3 plays a critical role in Th2 differentiation from naive $CD4^+$ cells,[282] and knockdown of GATA-3 expression using siRNA in human T-cells results in loss of anti-CD3/CD28-mediated Th2 cytokine expression.[284] This suggests that GATA-3 antisense may be a novel but excellent preventative therapy for asthma[285] (Figure 8.6).

NF-AT

Nuclear factor of activated T-cells (NF-AT) also regulates Th2 cytokine release by forming complexes with GATA-3 and AP-1 (Figure 8.6). The immunosuppressive drugs ciclosporin A (CsA), FK506 (tacrolimus) and pimecrolimus block calcineurin-dependent dephosphorylation of NF-AT thereby preventing its activation.[286] Systemic administration of CsA to patients with severe asthma has provided some improvement in lung function but has unacceptable side effects.[285] It is hoped that the development of MLD987, an inhaled derivative of these drugs, may reduce the side effects.[285] Alternative strategies for inhibiting NF-AT include using peptides that block the docking of calcineurin to NF-AT (inhibitors of NF-AT–calcineurin association, or INCA).[285] As described above, the numbers of CD4$^+$ and CD8$^+$ T-cells are also increased in COPD, and drugs that are directed against T-cell activation may also have a role in COPD.

STATs

The STAT (signal transducer and activator of transcription) proteins are the primary signal-specific mediators of cytokine-regulated gene expression activated by receptor-associated Janus kinases (JAKs) (Figure 8.6). For example, IL-4 and IL-12 drive Th2 and Th1 cell differentiation respectively through activation of STAT6 and STAT4.[286] Of the many STAT proteins, only STAT6 is unique to the asthma-related cytokines IL-4 and IL-13,[145] whereas the expression of STAT4 is enhanced in COPD.[140] This suggests that targeting JAK/STAT pathways could be an effective therapeutic strategy for asthma and COPD. Interestingly, a STAT1 decoy oligonucleotide (AVT-01) has proved successful in an animal model of asthma[287] and is now in phase IIa clinical trials.[145]

FOXP3

The characteristics of T$_{reg}$ cells have made these cells attractive candidates for immunotherapy.[288] The activity of T$_{reg}$ cells is under the control of the transcription factor forkhead box P3 (FOXP3). Stable overexpression or induction of FOXP3 by retinoic acid drives the conversion of naive T-cells to T$_{reg}$ cells, and this has been proposed to modulate asthmatic inflammation.[288] FOXP3 mRNA expression is also significantly decreased in the lungs of patients with COPD.[142]

PPARs

Peroxisome proliferator-activated receptors (PPARs) are nuclear receptors activated by polyunsaturated fatty acid derivatives, oxidized fatty acids and phospholipids.[289] PPARγ ligands decrease antigen-induced airway hyperresponsiveness, lung inflammation and eosinophilia, cytokine production and GATA-3 expression as well as serum levels of antigen-specific IgE in different animal models of asthma.[289] In contrast, rosiglitazone, a synthetic PPARγ agonist, can decrease TNF-α-mediated, but not cigarette smoke-mediated, cytokine release from monocytes. Cigarette smoke prevented PPARγ nuclear translocation, interaction with NF-κB and thus attenuation of cytokine release.[290]

No formal trials of PPARγ ligands have been reported for asthma to date. However, an intriguing case in a diabetic patient with asthma who was treated with pioglitazone has been reported.[291] This patient, who was prescribed pioglitazone for diabetes, experienced improvement in their asthma, which subsequently worsened upon drug withdrawal. Clinical studies are needed to evaluate the clinical effect of PPARγ ligands in both asthma and COPD.

Activation of PPARγ also alters dendritic cell (DC) maturation, and rosiglitazone reduces the proliferation of antigen-specific T-cells whilst increasing IL-10 production by these cells.[289] Interestingly, the panel of inflammatory genes regulated by PPARγ agonists is distinct from that regulated by corticosteroids, and the combination of both a PPARγ agonist and a corticosteroid may have a greater anti-inflammatory effect,[292] particularly since corticosteroids can induce PPARγ expression.[293]

8.13   Antioxidants in asthma and COPD

Oxidative stress has been implicated as a driving force behind the inflammatory response and lack of corticosteroid sensitivity in severe asthma and COPD.[62] Oxidative stress activates transcription factors, such as NF-κB and AP-1, which switch on multiple inflammatory genes, including CXC chemokines, thus leading to neutrophilic inflammation. Oxidative stress is further increased in acute exacerbations of asthma and COPD as a result of viral and/or bacterial infection of the respiratory tract.[62] Moreover, oxidative stress and its by-products may drive a Th2-dependent immune response.[294] The antioxidant butylated hydroxyanisole reduces respiratory syncytial virus-induced neutrophilic inflammation and airway hyperresponsiveness in a murine model.[295] Antioxidants including N-acetylcysteine (NAC), nacystelyn (NAL) and the SOD mimetic AEOL 10150 can restore corticosteroid functions that were reduced in response to cigarette smoke or other oxidative stresses in both primary human cells and in animal models,[62] but current antioxidants do not appear to affect the redox balance in the airways in humans. Therefore, smarter and more potent drugs are required to target the correct cellular compartment. Oxidative stress in combination with the high nitric oxide (NO) levels seen in asthma[296] will result in the formation of peroxynitrite, tyrosine nitration and lipid peroxidation products,[297] and this has been linked to corticosteroid insensitivity.[298] Nitric oxide synthase 2 (NOS2) inhibitors have recently been shown to be safe, but ineffective, in mild asthma,[299] but they may play an important role in treatment of patients with severe asthma and in smoking asthmatics who have increased levels of oxidative/nitrosative stress.[62]

Resveratrol (3,5,4'-trihydroxystilbene), a component of red wine, has anti-inflammatory and antioxidant properties.[62] Although resveratrol inhibits cytokine release by alveolar macrophages from COPD patients it is not clear if this is due to its antioxidant properties. Nevertheless, this compound may also be beneficial for patients with severe asthma.[300] Similarly, curcumin has many therapeutic properties dues to its antioxidant, anti-inflammatory and anticancer effects, albeit at micromolar concentrations.[200,277] Most importantly, however, curcumin did show nanomolar potency against restoration of steroid function in oxidant-stressed cells well below the micromolar concentrations required for propagation of its antioxidant and other therapeutic properties.[277] Furthermore, despite the low bioavailability of curcumin following oral application it is now in phase I clinical studies for several respiratory diseases.[301]

8.14   Immunomodulation and anti-allergy treatments in asthma and COPD

Anti-IgE

Since asthmatic patients are often atopic much effort has been directed at modulating the allergic response (Figure 8.1). IgE is the immunoglobulin that mediates the acute allergic response in mast cells and basophils through cross-linking of high-affinity IgE receptors, and may increase allergen uptake by dendritic cells. A humanized monoclonal antibody that binds to IgE (omalizumab) has been introduced for the treatment of severe allergic persistent asthma. Omalizumab is a useful add-on therapy in some patients who are affected by frequent exacerbations since it reduces the rate of exacerbations,[302] but it is expensive and its cost-effectiveness is debated.[303] Other more potent anti-IgE antibodies are in development and other strategies also being considered include the development of peptide-based vaccines or immunotherapeutics to induce IgE-specific antibodies. An antibody directed against the low-affinity IgE receptor (FceRII or CD23), lumiliximab, reduces IgE concentrations in atopic subjects.[304] A similar effect has been reported in mild asthma from the same group but the results have not been published in full.[305] Development of therapies directed at T-cell costimulatory molecules such as CD23, ICOS and OX40 is also progressing.[145]

Dendritic cells

Dendritic cells (DC) mount and maintain immune responses to inhaled allergen, and modulating their function represents a new approach to asthma treatment. The sphingosine-1 phosphate receptor antagonist, FTY720, strongly attenuates established lung inflammation in mice through inhibition of DC activation,[306] and is currently in clinical trials for the treatment of multiple sclerosis and transplant rejection.[306] Selective prostaglandin receptor agonists such as BW245C also suppress DC function, leading to decreased airway inflammation and bronchial hyperreactivity in a mouse model of asthma through the induction of FoxP3$^+$ T_{reg} cells.[307] A similar mechanism may account for the actions of the prostacyclin analogue, iloprost.[159]

Immunomodulatory therapies offer the opportunity to reverse the abnormal immune function observed in asthma by enhancing T_{reg} expression/function or altering T-cell class switching away from the Th2 response.[308] Sublingual immunotherapy (SLIT) has been used in asthma although questions remain about effective doses, treatment schedules and treatment duration.[309]

Specific subcutaneous immunotherapy increases IL-10 production from T_{reg} cells,[308,310] and allergen-specific T-cell peptides that enhance T_{reg} function and increase IL-10 release are now under development.[95] Treating T_{reg} cells from CSR subjects with vitamin D_3 in combination with dexamethasone restores the ability of these cells to release IL-10.[311] This, in turn, allows IL-10 to upregulate GR expression and reverses the dexamethasone-induced reduction in GR expression. Impressively, oral administration of vitamin D_3 (0.5 μg daily) for 7 days to corticosteroid resistant (CR) asthmatic patients enhanced *ex vivo* T_{reg} responses to dexamethasone.[311] This suggests that vitamin D_3 could potentially increase the therapeutic response to glucocorticoids in CR patients.

In addition, significantly fewer T_{reg} cells were found in the lungs of patients with COPD, with reduced gene expression for FOXP3, a transcription factor crucial for the development of T_{reg} cells, and less IL-10 secretion, which could allow for clonal expansion of elastin-specific Th1 cells.[142] By contrast, in cells recovered by BAL, increased numbers of $CD4^+CD25^+$ expressing cells were reported in smokers and COPD patients compared to non-smokers, with increased FOXP3 expression in these cells.[312] The reason for this discrepant result compared to those reported in lung tissue remains unclear. Invariant killer T-cells are not increased in COPD as assessed in sputum, BAL and in biopsies of central airways.[313]

The observation of increased numbers of B-cells and the presence of bronchus-associated lymphoid tissue in advanced COPD[13,314] (not usually present in healthy non-smokers) may reflect an adaptive immune response to chronic infection that is frequent at this stage. Lymphoid follicles consisting of B-cells and follicular dendritic cells with adjacent T-cells were demonstrated in both the parenchyma and bronchial walls of patients with emphysema,[315] and an oligoclonal, antigen-specific reaction of the B-cells is described. Plasma cells, which are derived from maturation of B-cells, were found to be in greater numbers in subepithelial and submucosal glands in COPD compared to asymptomatic smokers, and a majority of these cells were expressing IL-4 and IL-5.[104] The B-cell increase may also reflect a role for autoimmune responses, and this is supported by the reduced numbers of T_{reg} cells reported in lungs of COPD patients.[142] B-cells in COPD lung may be producing antibodies to various endogenous proteins such as elastin.[142]

Further evidence for a recruitment of DCs by cigarette smoke exposure comes from studies of mice where chronic cigarette exposure led to an increase in $CD11c^+$ DCs, associated with increased levels of CCL2 and CCL20.[316] Mice deficient in CCR6 expressed on pulmonary DCs and B-cells showed less emphysema after cigarette smoke exposure,[130] possibly through the inhibition of MMP-12 release from dendritic cells.[317] Other mechanisms of the initiation and perpetuation of airway inflammation and emphysema by DCs following cigarette smoke exposure remain to be studied.

Another mechanism by which dendritic cells could be involved in COPD is through inhibition of Th1 immunity and preferential induction of Th2 responses. Cigarette smoke extract inhibited DC-mediated priming of T-cells by human monocyte-derived DCs, with inhibition of IFN-γ and enhancement of IL-4 production.[318] However, the relevance of this is unclear as some studies have shown that IFN-γ levels are actually increased in COPD patients.[133,140]

Interferons

Human interferons (IFNs) are grouped into type I IFNs (IFN-α, IFN-β, IFN-ε, IFN-κ and IFN-ω), and type II IFN (IFN-γ). A new family of interferons, called type III IFN-lambdas (IFN-λs) and characterized by three elements – λ1, λ2 and λ3, also respectively named IL-29, IL-28A and IL-28B – has recently been described. These three highly homologous IFN-λ proteins demonstrate only limited ($\sim$20%) homology to cytokines from both type I IFNs and IL-10 families.[319]

Interferon-gamma

Interferon-gamma (IFN-γ) is synthesized principally by type 1 NK cells and T-cells. IFN-γ affects diverse aspects of innate immunity, such as the activation of macrophages, and has strong effects on acquired immune responses, promoting the development of type 1 while suppressing type 2 T-cell functions. Furthermore, IFN-γ strongly induces the nitric oxide synthase type 2 (iNOS) enzyme that leads to increased production of nitric oxide (NO), a potent antiviral defence. IFN-γ inhibits Th2/Tc2 lymphocyte differentiation and should therefore reduce airway inflammation in asthma. However, the subcutaneous administration of recombinant human IFN-γ has not been shown to be effective in the treatment of severe glucocorticoid-dependent asthma.[320]

Interferon-alpha/beta

Most types of virus-infected cells are capable of synthesizing IFN-α/β in cell culture. In addition to their antiviral effects, IFN-α/β are also known to contribute indirectly to the response by affecting cells of the immune system. IFN-α/β are crucial in the activation of NK cells and macrophages; they also directly affect the fate of CD8$^+$ T-cell proliferation and may therefore be critical for inducing effective B-cell responses. Intramuscular administration of IFN-α2a to oral glucocorticoid-dependent asthmatic patients (with or without Churg–Strauss syndrome) dramatically improves their asthma control.[321] Interestingly, intramuscular administration of IFN-α to hepatitis C virus (HCV)$^+$-asthmatic patients already being treated with inhaled glucocorticoids also improves their asthma control.[322] Taken collectively, these studies suggest a potential role for IFN-α treatment as a steroid-sparing strategy in asthmatic patients. *In vitro*, primary bronchial epithelial cells from asthmatic patients are more susceptible to rhinovirus (RV) infection compared to those obtained from normal subjects.[323] RV RNA expression and late RV release are increased 50- and 7-fold, respectively, in asthmatic cells compared with normal subjects, and RV infection induces late cell lysis in asthmatic cells but not in normal cells.[323] This is associated with RV-induced inhibition of apoptotic responses, caspase 3/7 activity, and IFN-β production in the asthmatic cells.[323] In RV-infected asthmatic cells, exogenous IFN-β induces apoptosis and reduces RV replication, demonstrating a causal link between deficient IFN-β, impaired apoptosis and increased virus replication.[323] There are ongoing phase I clinical trials on the administration by inhalation of recombinant human IFN-β to asthmatic patients (see www.synairgen.com).

Lambda interferons

Human IFN-λs bind to a unique heterodimeric receptor (IFN-λR), composed of IFN-λR1 (also designated CRF2–12) and IL10-R2 (also designated CRF2–4) shared with other class II cytokine-receptor ligands including IL-10, IL-22 and IL-26. A defect in the production of IFN-λ in response to RV infection has been described in bronchial epithelial cells of asthmatic patients.[324] This suggests that a treatment with human recombinant IFN-λ may be useful in the treatment of RV-induced asthmatic exacerbations, where there is a relative steroid resistance.[325]

Immunostimulatory oligodeoxynucleotides

The potential of non-selective skewing of the T-cell response in asthma using non-pathogenic bacterial products, such as immunostimulatory oligodeoxynucleotides (ISS-ODNs) including CpG oligodeoxynucleotides, which target Toll-like receptor-9 (TLR-9), is under active investigation.[326] However, early indications in asthma are not encouraging despite evidence of a robust increase in IFN-γ and IFN-γ-inducible genes.[327] The long-term consequences of this approach also need to be carefully evaluated, particularly as they would probably need to be used in young children before the onset of asthma.

8.15   Conclusions

Several new treatments are now under development for asthma and COPD but many of them are highly specific, targeting a single receptor, enzyme or mediator, and are unlikely to have a major clinical impact. They also have a high barrier to overcome in that combination therapy is efficacious and it is likely that once-a-day fast-onset LABA/steroid combinations will be available soon. Due to the overexpression of IL-13 in asthma and its role in many immuno-inflammatory processes in asthma it is possible that biologicals targeted against the IL-13 receptor may buck this trend. A similar case may be made for inhaled p38 MAPK and IKK2 inhibitors in COPD. Although we have not discussed these issues here, drug delivery and comorbidities will impact on the pharmacopoeia used to treat all patients with asthma and COPD.

Prospects for a cure in asthma are currently remote but might arise from the development of vaccines and immune therapies directed against T_{reg} and Th17 cells such as vitamin D_3/steroid combinations. It is important to recognize that distinct subgroups of patients may respond better to particular therapies such as those targeting the LT pathway although it is unlikely that these will be successful as monotherapies. Similarly, drugs reversing the lung destruction and airway remodelling seen in COPD are unlikely to be available in the near future.

There are several approaches that can be taken to treat these patients with severe and treatment-refractory disease. The type of inflammation in these patients may be distinct, and targeting this inflammation with selective therapeutic agents such as inhaled p38 MAPK and IKK2 inhibitors may be beneficial. More selective targeting of drugs to patients with particular subtypes of asthma might be possible in the future with the development of discriminatory handprints of clinical phenotypes, biomarkers and genetic profiles. Rapid tests that distinguish these subtypes may make the advent of selective therapy closer and more effective.

An alternative approach is to try to restore steroid sensitivity rather than prevent inflammation per se. Understanding the multiple mechanisms underlying CSR asthma and COPD may indicate patient-specific abnormalities in signalling pathways that could be targeted to restore asthma control and these would include inhaled p38 MAPK and PI3K inhibitors resulting in a reduced need for inhaled or systemic corticosteroids.

Finally, the fact that combination therapies are more effective than a single therapy approach, as has been previously observed in the treatment of rheumatoid arthritis, emphasizes the need to examine multi-drug approaches to asthma tailored to the genotype/phenotype of the particular asthma and COPD subtypes.

Acknowledgements

We apologize to any authors not cited, but due to restrictions on the number of references we are unable to cite all the important original articles in this area and have cited key reviews in particular areas. We would like to thank members of the Department of Airways Disease for helpful discussions. Work in the authors' laboratories in this area is funded by Asthma UK, the Medical Research Council (UK), the Royal Society, the University of Ferrara and the Wellcome Trust.

References

1. Masoli M, Fabian D, Holt S, Beasley, R. The global burden of asthma: executive summary of the GINA Dissemination Committee report. Allergy 2004;59:469–78.
2. Lopez AD, Mathers CD, Ezzati M, Jamison DT, Murray CJ. Global and regional burden of disease and risk factors, 2001: systematic analysis of population health data. Lancet 2006;367:1747–57.
3. Barnes PJ, Kleinert S. COPD – a neglected disease. Lancet 2004;364:564–5.
4. Rabe KF, Hurd S, Anzueto A, et al. Global strategy for the diagnosis, management, and prevention of chronic obstructive pulmonary disease: GOLD executive summary. Am J Respir Crit Care Med 2007;176:532–55.
5. Nilunger L, Diderichsen F, Burstrom B, Ostlin P. Using risk analysis in Health Impact Assessment: the impact of different relative risks for men and women in different socio-economic groups. Health Policy 2004;67:215–24.
6. Barnes PJ, Jonsson B, Klim JB. The costs of asthma. Eur Respir J 1996;9:636–42.
7. Chung KF, Godard P, Adelroth E, et al. Difficult/therapy-resistant asthma: the need for an integrated approach to define clinical phenotypes, evaluate risk factors, understand pathophysiology and find novel therapies. ERS Task Force on Difficult/Therapy-Resistant Asthma. Eur Respir J 1999;13:1198–208.

8. Global Initiative for Asthma (GINA). Global Strategy for Asthma Management and Prevention. NHLBI/WHO Workshop report. 2002. NIH Publication 02-3659. Last update 2007. http://www.ginasthma.com (accessed 16 April 2008).

9. Barnes PJ. Immunology of asthma and chronic obstructive pulmonary disease. Nat Rev Immunol 2008;8:183–92.

10. Bateman ED, Hurd SS, Barnes PJ, et al. Global strategy for asthma management and prevention: GINA executive summary. Eur Respir J 2008;31:143–78.

11. Global Initiative for Chronic Obstructive Lung Disease. Global Strategy for the Diagnosis, Management and Prevention of Chronic Obstructive Pulmonary Disease (GOLD). NHLBI/WHO workshop report. Bethesda, National Heart, Lung and Blood Institute, April 2001; NIH Publication No 2701:1-100. Last update 2007. http://www.goldcopd.com (accessed 1 September 2008).

12. Barnes PJ. Chronic obstructive pulmonary disease. N Engl J Med 2000;343:269–80.

13. Hogg JC, Chu F, Utokaparch S, et al. The nature of small-airway obstruction in chronic obstructive pulmonary disease. N Engl J Med 2004;350:2645–53.

14. Di Stefano A, Caramori G, Ricciardolo FL, Capelli A, Adcock IM, Donner CF. Cellular and molecular mechanisms in chronic obstructive pulmonary disease: an overview. Clin Exp Allergy 2004;34:1156–67.

15. Papi A, Bellettato CM, Braccioni F, et al. Infections and airway inflammation in chronic obstructive pulmonary disease severe exacerbations. Am J Respir Crit Care Med 2006;173:1114–21.

16. Retamales I, Elliott WM, Meshi B, et al. Amplification of inflammation in emphysema and its association with latent adenoviral infection. Am J Respir Crit Care Med 2001;164:469–73.

17. Barnes PJ. Alveolar macrophages as orchestrators of COPD. COPD 2004;1:59–70.

18. Wenzel SE. Asthma: defining of the persistent adult phenotypes. Lancet 2006;368:804–13.

19. Holgate ST. Pathogenesis of asthma. Clin Exp Allergy 2008;38:872–97.

20. Chanez P, Vignola AM, O'Shaugnessy T, et al. Corticosteroid reversibility in COPD is related to features of asthma. Am J Respir Crit Care Med 1997;155:1529–34.

21. Barnes PJ. Inhaled glucocorticoids for asthma. N Engl J Med 1995;332:868–75.

22. Ito K, Chung KF, Adcock IM. Update on glucocorticoid action and resistance. J Allergy Clin Immunol 2006;117:522–43.

23. Suissa S, Ernst P. Inhaled corticosteroids: impact on asthma morbidity and mortality. J Allergy Clin Immunol 2001;107:937–44.

24. Schacke H, Docke WD, Asadullah K. Mechanisms involved in the side effects of glucocorticoids. Pharmacol Ther 2002;96:23–43.

25. Rabe KF, Adachi M, Lai CK, et al. Worldwide severity and control of asthma in children and adults: the global asthma insights and reality surveys. J Allergy Clin Immunol 2004;114:40–7.

26. Jeffery PK, Venge P, Gizycki MJ, Egerod I, Dahl R, Faurschou P. Effects of salmeterol on mucosal inflammation in asthma: a placebo-controlled study. Eur Respir J 2002;20:1378–85.

27. Maneechotesuwan K, Essilfie-Quaye S, Meah S, et al. Formoterol attenuates neutrophilic airway inflammation in asthma. Chest 2005;128:1936–42.

28. Chung KF, Adcock IM. Combination therapy of long-acting beta2-adrenoceptor agonists and corticosteroids for asthma. Treat Respir Med 2004;3:279–89.

29. Postma DS, Kerstjens HA, ten Hacken NH. Inhaled corticosteroids and long-acting beta-agonists in adult asthma: a winning combination in all? N-S Arch Pharmacol 2008;378:203–15.

30. Appleton S, Smith B, Veale A, Bara A. Long-acting beta2-agonists for chronic obstructive pulmonary disease. Cochrane Database Syst Rev 2000;(2):CD001104.

31. Johnson M, Rennard S. Alternative mechanisms for long-acting beta(2)-adrenergic agonists in COPD. Chest 2001;120:258–70.

32. Ayers ML, Mejia R, Ward J, Lentine T, Mahler DA. Effectiveness of salmeterol versus ipratropium bromide on exertional dyspnoea in COPD. Eur Respir J 2001;17:1132–7.

33. Jarvis B, Markham A. Inhaled salmeterol: a review of its efficacy in chronic obstructive pulmonary disease. Drugs Aging 2001;18:441–72.

34. Rennard SI, Anderson W, ZuWallack R, et al. Use of a long-acting inhaled beta2-adrenergic agonist, salmeterol xinafoate, in patients with chronic obstructive pulmonary disease. Am J Respir Crit Care Med 2001;163:1087–92.

35. D'Urzo AD, De Salvo MC, Ramirez-Rivera A, et al. In patients with COPD, treatment with a combination of formoterol and ipratropium is more effective than a combination of salbutamol and ipratropium: a 3-week, randomized, double-blind, within-patient, multicenter study. Chest 2001;119:1347–56.

36. Dahl R, Greefhorst LA, Nowak D, et al. Inhaled formoterol dry powder versus ipratropium bromide in chronic obstructive pulmonary disease. Am J Respir Crit Care Med 2001;164:778–84.

37. Calverley PM, Anderson JA, Celli B, et al. Salmeterol and fluticasone propionate and survival in chronic obstructive pulmonary disease. N Engl J Med 2007;356:775–89.

38. Calverley P, Pauwels R, Vestbo J, et al. Combined salmeterol and fluticasone in the treatment of chronic obstructive pulmonary disease: a randomised controlled trial. Lancet 2003;361:449–56.

39. Calverley PM, Boonsawat W, Cseke Z, Zhong N, Peterson S, Olsson H. Maintenance therapy with budesonide and formoterol in chronic obstructive pulmonary disease. Eur Respir J 2003;22:912–19.

40. Szafranski W, Cukier A, Ramirez A, et al. Efficacy and safety of budesonide/formoterol in the management of chronic obstructive pulmonary disease. Eur Respir J 2003;21:74–81.

41. Martinez FD. Safety of long-acting beta-agonists – an urgent need to clear the air. N Engl J Med 2005;353:2637–9.

42. Salpeter SR, Buckley NS, Ormiston TM, Salpeter EE. Meta-analysis: effect of long-acting beta-agonists on severe asthma exacerbations and asthma-related deaths. Ann Intern Med 2006;144:904–12.

43. Barnes NC, Qiu YS, Pavord ID, et al. Antiinflammatory effects of salmeterol/fluticasone propionate in chronic obstructive lung disease. Am J Respir Crit Care Med 2006;173:736–43.

44. Tennant RC, Erin EM, Barnes PJ, Hansel TT. Long-acting beta 2-adrenoceptor agonists or tiotropium bromide for patients with COPD: is combination therapy justified? Curr Opin Pharmacol 2003;3:270–6.

45. Barr RG, Bourbeau J, Camargo CA, Ram FS. Tiotropium for stable chronic obstructive pulmonary disease: A meta-analysis. Thorax 2006;61:854–62.

46. Caramori G, Adcock I. Pharmacology of airway inflammation in asthma and COPD. Pulm Pharmacol Ther 2003;16:247–77.

47. Racke K, Matthiesen S. The airway cholinergic system: physiology and pharmacology. Pulm Pharmacol Ther 2004;17:181–98.

48. Barnes PJ. The role of anticholinergics in chronic obstructive pulmonary disease. Am J Med 2004;117(Suppl. 12A):24S–32S.

49. Tashkin DP, Celli B, Decramer M, et al. Bronchodilator responsiveness in patients with COPD. Eur Respir J 2008;31:742–50.

50. Bateman ED, Boushey HA, Bousquet J, et al. Can guideline-defined asthma control be achieved? The Gaining Optimal Asthma ControL study. Am J Respir Crit Care Med 2004;170:836–44.

51. Moore WC, Bleecker ER, Curran-Everett D et al. Characterization of the severe asthma phenotype by the National Heart, Lung, and Blood Institute's Severe Asthma Research Program. J Allergy Clin Immunol 2007;119:405–13.
52. Anon. The ENFUMOSA cross-sectional European multicentre study of the clinical phenotype of chronic severe asthma. European Network for Understanding Mechanisms of Severe Asthma. Eur Respir J 2003;22:470–7.
53. Kamel N, Compton C, Middelveld R, Higenbottam T, Dahlen SE. The Innovative Medicines Initiative (IMI): a new opportunity for scientific collaboration between academia and industry at the European level. Eur Respir J 2008;31:924–26.
54. Bourdin A, Neveu D, Vachier I, Paganin F, Godard P, Chanez P. Specificity of basement membrane thickening in severe asthma. J Allergy Clin Immunol 2007;119:1367–74.
55. Cohen L, Xueping E, Tarsi J, et al. Epithelial cell proliferation contributes to airway remodeling in severe asthma. Am J Respir Crit Care Med 2007;176:138–45.
56. Brasier AR, Victor S, Boetticher G, et al. Molecular phenotyping of severe asthma using pattern recognition of bronchoalveolar lavage-derived cytokines. J Allergy Clin Immunol 2008;121:30–7.
57. Haldar P, Pavord ID, Shaw DE, et al. Cluster analysis and clinical asthma phenotypes. Am J Respir Crit Care Med 2008;178:218–24.
58. Dragonieri S, Schot R, Mertens BJ, et al. An electronic nose in the discrimination of patients with asthma and controls. J Allergy Clin Immunol 2007;120:856–62.
59. Wenzel SE, Schwartz LB, Langmack EL, et al. Evidence that severe asthma can be divided pathologically into two inflammatory subtypes with distinct physiologic and clinical characteristics. Am J Respir Crit Care Med 1999;160:1001–8.
60. Barnes PJ. Mechanisms in COPD: differences from asthma. Chest 2000;117(2 Suppl.):10S–14S.
61. Barnes PJ, Ito K, Adcock IM. Corticosteroid resistance in chronic obstructive pulmonary disease: inactivation of histone deacetylase. Lancet 2004;363:731–3.
62. Kirkham P, Rahman I. Oxidative stress in asthma and COPD: antioxidants as a therapeutic strategy. Pharmacol Ther 2006;111:476–94.
63. Barnes PJ. Mediators of chronic obstructive pulmonary disease. Pharmacol Rev 2004;56:515–48.
64. Johnson M. Molecular mechanisms of beta(2)-adrenergic receptor function, response, and regulation. J Allergy Clin Immunol 2006;117:18–24.
65. Matera MG, Cazzola M. Ultra-long-acting beta2-adrenoceptor agonists: an emerging therapeutic option for asthma and COPD? Drugs 2007;67:503–15.
66. Derendorf H. Pharmacokinetic and pharmacodynamic properties of inhaled ciclesonide. J Clin Pharmacol 2007;47:782–9.
67. Usmani OS, Ito K, Maneechotesuwan K, et al. Glucocorticoid receptor nuclear translocation in airway cells after inhaled combination therapy. Am J Respir Crit Care Med 2005;172:704–12.
68. Reichardt HM, Tuckermann JP, Gottlicher M, et al. Repression of inflammatory responses in the absence of DNA binding by the glucocorticoid receptor. EMBO J 2001;20:7168–73.
69. Schacke H, Berger M, Rehwinkel H, Asadullah K. Selective glucocorticoid receptor agonists (SEGRAs): Novel ligands with an improved therapeutic index. Mol Cell Endocrinol 2007;275:109–17.
70. Miner JN, Ardecky B, Benbatoul K, et al. Antiinflammatory glucocorticoid receptor ligand with reduced side effects exhibits an altered protein-protein interaction profile. Proc Natl Acad Sci U S A 2007;104:19244–9.

71. Nevin BJ, Broadley KJ. Comparative effects of inhaled budesonide and the NO-donating budes-onide derivative, NCX 1020, against leukocyte influx and airway hyperreactivity following lipopolysaccharide challenge. Pulm Pharmacol Ther 2004;17:219–32.

72. Paul-Clark MJ, Roviezzo F, Flower R, et al. Glucocorticoid receptor nitration leads to enhanced anti-inflammatory effects of novel steroid ligands. J Immunol 2003;171:3245–52.

73. Lagente V, Advenier C. New nitric oxide-donating drugs for the treatment of airway diseases. Curr Opin Investig Drugs 2004;5:537–41.

74. Dahlen SE. Treatment of asthma with antileukotrienes: first line or last resort therapy? Eur J Pharmacol 2006;533:40–56.

75. Jayaram L, Duong M, Pizzichini MM, et al. Failure of montelukast to reduce sputum eosinophilia in high-dose corticosteroid-dependent asthma. Eur Respir J 2005;25:41–6.

76. Lazarus SC, Chinchilli VM, Rollings NJ, et al. Smoking affects response to inhaled cor-ticosteroids or leukotriene receptor antagonists in asthma. Am J Respir Crit Care Med 2007;175:783–90.

77. Coreno A, Skowronski M, Kotaru C, McFadden ER Jr. Comparative effects of long-acting beta2-agonists, leukotriene receptor antagonists, and a 5-lipoxygenase inhibitor on exercise-induced asthma. J Allergy Clin Immunol 2000;106:500–6.

78. Montuschi P, Kharitonov SA, Ciabattoni G, Barnes PJ. Exhaled leukotrienes and prostaglandins in COPD. Thorax 2003;58:585–8.

79. Profita M, Giorgi RD, Sala A, et al. Muscarinic receptors, leukotriene B4 production and neutrophilic inflammation in COPD patients. Allergy 2005;60:1361–9.

80. Biernacki WA, Kharitonov SA, Barnes PJ. Increased leukotriene B4 and 8-isoprostane in exhaled breath condensate of patients with exacerbations of COPD. Thorax 2003;58:294–8.

81. Crooks SW, Stockley RA. Leukotriene B4. Int J Biochem Cell Biol 1998;30:173–8.

82. Drazen JM. Leukotrienes as mediators of airway obstruction. Am J Respir Crit Care Med 1998;158:S193–S200.

83. Gompertz S, Stockley RA. A randomized, placebo-controlled trial of a leukotriene synthesis inhibitor in patients with COPD. Chest 2002;122:289–94.

84. Marian E, Baraldo S, Visentin A, et al. Up-regulated membrane and nuclear leukotriene B4 receptors in COPD. Chest 2006;129:1523–30.

85. Medina-Tato DA, Watson ML, Ward SG. Leukocyte navigation mechanisms as targets in airway diseases. Drug Discov Today 2006;11:866–79.

86. Beeh KM, Kornmann O, Buhl R, Culpitt SV, Giembycz MA, Barnes PJ. Neutrophil chemotactic activity of sputum from patients with COPD: role of interleukin 8 and leukotriene B4. Chest 2003;123:1240–7.

87. Evans DJ, Barnes PJ, Spaethe SM, van Alstyne EL, Mitchell MI, O'Connor BJ. Effect of a leukotriene B4 receptor antagonist, LY293111, on allergen induced responses in asthma. Thorax 1996;51:1178–84.

88. Gronke L, Beeh KM, Cameron R, et al. Effect of the oral leukotriene B4 receptor antago-nist LTB019 on inflammatory sputum markers in patients with chronic obstructive pulmonary disease. Pulm Pharmacol Ther 2008;21:409–17.

89. Peters-Golden M, Henderson WR Jr. Leukotrienes. N Engl J Med 2007;357:1841–54.

90. Pettipher R, Hansel TT, Armer R. Antagonism of the prostaglandin D2 receptors DP1 and CRTH2 as an approach to treat allergic diseases. Nat Rev Drug Discov 2007;6:313–25.

91. Rolin S, Masereel B, Dogne JM. Prostanoids as pharmacological targets in COPD and asthma. Eur J Pharmacol 2006;533:89–100.

92. Skogvall S Dalence-Guzman MF, Berglund M, et al. Discovery of a potent and long-acting bronchorelaxing capsazepinoid, RESPIR 4-95. Pulm Pharmacol Ther 2008;21:125–33.

93. Levy BD, Lukacs NW, Berlin AA, et al. Lipoxin A4 stable analogs reduce allergic airway responses via mechanisms distinct from CysLT1 receptor antagonism. FASEB J 2007;21:3877–84.

94. Vachier I, Bonnans C, Chavis C, et al. Severe asthma is associated with a loss of LX4, an endogenous anti-inflammatory compound. J Allergy Clin Immunol 2005;115:55–60.

95. Barnes PJ. New therapies for asthma. Trends Mol Med 2006;12:515–20.

96. Viola A, Luster AD. Chemokines and their receptors: drug targets in immunity and inflammation. Annu Rev Pharmacol Toxicol 2008;48:171–97.

97. Ying S, Robinson DS, Meng Q, et al. Enhanced expression of eotaxin and CCR3 mRNA and protein in atopic asthma. Association with airway hyperresponsiveness and predominant co-localization of eotaxin mRNA to bronchial epithelial and endothelial cells. Eur J Immunol 1997;27:3507–16.

98. Ravensberg AJ, Ricciardolo FL, van Schadewijk A, et al. Eotaxin-2 and eotaxin-3 expression is associated with persistent eosinophilic bronchial inflammation in patients with asthma after allergen challenge. J Allergy Clin Immunol 2005;115:779–85.

99. Gauvreau GM, Boulet LP, Cockcroft DW, et al. Antisense therapy against CCR3 and the common beta chain attenuates allergen-induced eosinophilic responses. Am J Respir Crit Care Med 2008;177:952–8.

100. Das AM, Vaddi KG, Solomon KA, et al. Selective inhibition of eosinophil influx into the lung by small molecule CC chemokine receptor 3 antagonists in mouse models of allergic inflammation. J Pharmacol Exp Ther 2006;318:411–17.

101. Wegmann M, Goggel R, Sel S, et al. Effects of a low-molecular-weight CCR-3 antagonist on chronic experimental asthma. Am J Respir Cell Mol Biol 2007;36:61–7.

102. Chung KF, Adcock IM. Multifaceted mechanisms in COPD: inflammation, immunity, and tissue repair and destruction. Eur Respir J 2008;31:1334–56.

103. Zhu J, Qiu YS, Majumdar S, et al. Exacerbations of bronchitis: bronchial eosinophilia and gene expression for interleukin-4, interleukin-5, and eosinophil chemoattractants. Am J Respir Crit Care Med 2001;164:109–16.

104. Zhu J, Qiu Y, Valobra M, et al. Plasma cells and IL-4 in chronic bronchitis and chronic obstructive pulmonary disease. Am J Respir Crit Care Med 2007;175:1125–33.

105. Panina-Bordignon P, Papi A, Mariani M, et al. The C-C chemokine receptors CCR4 and CCR8 identify airway T cells of allergen-challenged atopic asthmatics. J Clin Invest 2001;107:1357–64.

106. Kallinich T, Schmidt S, Hamelmann E, et al. Chemokine-receptor expression on T cells in lung compartments of challenged asthmatic patient. Clin Exp Allergy 2005;35:26–33.

107. Donnelly LE, Barnes PJ. Chemokine receptors as therapeutic targets in chronic obstructive pulmonary disease. Trends Pharmacol Sci 2006;27:546–53.

108. Keatings VM, Collins PD, Scott DM, Barnes PJ. Differences in interleukin-8 and tumor necrosis factor-alpha in induced sputum from patients with chronic obstructive pulmonary disease or asthma. Am J Respir Crit Care Med 1996;153:530–4.

109. Yamamoto C, Yoneda T, Yoshikawa M, et al. Airway inflammation in COPD assessed by sputum levels of interleukin-8. Chest 1997;112:505–10.

110. Gompertz S, O'Brien C, Bayley DL, Hill SL, Stockley RA. Changes in bronchial inflammation during acute exacerbations of chronic bronchitis. Eur Respir J 2001;17:1112–19.

111. Yang XD, Corvalan JR, Wang P, Roy CM, Davis CG. Fully human anti-interleukin-8 monoclonal antibodies: potential therapeutics for the treatment of inflammatory disease states. J Leukoc Biol 1999;66:401–10.

112. Mahler DA, Huang S, Tabrizi M, Bell GM. Efficacy and safety of a monoclonal antibody recognizing interleukin-8 in COPD: a pilot study. Chest 2004;126:926–34.

113. Qiu Y, Zhu J, Bandi V, et al. Biopsy neutrophilia, neutrophil chemokine and receptor gene expression in severe exacerbations of chronic obstructive pulmonary disease. Am J Respir Crit Care Med 2003;168:968–75.
114. Qiu Y, Zhu J, Bandi V, Guntupalli KK, Jeffery PK. Bronchial mucosal inflammation and upregulation of CXC chemoattractants and receptors in severe exacerbations of asthma. Thorax 2007;62:475–82.
115. Traves SL, Culpitt SV, Russell RE, Barnes PJ, Donnelly LE. Increased levels of the chemokines GROalpha and MCP-1 in sputum samples from patients with COPD. Thorax 2002;57:590–5.
116. Jones CE, Chan K. Interleukin-17 stimulates the expression of interleukin-8, growth-related oncogene-alpha, and granulocyte-colony-stimulating factor by human airway epithelial cells. Am J Respir Cell Mol Biol 2002;26:748–53.
117. Prause O, Laan M, Lötvall J, Linden A. Pharmacological modulation of interleukin-17-induced GCP-2-, GRO-alpha- and interleukin-8 release in human bronchial epithelial cells. Eur J Pharmacol 2003;462:193–8.
118. Schulz, C, Kratzel K, Wolf K, Schroll S, Kohler M, Pfeifer M. Activation of bronchial epithelial cells in smokers without airway obstruction and patients with COPD. Chest 2004;125:1706–13.
119. Imaizumi T, Albertine KH, Jicha DL, McIntyre TM, Prescott SM, Zimmerman GA. Human endothelial cells synthesize ENA-78: relationship to IL-8 and to signaling of PMN adhesion. Am J Respir Cell Mol Biol 1997;17:181–92.
120. Tanino M, Betsuyaku T, Takeyabu K, Tanino Y, Yamaguchi E, Miyamoto K, Nishimura M. Increased levels of interleukin-8 in BAL fluid from smokers susceptible to pulmonary emphysema. Thorax 2002;57:405–11.
121. Costa C, Rufino R, Traves SL, et al. CXCR3 and CCR5 chemokines in induced sputum from patients with COPD. Chest 2008;133:26–33.
122. Fujimoto K, Yasuo M, Urushibata K, Hanaoka M, Koizumi T, Kubo K. Airway inflammation during stable and acutely exacerbated chronic obstructive pulmonary disease. Eur Respir J 2005;25:640–6.
123. Bracke KR, D'hulst AI, Maes T, et al. Cigarette smoke-induced pulmonary inflammation, but not airway remodelling, is attenuated in chemokine receptor 5-deficient mice. Clin Exp Allergy 2007;37:1467–79.
124. Dragic T, Trkola A, Thompson DA, et al. A binding pocket for a small molecule inhibitor of HIV-1 entry within the transmembrane helices of CCR5. Proc Natl Acad Sci U S A 2000;97:5639–44.
125. Schols D. HIV co-receptor inhibitors as novel class of anti-HIV drugs. Antiviral Res 2006;71:216–26.
126. Proudfoot AE, Power CA, Hoogewerf AJ, et al. Extension of recombinant human RANTES by the retention of the initiating methionine produces a potent antagonist. J Biol Chem 1996;271:2599–603.
127. Simmons G, Clapham PR, Picard L, et al. Potent inhibition of HIV-1 infectivity in macrophages and lymphocytes by a novel CCR5 antagonist. Science 1997;276:276–9.
128. Lederman MM, Veazey RS, Offord R, et al. Prevention of vaginal SHIV transmission in rhesus macaques through inhibition of CCR5. Science 2004;306:485–7.
129. Demedts IK, Bracke KR, Van PG, et al. Accumulation of dendritic cells and increased CCL20 levels in the airways of patients with chronic obstructive pulmonary disease. Am J Respir Crit Care Med 2007;175:998–1005.
130. Bracke KR, D'hulst AI, Maes T, et al. Cigarette smoke-induced pulmonary inflammation and emphysema are attenuated in CCR6-deficient mice. J Immunol 2006;177:4350–9.

131. Ying S, O'Connor B, Ratoff J, et al. Expression and cellular provenance of thymic stromal lymphopoietin and chemokines in patients with severe asthma and chronic obstructive pulmonary disease. J Immunol 2008;181:2790–8.

132. Saetta M, Mariani M, Panina-Bordignon P, et al. Increased expression of the chemokine receptor CXCR3 and its ligand CXCL10 in peripheral airways of smokers with chronic obstructive pulmonary disease. Am J Respir Crit Care Med 2002;165:1404–9.

133. Grumelli S, Corry DB, Song LZ, et al. An immune basis for lung parenchymal destruction in chronic obstructive pulmonary disease and emphysema. PLoS Med 2004;1:e8.

134. Freeman CM, Curtis JL, Chensue SW. CC chemokine receptor 5 and CXC chemokine receptor 6 expression by lung CD8+ cells correlates with chronic obstructive pulmonary disease severity. Am J Pathol 2007;171:767–76.

135. Godessart N. Chemokine receptors: attractive targets for drug discovery. Ann NY Acad Sci 2005;1051:647–57.

136. Gao P, Zhou XY, Yashiro-Ohtani Y, et al. The unique target specificity of a nonpeptide chemokine receptor antagonist: selective blockade of two Th1 chemokine receptors CCR5 and CXCR3. J Leukoc Biol 2003;73:273–80.

137. Lever R, Page CP. Novel drug development opportunities for heparin. Nat Rev Drug Discov 2002;1:140–8.

138. Turato G, Zuin R, Miniati M, et al. Airway inflammation in severe chronic obstructive pulmonary disease: relationship with lung function and radiologic emphysema. Am J Respir Crit Care Med 2002;166:105–110.

139. Barczyk A, Pierzchala W, Kon OM, Cosio B, Adcock IM, Barnes PJ. Cytokine production by bronchoalveolar lavage T lymphocytes in chronic obstructive pulmonary disease. J Allergy Clin Immunol 2006;117:1484–92.

140. Di Stefano A, Caramori G, Capelli A, et al. STAT4 activation in smokers and patients with chronic obstructive pulmonary disease. Eur Respir J 2004;24:78–85.

141. Sullivan AK, Simonian PL, Falta MT, et al. Oligoclonal CD4+ T cells in the lungs of patients with severe emphysema. Am J Respir Crit Care Med 2005;172:590–6.

142. Lee SH, Goswami S, Grudo A, et al. Antielastin autoimmunity in tobacco smoking-induced emphysema. Nat Med 2007;13:567–9.

143. Therien AG, Bernier V, Weicker S, et al. Adenovirus IL-13-induced airway disease in mice: a corticosteroid-resistant model of severe asthma. Am J Respir Cell Mol Biol 2008;39:26–35.

144. Borish LC, Nelson HS, Corren J, et al. Efficacy of soluble IL-4 receptor for the treatment of adults with asthma. J Allergy Clin Immunol 2001;107:963–70.

145. Caramori G, Groneberg D, Ito K, Casolari P, Adcock IM, Papi A. New drugs targeting Th2 lymphocytes in asthma. J Occup Med Toxicol 2008;3(Suppl. 1):S6.

146. Wenzel SE, Balzar S, Ampleford E, et al. IL4R alpha mutations are associated with asthma exacerbations and mast cell/IgE expression. Am J Respir Crit Care Med 2007;175:570–6.

147. Boutten A, Bonay M, Laribe S, et al. Decreased expression of interleukin 13 in human lung emphysema. Thorax 2004;59:850–4.

148. Miotto D, Ruggieri MP, Boschetto P, et al. Interleukin-13 and -4 expression in the central airways of smokers with chronic bronchitis. Eur Respir J 2003;22:602–8.

149. Zheng T, Zhu Z, Wang Z, et al. Inducible targeting of IL-13 to the adult lung causes matrix metalloproteinase- and cathepsin-dependent emphysema. J Clin Invest 2000;106:1081–93.

150. Hoshino T, Kato S, Oka N, et al. Pulmonary inflammation and emphysema: role of the cytokines IL-18 and IL-13. Am J Respir Crit Care Med 2007;176:49–62.

151. Wang Z, Zheng T, Zhu Z, et al. Interferon gamma induction of pulmonary emphysema in the adult murine lung. J Exp Med 2000;192:1587–600.
152. Kips JC, O'Connor BJ, Langley SJ, et al. Effect of SCH55700, a humanized anti-human interleukin-5 antibody, in severe persistent asthma: a pilot study. Am J Respir Crit Care Med 2003;167:1655–9.
153. Leckie MJ, ten Brinke A, Khan J, et al. Effects of an interleukin-5 blocking monoclonal antibody on eosinophils, airway hyper-responsiveness, and the late asthmatic response. Lancet 2000;356:2144–8.
154. Flood-Page P, Menzies-Gow A, Phipps S, et al. Anti-IL-5 treatment reduces deposition of ECM proteins in the bronchial subepithelial basement membrane of mild atopic asthmatics. J Clin Invest 2003;112:1029–36.
155. Rothenberg ME, Klion AD, Roufosse FE, et al. Treatment of patients with the hypereosinophilic syndrome with mepolizumab. N Engl J Med 2008;358:1215–28.
156. Busse WW, Ring J, Huss-Marp J, Kahn JE. A review of treatment with mepolizumab, an anti-IL-5 mAb, in hypereosinophilic syndromes and asthma. J Allergy Clin Immunol. 2010;125:803–813.
157. Tamaoki J, Kondo M, Sakai N, et al. Effect of suplatast tosilate, a Th2 cytokine inhibitor, on steroid-dependent asthma: a double-blind randomised study. Tokyo Joshi-Idai Asthma Research Group. Lancet 2000;356:273–8.
158. Tohda Y, Kubo H, Haraguchi R, Iwanaga T, Fukuoka M. Effects of suplatast tosilate (IPD Capsules) on the production of active oxygen by neutrophils and of IL-8 by mononuclear cells. Int Immunopharmacol 2001;1:1183–7.
159. Hammad H, Lambrecht BN. Dendritic cells and epithelial cells: linking innate and adaptive immunity in asthma. Nat Rev Immunol 2008;8:193–204.
160. Liu YJ, Soumelis V, Watanabe N, et al. TSLP: an epithelial cell cytokine that regulates T cell differentiation by conditioning dendritic cell maturation. Annu Rev Immunol 2007;25:193–219.
161. Zhang K, Shan L, Rahman MS, Unruh H, Halayko AJ, Gounni AS. Constitutive and inducible thymic stromal lymphopoietin expression in human airway smooth muscle cells: role in chronic obstructive pulmonary disease. Am J Physiol Lung Cell Mol Physiol 2007;293:L375–L382.
162. Lim S, Crawley E, Woo P, Barnes PJ. Haplotype associated with low interleukin-10 production in patients with severe asthma. Lancet 1998;352:113.
163. Tomita K, Lim S, Hanazawa T, et al. Attenuated production of intracellular IL-10 and IL-12 in monocytes from patients with severe asthma. Clin Immunol 2002;102:258–66.
164. Bryan SA, O'Connor BJ, Matti S, et al. Effects of recombinant human interleukin-12 on eosinophils, airway hyper-responsiveness, and the late asthmatic response. Lancet 2000;356:2149–53.
165. Barnes PJ. New treatments for chronic obstructive pulmonary disease. Curr Opin Pharmacol 2001;1:217–22.
166. Barnes PJ. Cytokine modulators as novel therapies for asthma. Annu Rev Pharmacol Toxicol 2002;42:81–98.
167. Numerof RP, Asadullah K. Cytokine and anti-cytokine therapies for psoriasis and atopic dermatitis. BioDrugs 2006;20:93–103.
168. Zhu J, Majumdar S, Qiu Y, et al. Interleukin-4 and interleukin-5 gene expression and inflammation in the mucus-secreting glands and subepithelial tissue of smokers with chronic bronchitis. Lack of relationship with CD8(+) cells. Am J Respir Crit Care Med 2001;164:2220–2228.
169. Bradding P, Roberts JA, Britten KM, et al. Interleukin-4, -5, and -6 and tumor necrosis factor-alpha in normal and asthmatic airways: evidence for the human mast cell as a source of these cytokines. Am J Respir Cell Mol Biol 1994;10:471–80.

170. Virchow JC Jr, Walker C, Hafner D, et al. T cells and cytokines in bronchoalveolar lavage fluid after segmental allergen provocation in atopic asthma. Am J Respir Crit Care Med 1995;151:960–8.
171. Li L, Das AM, Torphy TJ, Griswold DE. What's in the pipeline? Prospects for monoclonal antibodies (mAbs) as therapies for lung diseases. Pulm Pharmacol Ther 2002;15:409–16.
172. Erin EM, Leaker BR, Nicholson GC, et al. The effects of a monoclonal antibody directed against tumor necrosis factor-alpha in asthma. Am J Respir Crit Care Med 2006;174:753–62.
173. Berry MA, Hargadon B, Shelley M, et al. Evidence of a role of tumor necrosis factor alpha in refractory asthma. N Engl J Med 2006;354:697–708.
174. Howarth PH, Babu KS, Arshad HS, et al. Tumour necrosis factor (TNFalpha) as a novel therapeutic target in symptomatic corticosteroid dependent asthma. Thorax 2005;60:1012–18.
175. Morjaria JB, Chauhan AJ, Babu KS, Polosa R, Davies DE, Holgate ST. The role of a soluble TNFalpha receptor fusion protein (etanercept) in corticosteroid refractory asthma: a double blind, randomised, placebo controlled trial. Thorax 2008;63:584–91.
176. Rennard SI, Fogarty C, Kelsen S, et al. The safety and efficacy of infliximab in moderate-to-severe chronic obstructive pulmonary disease. Am J Respir Crit Care Med 2007;175:926–34.
177. Suissa S, Ernst P, Hudson M. TNF-alpha antagonists and the prevention of hospitalisation for chronic obstructive pulmonary disease. Pulm Pharmacol Ther 2008;21:234–8.
178. Noguera A, Busquets X, Sauleda J, Villaverde JM, Macnee W, Agusti AG. Expression of adhesion molecules and G proteins in circulating neutrophils in chronic obstructive pulmonary disease. Am J Respir Crit Care Med 1998;158:1664–8.
179. Yamagata T, Sugiura H, Yokoyama T, et al. Overexpression of CD-11b and CXCR1 on circulating neutrophils: its possible role in COPD. Chest 2007;132:890–9.
180. Pignatti P, Moscato G, Casarini S, et al. Downmodulation of CXCL8/IL-8 receptors on neutrophils after recruitment in the airways. J Allergy Clin Immunol 2005;115:88–94.
181. Hidalgo A, Peired AJ, Wild MK, Vestweber D, Frenette PS. Complete identification of E-selectin ligands on neutrophils reveals distinct functions of PSGL-1, ESL-1, and CD44. Immunity 2007;26:477–89.
182. Di Stefano A, Maestrelli P, Roggeri A, et al. Upregulation of adhesion molecules in the bronchial mucosa of subjects with chronic obstructive bronchitis. Am J Respir Crit Care Med 1994;149:803–10.
183. Yoshikawa T, Dent G, Ward J, et al. Impaired neutrophil chemotaxis in chronic obstructive pulmonary disease. Am J Respir Crit Care Med 2007;175:473–9.
184. Yasuda M, Nakano K, Yasumoto K, Tanaka Y. CD44: functional relevance to inflammation and malignancy. Histol Histopathol 2002;17:945–50.
185. Kipnis A, Basaraba RJ, Turner J, Orme IM. Increased neutrophil influx but no impairment of protective immunity to tuberculosis in mice lacking the CD44 molecule. J Leukoc Biol 2003;74:992–7.
186. Araya J, Cambier S, Markovics JA, et al. Squamous metaplasia amplifies pathologic epithelial-mesenchymal interactions in COPD patients. J Clin Invest 2007;117:3551–62.
187. Pilette C, Colinet B, Kiss R, et al. Increased galectin-3 expression and intraepithelial neutrophils in small airways in severe chronic obstructive pulmonary disease. Eur Respir J 2007;29:914–22.
188. de Boer WI, Sont JK, van Schadewijk A, Stolk J, van Krieken JH, Hiemstra PS. Monocyte chemoattractant protein 1, interleukin 8, and chronic airways inflammation in COPD. J Pathol 2000;190:619–26.
189. Takizawa H, Tanaka M, Takami K, et al. Increased expression of transforming growth factor-beta1 in small airway epithelium from tobacco smokers and patients with chronic obstructive pulmonary disease (COPD). Am J Respir Crit Care Med 2001;163:1476–83.

190. Takizawa H, Tanaka M, Takami K, et al. Increased expression of transforming growth factor-beta1 in small airway epithelium from tobacco smokers and patients with chronic obstructive pulmonary disease (COPD). Am J Respir Crit Care Med 2001;163:1476–83.

191. Vignola AM, Chanez P, Chiappara G, et al. Transforming growth factor-beta expression in mucosal biopsies in asthma and chronic bronchitis. Am J Respir Crit Care Med 1997;156:591–9.

192. Kranenburg AR, Willems-Widyastuti A, Mooi WJ, et al. Chronic obstructive pulmonary disease is associated with enhanced bronchial expression of FGF-1, FGF-2, and FGFR-1. J Pathol 2005;206:28–38.

193. Pierrou S, Broberg P, O'Donnell RA, et al. Expression of genes involved in oxidative stress responses in airway epithelial cells of smokers with chronic obstructive pulmonary disease. Am J Respir Crit Care Med 2007;175:577–86.

194. Ning W, Li CJ, Kaminski N, et al. Comprehensive gene expression profiles reveal pathways related to the pathogenesis of chronic obstructive pulmonary disease. Proc Natl Acad Sci U S A 2004;101:14895–900.

195. Wang H, Liu X, Umino T, et al. Effect of cigarette smoke on fibroblast-mediated gel contraction is dependent on cell density. Am J Physiol Lung Cell Mol Physiol 2003;284:L205–L213.

196. Murphy-Ullrich JE, Poczatek M. Activation of latent TGF-beta by thrombospondin-1: mechanisms and physiology. Cytokine Growth Factor Rev 2000;11:59–69.

197. Mu D, Bessho T, Nechev LV, et al. DNA interstrand cross-links induce futile repair synthesis in mammalian cell extracts. Mol Cell Biol 2000;20:2446–54.

198. Munger JS, Huang X, Kawakatsu H, et al. The integrin alpha v beta 6 binds and activates latent TGF beta 1: a mechanism for regulating pulmonary inflammation and fibrosis. Cell 1999;96:319–28.

199. Lee K-Y, Ho S-C, Lin H-C, et al. Neutrophil-derived elastase induces TGFβ secretion in human airway smooth muscle via NFκB pathway. Am J Respir Cell Mol Biol 2006;35:407–14.

200. Rahman I, Biswas SK, Kirkham PA. Regulation of inflammation and redox signaling by dietary polyphenols. Biochem Pharmacol 2006;72:1439–52.

201. Kurie JM, Shin HJ, Lee JS, et al. Increased epidermal growth factor receptor expression in metaplastic bronchial epithelium. Clin Cancer Res 1996;2:1787–93.

202. O'Donnell RA, Richter A, Ward J, et al. Expression of ErbB receptors and mucins in the airways of long term current smokers. Thorax 2004;59:1032–40.

203. Lapperre TS, Sont JK, van Schadewijk A, et al. Smoking cessation and bronchial epithelial remodelling in COPD: a cross-sectional study. Respir Res 2007;8:85.

204. Hodkinson PS, Mackinnon A, Sethi T. Targeting growth factors in lung cancer. Chest 2008;133:1209–16.

205. Peto R, Speizer FE, Cochrane AL, et al. The relevance in adults of air-flow obstruction, but not of mucus hypersecretion, to mortality from chronic lung disease. Results from 20 years of prospective observation. Am Rev Respir Dis 1983;128:491–500.

206. de Marco R, Accordini S, Cerveri I, et al. Incidence of chronic obstructive pulmonary disease in a cohort of young adults according to the presence of chronic cough and phlegm. Am J Respir Crit Care Med 2007;175:32–9.

207. Barnes PJ. Current and future therapies for airway mucus hypersecretion. Novartis Found Symp 2002;248:237–49.

208. Zheng JP, Kang J, Huang SJ, et al. Effect of carbocisteine on acute exacerbation of chronic obstructive pulmonary disease (PEACE Study): a randomised placebo-controlled study. Lancet 2008;371:2013–18.

209. Caramori G, Di Gregorio C, Carlstedt I, et al. Mucin expression in peripheral airways of patients with chronic obstructive pulmonary disease. Histopathology 2004;45:477–84.

210. Fahy JV. Goblet cell and mucin gene abnormalities in asthma. Chest 2002;122(6 Suppl.): 320S–326S.

211. Rose MC, Voynow JA. Respiratory tract mucin genes and mucin glycoproteins in health and disease. Physiol Rev 2006;86:245–78.

212. Bjornsson E, Hjelm E, Janson C, Fridell E, Boman G. Serology of chlamydia in relation to asthma and bronchial hyperresponsiveness. Scand J Infect Dis 1996;28:63–9.

213. Hahn DL. Infection as a cause of asthma. Ann Allergy 1994;73:276.

214. Von Hertzen L, Toyryla M, Gimishanov A, et al. Asthma, atopy and Chlamydia pneumoniae antibodies in adults. Clin Exp Allergy 1999;29:522–8.

215. Kraft M, Cassell GH, Henson JE, et al. Detection of Mycoplasma pneumoniae in the airways of adults with chronic asthma. Am J Respir Crit Care Med 1998;158:998–1001.

216. Larsen FO, Norn S, Mordhorst CH, Skov PS, Milman N, Clementsen P. Chlamydia pneumoniae and possible relationship to asthma. Serum immunoglobulins and histamine release in patients and controls. Acta Pathol Microbiol Immunol Scand 1998;106:928–34.

217. Mills GD, Lindeman JA, Fawcett JP, Herbison GP, Sears MR. Chlamydia pneumoniae serological status is not associated with asthma in children or young adults. Int J Epidemiol 2000;29:280–4.

218. Routes JM, Nelson HS, Noda JA, Simon FT. Lack of correlation between Chlamydia pneumoniae antibody titers and adult-onset asthma. J Allergy Clin Immunol 2000;105:391–2.

219. Yano T, Ichikawa Y, Komatu S, Arai S, Oizumi K. Association of Mycoplasma pneumoniae antigen with initial onset of bronchial asthma [see comments]. Am J Respir Crit Care Med 1994;149:1348–53.

220. Chu HW, Kraft M, Rex MD, Martin RJ. Evaluation of blood vessels and edema in the airways of asthma patients: regulation with clarithromycin treatment. Chest 2001;120:416–22.

221. Johnston SL, Blasi F, Black PN, Martin RJ, Farrell DJ, Nieman RB. The effect of telithromycin in acute exacerbations of asthma. N. Engl J Med 2006;354:1589–600.

222. Simpson JL, Powell H, Boyle MJ, Scott RJ, Gibson PG. Clarithromycin targets neutrophilic airway inflammation in refractory asthma. Am J Respir Crit Care Med 2008;177:148–55.

223. Beaty CD, Grayston JT, Wang SP, Kuo CC, Reto CS, Martin TR. Chlamydia pneumoniae, strain TWAR, infection in patients with chronic obstructive pulmonary disease. Am Rev Respir Dis 1991;144:1408–10.

224. Verkooyen RP, Van Lent NA, Mousavi Joulandan SA, et al. Diagnosis of Chlamydia pneumoniae infection in patients with chronic obstructive pulmonary disease by micro-immunofluorescence and ELISA. J Med Microbiol 1997;46:959–64.

225. Von Hertzen L, Alakarppa H, Koskinen R, et al. Chlamydia pneumoniae infection in patients with chronic obstructive pulmonary disease. Epidemiol Infect 1997;118:155–64.

226. Gencay M, Dereli D, Ertem E, et al. Prevalence of Chlamydia pneumoniae specific antibodies in different clinical situations and healthy subjects in Izmir, Turkey. Eur J Epidemiol 1998;14:505–9.

227. Gencay M, Rudiger JJ, Tamm M, Soler M, Perruchoud AP, Roth M. Increased frequency of Chlamydia pneumoniae antibodies in patients with asthma. Am J Respir Crit Care Med 2001;163:1097–100.

228. Theegarten D, Mogilevski G, Anhenn O, Stamatis G, Jaeschock R, Morgenroth K. The role of chlamydia in the pathogenesis of pulmonary emphysema. Electron microscopy and immunofluorescence reveal corresponding findings as in atherosclerosis. Virchows Arch 2000;437:190–3.

229. Wu L, Skinner SJ, Lambie N, Vuletic JC, Blasi F, Black PN. Immunohistochemical staining for Chlamydia pneumoniae is increased in lung tissue from subjects with chronic obstructive pulmonary disease. Am J Respir Crit Care Med 2000;162:1148–51.

230. Strachan, DP, Carrington D, Mendall M, Butland BK, Yarnell JW, Elwood P. Chlamydia pneumoniae serology, lung function decline, and treatment for respiratory disease. Am J Respir Crit Care Med 2000;161:493–7.

231. Feleszko W, Jaworska J, Hamelmann E. Toll-like receptors – novel targets in allergic airway disease (probiotics, friends and relatives). Eur J Pharmacol 2006;533:308–18.

232. Bellattato C, Adcock IM, Ito K, et al. Rhinovirus infection reduces glucocorticoid receptor nuclear translocation in airway epithelial cells. Eur Respir J 2003;22(Suppl.):565S.

233. Solit DB, Chiosis G. Development and application of Hsp90 inhibitors. Drug Discov Today 2008;13:38–43.

234. Bundschuh DS, Eltze M, Barsig J, Wollin L, Hatzelmann A, Beume R. In vivo efficacy in airway disease models of roflumilast, a novel orally active PDE4 inhibitor. J Pharmacol Exp Ther 2001;297:280–90.

235. Chung KF. Phosphodiesterase inhibitors in airways disease. Eur J Pharmacol 2006;533:110–17.

236. Bousquet J, Aubier M, Sastre J, et al. Comparison of roflumilast, an oral anti-inflammatory, with beclomethasone dipropionate in the treatment of persistent asthma. Allergy 2006;61: 72–8.

237. Gamble E, Grootendorst DC, Hattotuwa K, et al. Airway mucosal inflammation in COPD is similar in smokers and ex-smokers: a pooled analysis. Eur Respir J 2007;30:467–71.

238. Boswell-Smith V, Spina D. PDE4 inhibitors as potential therapeutic agents in the treatment of COPD-focus on roflumilast. Int J Chron Obstruct Pulmon Dis 2007;2:121–9.

239. Leclerc O, Lagente V, Planquois JM, et al. Involvement of MMP-12 and phosphodiesterase type 4 in cigarette smoke-induced inflammation in mice. Eur Respir J 2006;27:1102–9.

240. Gamble E, Grootendorst DC, Brightling CE, et al. Antiinflammatory effects of the phosphodiesterase-4 inhibitor cilomilast (Ariflo) in chronic obstructive pulmonary disease. Am J Respir Crit Care Med 2003;168:976–82.

241. Adcock IM, Chung KF, Caramori G, Ito K. Kinase inhibitors and airway inflammation. Eur J Pharmacol 2006;533:118–32.

242. Ito K, Caramori G, Adcock IM. Therapeutic potential of phosphatidylinositol 3-kinase inhibitors in inflammatory respiratory disease. J Pharmacol Exp Ther 2007;321:1–8.

243. Adcock IM, Lane SJ. Corticosteroid-insensitive asthma: molecular mechanisms. J Endocrinol 2003;178:347–55.

244. Li LB, Goleva E, Hall CF, Ou LS, Leung DY. Superantigen-induced corticosteroid resistance of human T cells occurs through activation of the mitogen-activated protein kinase kinase/extracellular signal-regulated kinase (MEK-ERK) pathway. J Allergy Clin. Immunol 2004;114:1059–69.

245. Tsitoura DC, Rothman PB. Enhancement of MEK/ERK signaling promotes glucocorticoid resistance in CD4+ T cells. J Clin Invest 2004;113:619–27.

246. Bhavsar P, Hew M, Khorasani N, et al. Relative corticosteroid insensitivity of alveolar macrophages in severe asthma compared to non-severe asthma. Thorax 2008;63:784–90.

247. Renda T, Baraldo S, Pelaia G, et al. Increased activation of p38 MAPK in COPD. Eur Respir J 2008;31:62–9.

248. Underwood DC, Osborn RR, Bochnowicz S, et al. SB 239063, a p38 MAPK inhibitor, reduces neutrophilia, inflammatory cytokines, MMP-9, and fibrosis in lung. Am J Physiol Lung Cell Mol Physiol 2000;279:L895–L902.

249. Medicherla S, Fitzgerald MF, Spicer D, et al. p38alpha-selective mitogen-activated protein kinase inhibitor SD-282 reduces inflammation in a subchronic model of tobacco smoke-induced airway inflammation. J Pharmacol Exp Ther 2008;324:921–9.
250. Kotlyarov A, Neininger A, Schubert C, et al. MAPKAP kinase 2 is essential for LPS-induced TNF-alpha biosynthesis. Nat Cell Biol 1999;1:94–7.
251. Sousa AR, Lane SJ, Soh C, Lee TH. In vivo resistance to corticosteroids in bronchial asthma is associated with enhanced phosphorylation of JUN N-terminal kinase and failure of prednisolone to inhibit JUN N-terminal kinase phosphorylation. J Allergy Clin Immunol 1999;104: 565–74.
252. Eynott PR, Nath P, Leung SY, Adcock IM, Bennett BL, Chung KF. Allergen-induced inflammation and airway epithelial and smooth muscle cell proliferation: role of Jun N-terminal kinase. Br J Pharmacol 2003;140:1373–80.
253. Nath P, Eynott P, Leung SY, Adcock IM, Bennett BL, Chung KF. Potential role of c-Jun NH2-terminal kinase in allergic airway inflammation and remodelling: effects of SP600125. Eur J Pharmacol 2005;506:273–83.
254. Williams AS, Issa R, Leung SY, et al. Attenuation of ozone-induced airway inflammation and hyper-responsiveness by c-Jun NH2 terminal kinase inhibitor SP600125. J Pharmacol Exp Ther 2007;322:351–9.
255. Costello PS, Turner M, Walters AE, et al. Critical role for the tyrosine kinase Syk in signalling through the high affinity IgE receptor of mast cells. Oncogene 1996;13:2595–605.
256. Yousefi S, Hoessli DC, Blaser K, Mills GB, Simon HU. Requirement of Lyn and Syk tyrosine kinases for the prevention of apoptosis by cytokines in human eosinophils. J Exp Med 1996;183:1407–14.
257. Yamamoto N, Takeshita K, Shichijo M, et al. The orally available spleen tyrosine kinase inhibitor 2-[7-(3,4-dimethoxyphenyl)-imidazo[1,2-c]pyrimidin-5-ylamino]nicotinamide dihydrochloride (BAY 61-3606) blocks antigen-induced airway inflammation in rodents. J Pharmacol Exp Ther 2003;306:1174–81.
258. Meltzer EO, Berkowitz RB, Grossbard EB. An intranasal Syk-kinase inhibitor (R112) improves the symptoms of seasonal allergic rhinitis in a park environment. J Allergy Clin Immunol 2005;115:791–96.
259. Finan PM, Thomas MJ. PI 3-kinase inhibition: a therapeutic target for respiratory disease. Biochem Soc Trans 2004;32:378–82.
260. Sasaki T, Irie-Sasaki J, Jones RG, et al. Function of PI3Kgamma in thymocyte development, T cell activation, and neutrophil migration. Science 2000;287:1040–6.
261. Marwick JA, Stevenson CS, Barnes PJ, Ito K, Adcock IM, Kirkham PA. Cigarette smoke reduces steroid sensitivity by reducing glucocorticoid receptor (GR) and GR co-repressor expression. Proc Am Thorac Soc 2008;5:A333.
262. Marone R, Cmiljanovic V, Giese B, Wymann MP. Targeting phosphoinositide 3-kinase: moving towards therapy. Biochim Biophys Acta 2008;1784:159–85.
263. Gagliardo R, Chanez P, Mathieu M, et al. Persistent activation of nuclear factor-kappaB signaling pathway in severe uncontrolled asthma. Am J Respir Crit Care Med 2003;168:1190–8.
264. Hart LA, Krishnan VL, Adcock IM, Barnes PJ, Chung KF. Activation and localization of transcription factor, nuclear factor-kappaB, in asthma. Am J Respir Crit Care Med 1998;158: 1585–92.
265. Hakonarson H, Bjornsdottir US, Halapi E, et al. Profiling of genes expressed in peripheral blood mononuclear cells predicts glucocorticoid sensitivity in asthma patients. Proc Natl Acad Sci U S A 2005;102:14789–94.

266. Caramori G, Romagnoli M, Casolari P, et al. Nuclear localisation of p65 in sputum macrophages but not in sputum neutrophils during COPD exacerbations. Thorax 2003;58:348–51.
267. Cosio BG, Tsaprouni L, Ito K, Jazrawi E, Adcock IM, Barnes PJ. Theophylline restores histone deacetylase activity and steroid responses in COPD macrophages. J Exp Med 2004;200:689–95.
268. Di Stefano A, Caramori G, Oates T, et al. Increased expression of nuclear factor-kappaB in bronchial biopsies from smokers and patients with COPD. Eur Respir J 2002;20:556–63.
269. Birrell MA, Hardaker E, Wong S, et al. Ikappa-B kinase-2 inhibitor blocks inflammation in human airway smooth muscle and a rat model of asthma. Am J Respir Crit Care Med 2005;172:962–71.
270. Cosio BG, Mann B, Ito K et al. Histone acetylase and deacetylase activity in alveolar macrophages and blood mononocytes in asthma. Am J Respir Crit Care Med 2004;170: 141–7.
271. Tliba O, Damera G, Banerjee A, et al. Cytokines induce an early steroid resistance in airway smooth muscle cells: novel role of IRF-1. Am J Respir Cell Mol Biol 2008;38:463–72.
272. Tudhope SJ, Catley MC, Fenwick PS, et al. The role of IkappaB kinase 2, but not activation of NF-kappaB, in the release of CXCR3 ligands from IFN-gamma-stimulated human bronchial epithelial cells. J Immunol 2007;179:6237–45.
273. Suzuki K, Verma IM. Phosphorylation of SNAP-23 by IkappaB kinase 2 regulates mast cell degranulation. Cell 2008;134:485–95.
274. Bilodeau S, Vallette-Kasic S, Gauthier Y, et al. Role of Brg1 and HDAC2 in GR trans-repression of the pituitary POMC gene and misexpression in Cushing disease. Genes Dev 2006;20:2871–86.
275. Ito K, Ito M, Elliott WM, et al. Decreased histone deacetylase activity in chronic obstructive pulmonary disease. N Engl J Med 2005;352:1967–76.
276. Ito K, Yamamura S, Essilfie-Quaye S, et al. Histone deacetylase 2-mediated deacetylation of the glucocorticoid receptor enables NF-kappaB suppression. J Exp Med 2006;203:7–13.
277. Meja KK, Rajendrasozhan S, Adenuga D, et al. Curcumin restores corticosteroid function in monocytes exposed to oxidants by maintaining HDAC2. Am J Respir Cell Mol. Biol. 2008;39:312–23.
278. Barnes PJ. How corticosteroids control inflammation: Quintiles Prize Lecture 2005. Br J Pharmacol 2006;148:245–54.
279. Caramori G, Lim S, Ito K, et al. Expression of GATA family of transcription factors in T-cells, monocytes and bronchial biopsies. Eur Respir J 2001;18:466–73.
280. Nakamura Y, Ghaffar O, Olivenstein R, et al. Gene expression of the GATA-3 transcription factor is increased in atopic asthma. J Allergy Clin Immunol 1999;103:215–22.
281. Erpenbeck VJ, Hagenberg A, Krentel H, et al. Regulation of GATA-3, c-maf and T-bet mRNA expression in bronchoalveolar lavage cells and bronchial biopsies after segmental allergen challenge. Int Arch Allergy Immunol 2006;139:306–16.
282. Ho IC, Pai SY. GATA-3 – not just for Th2 cells anymore. Cell Mol Immunol 2007;4:15–29.
283. Mantel PY, Kuipers H, Boyman O, et al. GATA3-driven Th2 responses inhibit TGF-beta1-induced FOXP3 expression and the formation of regulatory T cells. PLoS Biol 2007;5:e329.
284. Maneechotesuwan K, Xin Y, Ito K, et al. Regulation of Th2 cytokine genes by p38 MAPK-mediated phosphorylation of GATA-3. J Immunol 2007;178:2491–8.
285. Cousins DJ, McDonald J, Lee TH. Therapeutic approaches for control of transcription factors in allergic disease. J Allergy Clin Immunol 2008;121:803–9.
286. O'Shea JJ, Murray PJ. Cytokine signaling modules in inflammatory responses. Immunity 2008;28:477–87.

287. Quarcoo D, Weixler S, Groneberg D, et al. Inhibition of signal transducer and activator of transcription 1 attenuates allergen-induced airway inflammation and hyperreactivity. J Allergy Clin Immunol 2004;114:288–95.
288. Chatila TA, Li N, Garcia-Lloret M, Kim HJ, Nel AE. T-cell effector pathways in allergic diseases: transcriptional mechanisms and therapeutic targets. J Allergy Clin Immunol 2008;121: 812–23.
289. Belvisi MG, Hele DJ, Birrell MA. Peroxisome proliferator-activated receptor gamma agonists as therapy for chronic airway inflammation. Eur J Pharmacol 2006;533:101–9.
290. Caito S, Yang SR, Kode A, et al. Rosiglitazone and 15-deoxy-Delta12,14-prostaglandin J2, PPARgamma agonists, differentially regulate cigarette smoke-mediated pro-inflammatory cytokine release in monocytes/macrophages. Antioxid Redox Signal 2008;10:253–60.
291. Hashimoto Y, Nakahara K. Improvement of asthma after administration of pioglitazone. Diabetes Care 2002;25:401.
292. Ogawa S, Lozach J, Benner C, et al. Molecular determinants of crosstalk between nuclear receptors and toll-like receptors. Cell 2005;122:707–21.
293. Usami A, Ueki S, Ito W, et al. Theophylline and dexamethasone induce peroxisome proliferator-activated receptor-gamma expression in human eosinophils. Pharmacology 2006;77:33–7.
294. King MR, Ismail AS, Davis LS, Karp DR. Oxidative stress promotes polarization of human T cell differentiation toward a T helper 2 phenotype. J Immunol 2006;176:2765–72.
295. Castro SM, Guerrero-Plata A, Suarez-Real G, et al. Antioxidant treatment ameliorates respiratory syncytial virus-induced disease and lung inflammation. Am J Respir Crit Care Med 2006;174:1361–9.
296. Kharitonov SA, Barnes PJ. Effects of corticosteroids on noninvasive biomarkers of inflammation in asthma and chronic obstructive pulmonary disease. Proc Am Thorac Soc 2004;1:191–9.
297. Sugiura H, Komaki Y, Koarai A, Ichinose M. Nitrative stress in refractory asthma. J Allergy Clin Immunol 2008;121:355–60.
298. Kirkham, P. Oxidative stress and macrophage function: a failure to resolve the inflammatory response. Biochem Soc Trans 2007;35:284–7.
299. Singh D, Richards D, Knowles RG, et al. Selective inducible nitric oxide synthase inhibition has no effect on allergen challenge in asthma. Am J Respir Crit Care Med 2007;176: 988–93.
300. Culpitt SV, Rogers DF, Fenwick PS, et al. Inhibition by red wine extract, resveratrol, of cytokine release by alveolar macrophages in COPD. Thorax 2003;58:942–6.
301. Hsu CH, Cheng AL. Clinical studies with curcumin. Adv Exp Med Biol 2007;595:471–80.
302. Sthoeger ZM, Eliraz A, Asher I, Berkman N, Elbirt D. The beneficial effects of Xolair (omalizumab) as add-on therapy in patients with severe persistent asthma who are inadequately controlled despite best available treatment (GINA 2002 step IV) – the Israeli arm of the INNOVATE study. Isr Med Assoc J 2007;9:472–5.
303. Wu AC, Paltiel AD, Kuntz KM, Weiss ST, Fuhlbrigge AL. Cost-effectiveness of omalizumab in adults with severe asthma: results from the Asthma Policy Model. J Allergy Clin Immunol 2007;120:1146–52.
304. Poole JA, Meng J, Reff M, Spellman MC, Rosenwasser LJ. Anti-CD23 monoclonal antibody, lumiliximab, inhibited allergen-induced responses in antigen-presenting cells and T cells from atopic subjects. J Allergy Clin Immunol 2005;116:780–8.
305. Rosenwasser LJ, Meng J. Anti-CD23. Clin Rev Allergy Immunol 2005;29:61–72.
306. Idzko M, Hammad H, van Nimwegen M, et al. Local application of FTY720 to the lung abrogates experimental asthma by altering dendritic cell function. J Clin Invest 2006;116:2935–44.

307. Hammad H, Kool M, Soullie T, et al. Activation of the D prostanoid 1 receptor suppresses asthma by modulation of lung dendritic cell function and induction of regulatory T cells. J Exp Med 2007;204:357–67.

308. Akdis CA, Blaser K, Akdis M. Mechanisms of allergen-specific immunotherapy. Chem Immunol Allergy 2006;91:195–203.

309. Frew AJ. Sublingual immunotherapy. N Engl J Med 2008;358:2259–64.

310. Radulovic S, Jacobson MR, Durham SR, Nouri-Aria KT. Grass pollen immunotherapy induces Foxp3-expressing CD4(+)CD25(+) cells in the nasal mucosa. J Allergy Clin Immunol 2008;121:1467–72.

311. Xystrakis E, Kusumakar S, Boswell S, et al. Reversing the defective induction of IL-10-secreting regulatory T cells in glucocorticoid-resistant asthma patients. J Clin Invest 2006;116:146–55.

312. Smyth LJ, Starkey C, Vestbo J, Singh D. CD4-regulatory cells in COPD patients. Chest 2007;132:156–63.

313. Vijayanand P, Seumois G, Pickard C, et al. Invariant natural killer T cells in asthma and chronic obstructive pulmonary disease. N Engl J Med 2007;356:1410–22.

314. Gosman MM, Willemse BW, Jansen DF, et al. Increased number of B-cells in bronchial biopsies in COPD. Eur Respir J 2006;27:60–4.

315. van der Strate BW, Postma DS, Brandsma CA, et al. Cigarette smoke-induced emphysema: a role for the B cell? Am J Respir Crit Care Med 2006;173:751–8.

316. D'hulst AI, Maes T, Bracke KR, et al. Cigarette smoke-induced pulmonary emphysema in scid-mice. Is the acquired immune system required? Respir Res 2005;6:147.

317. Bracke K, Cataldo D, Maes T, et al. Matrix metalloproteinase-12 and cathepsin D expression in pulmonary macrophages and dendritic cells of cigarette smoke-exposed mice. Int Arch Allergy Immunol 2005;138:169–79.

318. Vassallo R, Tamada K, Lau JS, Kroening PR, Chen L. Cigarette smoke extract suppresses human dendritic cell function leading to preferential induction of Th-2 priming. J Immunol 2005;175:2684–91.

319. Tayal V, Kalra BS. Cytokines and anti-cytokines as therapeutics – an update. Eur J Pharmacol 2008;579:1–12.

320. Boguniewicz M, Martin RJ, Martin D, et al. The effects of nebulized recombinant interferon-gamma in asthmatic airways. J Allergy Clin Immunol 1995;95:133–5.

321. Simon HU, Seelbach H, Ehmann R, Schmitz M. Clinical and immunological effects of low-dose IFN-alpha treatment in patients with corticosteroid-resistant asthma. Allergy 2003;58:1250–5.

322. Kanazawa H, Mamoto T, Hirata K, Yoshikawa J. Interferon therapy induces the improvement of lung function by inhaled corticosteroid therapy in asthmatic patients with chronic hepatitis C virus infection: a preliminary study. Chest 2003;123:600–3.

323. Wark PA, Johnston SL, Bucchieri F, et al. Asthmatic bronchial epithelial cells have a deficient innate immune response to infection with rhinovirus. J Exp. Med 2005;201:937–47.

324. Contoli M, Message SD, Laza-Stanca V, et al. Role of deficient type III interferon-lambda production in asthma exacerbations. Nat Med 2006;12:1023–6.

325. Caramori G, Ito K, Contoli M, et al. Molecular mechanisms of respiratory virus-induced asthma and COPD exacerbations and pneumonia. Curr Med Chem 2006;13:2267–90.

326. Krieg AM. Therapeutic potential of Toll-like receptor 9 activation. Nat Rev Drug Discov 2006;5:471–84.

327. Gauvreau GM, Hessel EM, Boulet LP, Coffman RL, O'Byrne PM. Immunostimulatory sequences regulate interferon-inducible genes but not allergic airway responses. Am J Respir Crit Care Med 2006;174:15–20.

9

Novel biologicals alone and in combination in asthma and allergy

Sharmilee M. Nyenhuis and William W. Busse

Division of Allergy and Immunology, Department of Medicine, University of Wisconsin, Madison, USA

9.1   Introduction

Asthma is a common disease that is characterized by chronic airway inflammation and airway hyperresponsiveness.[1] The prevalence of asthma is increasing worldwide, with the highest prevalence in industrialized countries, where it affects about 15% of the adult population.[2] The majority of these patients have mild-to-moderate persistent asthma that can be well controlled by environmental avoidance measures and appropriate use of controller and reliever medications. It is estimated, however, that 5–10% of patients with asthma have severe disease that is largely recalcitrant to typical treatment modalities, including, in some cases, the administration of systemic corticosteroids. In addition, chronic systemic corticosteroids can lead to significant adverse effects, such as osteoporosis, hypertension, weight gain and diabetes, which can impede usage of these drugs in the treatment of severe asthma. Moreover, this subgroup of asthma patients has the greatest impairment of lifestyle, highest morbidity, and accounts for a disproportionate amount of healthcare cost associated with the disease.[3–5] Consequently, treatment options are limited in these patients and there is a growing need for new therapeutic approaches to help achieve better disease control. As more information is gained about the pathogenesis of this disease, new targets for therapy are being identified that will lead to the development of novel therapies for this heterogeneous disease.

Advances in Combination Therapy for Asthma and COPD, First Edition. Edited by Jan Lötvall.
© 2012 John Wiley & Sons, Ltd. Published 2012 by John Wiley & Sons, Ltd.

9.2   Targets of therapy

Asthma and other allergic diseases are often associated with atopy, which can be characterized by a persistent IgE response to common environmental allergens at mucosal surfaces. In addition, atopy can be attributed to immune deviation from type 1 (Th1) to type 2 (Th2) helper T-cells. This occurrence may be due to several factors such as decreased exposure to bacterial infections and endotoxins that stimulate Th1 cells, an uninhibited Th2 response that is normally present at birth, and the presentation of a restricted panel of antigens in the presence of the appropriate cytokines. Cytokines produced by the Th2 subset lymphocytes – interleukin-3 (IL-3), IL-4, IL-5, IL-13 and granulocyte-macrophage colony-stimulating factor (GM-CSF) – promote the production of IgE as well as enhancing eosinophil differentiation, migration and mediator release.[6] The induction of allergen-specific IgE also leads to the binding of surface Fc (fragment, crystallizable) receptors on mast cells and basophils, which can then cause cell activation and release of inflammatory mediators. Furthermore, eosinophils are thought to play a role in the pathogenesis of atopic asthma by the generation of basic enzymes and leukotrienes, to produce cytotoxic effects.

The airways of asthma subjects are infiltrated with numerous inflammatory cells, eosinophils, Th2 lymphocytes, and mast cells.[7] Cellular differences have been identified in the inflammatory pattern of severe asthma that support the heterogeneity of this disease.[8] Jatakanon and colleagues have detected higher concentrations of neutrophils in the sputum of severe asthma subjects when compared to normal subjects and milder asthma patients, implying a greater involvement of neutrophilic inflammation in the pathogenesis of severe asthma.[9] In contrast, eosinophils were found to be most prominent in the moderate asthma subjects (not receiving glucocorticoids) compared to the normal controls and severe asthma subjects.[10] Furthermore, genetic differences have been found, with mutations in the IL-4 gene and the IL-4 receptor being linked to severe asthma, a loss of lung function, and a high level of severe (intensive care unit/intubation) exacerbations.[11–13]

Suppression of these inflammatory factors may be approached in a myriad of ways, such as blocking antibodies to the cytokines or their receptors, using soluble receptors to remove secreted cytokines, deploying receptor antagonists or blocking signal transduction pathways (Figure 9.1).[14] Many such blocking antibodies and antagonists have been developed and, with the exception of one, anti-IgE, are still undergoing study in clinical trials and have yet to be approved by the US Food and Drug Administration (FDA) or recommended for use by Expert Panel Report-3 in the treatment of asthma and allergic disease.[15]

9.3   Interleukin-4

Interleukin-4 (IL-4) is a pleotropic cytokine with both agonistic and antagonistic effects on many cell types, including T-lymphocytes, B-lymphocytes, fibroblasts, monocytes, granulocytes and endothelial cells.[16] IL-4 has numerous biological activities that can mediate allergic inflammation.[6] It can upregulate vascular cell adhesion molecule-1

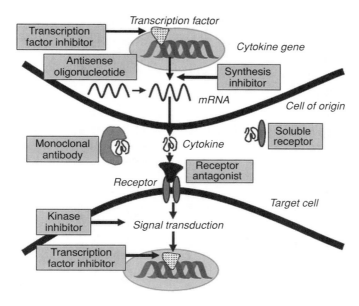

Figure 9.1   Strategies used to inhibit cytokine synthesis. Reprinted by permission from Macmillan Publishers Ltd:[Nature] (402: B31–38), (1999).

(VCAM-1) expression on endothelial cells to facilitate eosinophil and lymphocyte recruitment.[17] In addition, IL-4 induces the expression of eosinophil-associated cytokines and chemokines by epithelial cells to inhibit eosinophil apoptosis.[18] IL-4 can also trigger a switch in immunoglobulin isotype production to IgE by inducing immunoglobulin heavy chain gene rearrangement. The regulation of IgE production is clinically important as this antibody plays a major role in the mediation of immediate type I allergic responses.[19] Other mechanisms by which IL-4 can contribute to the pathogenesis of asthma include the induction of mucin gene expression to increase mucus production.[20] A distinctive biological action of IL-4 is its ability to drive the differentiation of naive Th0 lymphocytes into the Th2-like differentiation. When IL-4 is present, Th0 lymphocytes differentiate into the Th2-like cells with a cytokine profile of IL-4, IL-5, IL-9 and IL-13.[17]

The biological actions of IL-4 are mediated through binding to its receptor, which is made up of two subunits: IL-4Rα (IL-4 specific), which can complex with either the γ chain, which is shared among the receptors for IL-2, IL-7, IL-9 and IL-15, or with the α subunit of the IL-13 receptor.[21] In atopic asthma, increased levels of IL-4 in bronchial biopsy samples have been shown, with severe asthma subjects expressing persistently high levels of IL-4.[22,23] Furthermore, in lung tissue from atopic patients with asthma an increase in IL-4Rα mRNA expression in epithelial, subepithelial and endothelial cell layers, as well as in CD3+ T-cells and mast cells, has been shown (Figure 9.2).[18]

Given its central role in IgE production and Th2-like differentiation, multiple strategies have been devised to interfere with the functional activities of IL-4, including

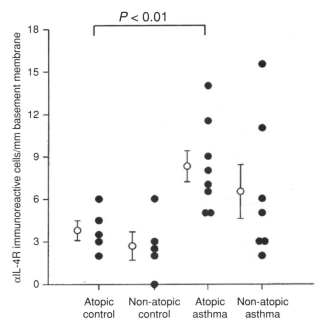

Figure 9.2   Immunocytochemistry of bronchial biopsy specimens showing the number of αIL-4R immunoreactive cells in the bronchial mucosa of atopic and non-atopic controls compared with atopic and non-atopic asthma subjects. Individual data points (filled circles) are given with the mean (open circles) and SEM (bars). Reprinted from Journal of Allergy and Clinical Immunology, 102, Kotsimbos TC, Ghaffar O, Minshall EM, et al. Expression of the IL-4 receptor a-subunit is increased in bronchial biopsy specimens from atopic and nonatopic asthmatic subjects. 859–66 (1998), with permission from Elsevier.

agents that limit IL-4 activity, production of IL-4 or accessibility of IL-4 to its specific receptor. Interferon-γ (IFN-γ) inhibits IgE production by interfering with the IL-4-mediated switch to ε-gene expression; the use in severe asthma subjects by Boguniewicz and colleagues resulted in no improvement in forced expiratory volume in 1 second (FEV_1) or to decrease the dose of prednisone when compared to placebo.[24,25] Experience with other agents that interfere with the functional activities of IL-4, such as a monoclonal anti-IL-4 antibody, an antibody directed against the IL-4R to prevent binding of IL-4 to its receptor, and soluble IL-4R, which suppresses IL-4 mediated T- and B-cell function, have given varied results.[16,19] Use of a monoclonal anti-IL-4 antibody was reasonably effective in regulating primary and secondary IgE responses; however, achieving this response efficacy required high concentrations, making the use of anti-IL-4 antibodies for *in vivo* treatment impractical.[19]

Secreted forms of IL-4Rα lack the transmembrane and cytoplasmic domains yet effectively bind to IL-4, resulting in inhibition of IL-4-induced B-cell proliferation, IgE production and T-cell proliferation *in vivo*.[26] Initial studies by Borish and colleagues to assess the tolerability and efficacy of a soluble recombinant IL-4 receptor

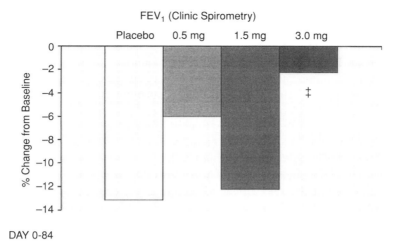

FEV$_1$ (Clinic Spirometry)

DAY 0-84

Figure 9.3 Mean percentage change from baseline forced expiratory volume in 1 second (FEV$_1$). Treatment with 3.0 mg of IL-4R after discontinuation of inhaled corticosteroids prevented decline in clinic-measured FEV$_1$ ($^‡P = 0.05$) over the 3-month treatment period. Reprinted from Journal of Allergy and Clinical Immunology, 107, Borish LC, Nelson HS, and Corren J. Efficacy of soluble IL-4 receptor for the treatment of adults with asthma. 963–70 (2001), with permission from Elsevier.

(sIL-4R) for moderate persistent asthma revealed that the drug was well tolerated.[27] In addition, asthma subjects receiving sIL-4R did not have a reduction in FEV$_1$ or increase in asthma symptoms following an acute withdrawal of inhaled corticosteroids (Figure 9.3).[17] However, in a subsequent large-scale trial, administration of the sIL-4R had little or no clinical efficacy in asthma. This lack of effect may have been due to the partial agonist function of sIL-4R to augment IL-13 activity at lower but physiological concentrations of IL-13.[26] Other approaches for blocking IL-4 receptor may include interrupting downstream IL-4 receptor signalling by targeting transcription factors such as Stat6, GATA-3 or FOG-1.[28]

9.4 Interleukin-5

Eosinophils have been a major target in the development of biological therapy in asthma as they are prominent in sputum, bronchoalveolar lavage (BAL) and mucosal biopsy samples of asthma subjects.[29] Eosinophils can cause airway hyperresponsiveness, increase mucus secretion and increase vasopermeability by the release of mediators such as eosinophil-derived neurotoxin (EDN) and eosinophil cationic protein (ECP).[30] Moreover, eosinophilia correlates with asthma severity, suggesting that the eosinophil is the major effector cell driving airway inflammation in asthma.[29]

Eosinophil production is regulated by IL-3, IL-5 and GM-CSF, but only IL-5 is specific for the eosinophil/basophil lineage (CD34$^+$).[30] IL-5 is a T-helper (Th) type 2 cytokine responsible for eosinophil production, activation and terminal differentiation, and has a multitude of other functions ranging from upregulating the expression of its own specific receptor α chain, enhancing chemotaxis and delaying apoptosis.[31] Its role in eosinophilic airway inflammation has been evaluated. Increased concentrations of IL-5 in serum, BAL fluid and bronchial biopsy samples are found in asthma.[22,32,33] IL-5 has also been implicated as a major proinflammatory cytokine in the late asthmatic reaction (LAR), with raised serum levels of IL-5 and blood eosinophils associated with a fall in FEV_1, the hallmark of the LAR.[34] Furthermore, Shi and colleagues demonstrated that IL-5 had a direct effect on airway hyperresponsiveness and sputum eosinophilia when inhaled by asthma subjects.[35] The linkages of IL-5 to features of asthma led to the development of a monoclonal antibody to IL-5, and subsequent studies to examine its effects in animal models of allergic asthma resulted in promising findings.

However, when Leckie and colleagues examined the use of humanized IL-5 monoclonal antibody in mild allergic asthma, the results were surprising.[36] The study was designed to assess the tolerability and activity of IL-5 monoclonal antibody against the late asthmatic response (LAR) to inhaled antigen. The drug was well tolerated with no clinically relevant adverse events. However, there was a reduction of blood eosinophils in the treatment groups compared to a control (Figure 9.4).[36] The reduction of blood eosinophils was maintained for up to 16 weeks after a 10 mg/kg dose and for up to 30 days after the 2.5 mg/kg dose.[36] In addition, there was a dose-dependent

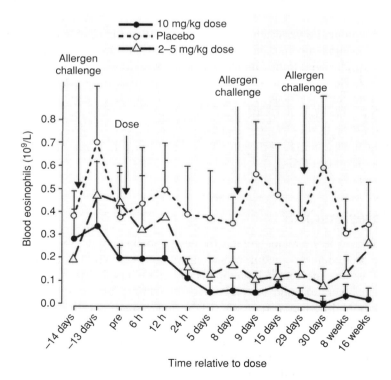

Figure 9.4   Effect of monoclonal antibody to IL-5 on blood eosinophil number. Reprinted from The Lancet, 356, Leckie MJ, ten Brinke A, Khan J, et al. 2144–8, (2000), with permission from Elsevier.

decrease in sputum eosinophils after allergen challenge, which lasted for 30 days after the dose. Despite these significant decreases in blood and sputum eosinophils, no significant change was found in the LAR or airway responsiveness to histamine either before or after allergen challenge. This study raised serious questions about the role of eosinophils and IL-5 in asthma.

Flood-Page and colleagues then evaluated if any changes in the bone marrow or airway tissue occurred with the use of IL-5 monoclonal antibody (mepolizumab). Again, the use of anti-IL-5 caused a significant decrease in the number of eosinophils in the peripheral blood, bone marrow and bronchial mucosa of subjects in the treatment group.[31] In spite of the significant decrease of eosinophils in the mepolizumab group, only a 50% decline in eosinophils occurred in the bone marrow and airway tissue. In addition with mepolizumab, no significant reduction in the amount of eosinophil major basic protein (MBP) was found in the airway tissue. Finally, no significant changes occurred in morning peak expiratory flow rate (PEFR), FEV_1 or airway hyperresponsiveness (Table 9.1).[31]

Interleukin-5 monoclonal antibodies were also evaluated in more severe persistent asthma by Kips and colleagues. They assessed the safety and biological activity of one dose of SCH55700, anti-IL-5 humanized monoclonal antibody, in a group of asthma subjects with severe disease. The drug was well tolerated and reduced the number of circulating blood eosinophils in the severe asthma group despite the use of ongoing high-dose inhaled corticosteroids (ICS) or oral corticosteroids (OCS), suggesting that even high doses of ICS do not entirely block Il-5-dependent peripheral blood eosinophilia.[37] In contrast to previous studies, a small, but significant improvement in FEV_1 occurred within 24 hours of receiving a 0.3 mg/kg dose; no other clinical improvements were seen.[37]

The results from these previous studies led to more questions regarding the role of IL-5 and eosinophils in asthma. Consequently, an International Mepolizumab Study Group was formed to investigate further the clinical efficacy of the anti-IL-5 antibody, mepolizumab. The Study Group designed a multicentre, randomized, double-blind, placebo-controlled study to examine the safety and efficacy of mepolizumab in moderately severe asthma with persistent symptoms despite ICS treatment.[38] The study design included a 12-week treatment period during which subjects received placebo, mepolizumab (250 mg) or mepolizumab (750 mg), once a month for 3 months. There was also an 8-week follow-up period, making this the longest clinical trial to evaluate the clinical efficacy of mepolizumab.[38] As previously shown, this study found mepolizumab to be well tolerated. Although significant reductions in peripheral blood eosinophils and sputum eosinophilia occurred, the effects on lung function were negligible with no significant improvement of either the FEV_1 or asthma symptom scores (Figure 9.3).[38] Although a 50% reduction in exacerbations was noted with mepolizumab (750 mg), the study was not sufficiently powered to determine the statistical significance of this trend.[38] The reduction in exacerbations in the mepolizumab (750 mg) group may relate to the significant reduction in sputum eosinophils and parallels the observations by Green and colleagues, who found the frequency of asthma exacerbations to be significantly decreased when treatment was directed to reduce sputum eosinophils to less than 3%.[39]

Table 9.1 Clinical measurement of asthma before and after treatment with mepolizumab or placebo.

	Mepolizumb		Placebo		Median Difference	p Value Between Groups
	Pre	Post	Pre	Pre		
FEV_1, L/sec	3.05 (2.69–3.28)	3.1 (2.82–3.85)	3.1 (2.65–3.51)	3.05 (2.65–3.45)	0.15	0.22
Morning PEFR, L/min	433 (402–497)	436* (417–503)	459.5 (408–481)	448 (370–490)	21	0.09
Histamine PC_{20}, mg/ml	1.75 (1.23–3.78)	2.2 (1.24–32)	1.59 (1.05–2.1)	2.23 (1.85–4.22)	1.21	0.49

Definition of abbreviations: PC_{20} = provocative concentration of histamine causing a 20% fall in FEV_1; PEFR = peak expiratory flow rate.
Results expressed as medians (interquartile range).
*p < 0.05 when compared with baseline.

Source: Reprinted with permission from Eosinophil's Role Remains Uncertain as Anti-Interleukin-5 only Partially Depletes Numbers in Asthmatic Airway. Flood-Page PT, Menzies-Gow AN, Kay AB, and Robinson DS. American Journal of Respiratory and Critical Care Medicine, 167;199–204. (2003) © The American Thoracic Society.

More recently, Jayaram and colleagues also studied the impact of controlling sputum eosinophils on asthma exacerbations in moderate-to-severe asthma subjects.[40] Their results reinforced the findings of Green and colleagues, and showed a reduction in the number of asthma exacerbations and a reduction in the severity of both eosinophilic and non-eosinophilic exacerbations without the need for an increase in the total corticosteroid dose.[39] Further studies with anti-IL-5 will need to be undertaken to provide a definitive answer regarding any possible role it may have in controlling exacerbations in those patients with persistent airway eosinophilia.

The International Mepolizumab Study Group has speculated upon the reasons why there is an apparent lack of clinical response seen with the use of anti-IL-5 in mild, moderate and even severe asthma. One possible explanation is that tissue eosinophils may be unresponsive to IL-5.[38] Preincubation of eosinophils with IL-5 *in vitro* leads to long-term downregulation of the IL-5 receptor α-chain expression as well as reduced responsiveness to IL-5.[38,41,42] These findings suggest that eosinophils in airway tissue may not be dependent on IL-5 alone for their survival and eventual function. Other cytokines, such as IL-3, GM-CSF and IL-13, may play a larger role in tissue eosinophil survival and function than previously thought. However, there may be specific cytokines to regulate the function of airway eosinophils as clinical responses to anti-IL-5 are found in hypereosinophilic syndromes where eosinophils may be directly responsible for the pathogenesis of the disease.[43,44]

9.5   Interleukin-13

The pathophysiology of asthma is felt to be mediated in part by CD4[+] T-lymphocytes producing a type 2 cytokine profile, with important roles for IL-4 and IL-5 as previously discussed. Another type 2 cytokine, IL-13, was first recognized for its effects on B-cells and monocytes, in which it upregulated major histocompatibility complex (MHC) class II expression, promoted IgE class switching and inhibited inflammatory cytokine production.[45] These properties were, however, thought to be functionally redundant of IL-4 and there were no effector functions unique to IL-13. IL-13 is closely related to IL-4 as it binds to the α subunit of the IL-4 receptor and, in addition, IL-13 binds to at least one of two known IL-13-specific binding chains, IL-13Rα1 and IL-13Rα2.[45]

But as more information has been gained about the type 2 cytokines, IL-13 has been found to have its own specific effector functions and, further, has been identified as a central mediator in allergic asthma.[45,46] Grünig and colleagues found that if an IL-13-selective antibody was administered in ovalbumin (OVA)-sensitized mice, there was amelioration of the asthma phenotype independent of IL-4.[47] In addition, Wills-Karp and co-workers showed that when an IL-13-selective antibody was given to OVA-sensitized mice immediately before antigen challenge, there was complete reversal of airway hyperresponsiveness (AHR) after the full development of the phenotype of allergic asthma; this contrasts with the inability of IL-4 ablation to achieve complete reversal of AHR.[46] To assess further the role of IL-13 in airway inflammation, Zhu and colleagues targeted IL-13 to the murine lung and then characterized the phenotype it produced.[48] IL-13 induced tissue inflammation, mucus hyperproduction, goblet cell hyperplasia, subepithelial fibrosis, airway obstruction and AHR upon methacholine challenge. The role of IL-13 in murine asthma models is now well appreciated, with emerging data in human asthma supporting the findings from these models.

In humans, elevated levels of IL-13 mRNA and protein have been noted in asthma. Polymorphisms specific to the coding region of the IL-13 gene have also been associated with asthma.[49,50] Elevated IL-13 levels have been found in both mild and moderate asthma as well as corticosteroid-naive asthma subjects. Recently, Saha and colleagues reported that severe asthma subjects, as defined by Global Initiative for Asthma (GINA) guidelines, demonstrated significantly increased IL-13 expression in sputum and bronchial samples when compared to healthy controls.[51] Furthermore, IL-13 expression in the bronchial samples of severe asthma subjects correlated positively with the intensity of eosinophilic airway inflammation, and the sputum IL-13 concentration was related to subjective asthma control as determined by use of Asthma Control Questionnaire (ACQ) ($P = 0.04$).[51] With IL-13 overexpression seen in a wide range of asthma phenotypes (mild–severe), it is likely that IL-13 may be an important target for therapeutic intervention. Wenzel and colleagues have shown an attenuation of the late asthmatic response after experimental allergen challenge in atopic asthma subjects with the use of pitrakinra, an IL-4 variant that blocks the binding of both IL-4 and IL-13 to the IL-4Rα complex.[52] Currently, anti-IL-13 monoclonal antibodies for use in humans are in the development phase and information is eagerly awaited from studying the effects of blocking this central mediator of asthma.

9.6   Tumor necrosis factor-α

Tumor necrosis factor-α (TNF-α) is a proinflammatory cytokine with a diverse set of cellular responses that includes cellular differentiation, activation and apoptosis.[53] TNF-α also has an important role in the regulation of innate immunity.[54] There is evidence to support the idea that TNF-α is a critical cytokine in the pathogenesis of airway inflammation in asthma. Elevated levels of TNF-α mRNA and protein have been found in BAL fluid from asthma subjects, and upregulated TNF expression has been detected in alveolar macrophages, mast cells and bronchial epithelial cells.[55–58] In addition, when inhaled recombinant TNF-α was administered to normal subjects, airway hyperresponsiveness (AHR) and airway neutrophilia developed.[59] The mechanisms regulating AHR are not fully elucidated and may be either a direct effect on the airway smooth muscle or an indirect effect via the release of cysteinyl leukotrienes, LTC$_4$ and LTD$_4$.[60] TNF-α exerts other actions relevant to asthma such as chemoattraction of neutrophils and eosinophils by the upregulation of E-selectin, VCAM-1 and intercellular adhesion molecule-1 (ICAM-1), activation of T-cells and stimulation of cytotoxic cellular products.[61–63] In the pathogenesis of severe asthma, TNF-α may play a larger role by recruiting neutrophils, inducing glucocorticoid resistance, and stimulating fibroblast growth leading to transforming growth factor-β (TGF-β) expression.[59,64,65] Furthermore, Berry and colleagues have recently found that increased membrane-bound TNF-α (mTNF-α) and TNF-α receptor 1 on peripheral blood cells were found only in patients with severe disease.[66] These findings suggest that certain asthma phenotypes, i.e., those with severe refractory disease, may be particularly responsive to therapies that target TNF-α.

Anti-TNF-α therapies, such as etanercept (a soluble TNF-α receptor–IgG1Fc fusion protein), infliximab (a recombinant human-murine chimeric monoclonal antibody) and adalimumab (a fully human monocloncal antibody) have been effective in the treatment of chronic inflammatory disorders involving neutrophils, such as rheumatoid arthritis, ankylosing spondylitis, Crohn's disease, sarcoidosis and Behçet's disease.[67] Targeting TNF-α in murine models of asthma has resulted in a significant reduction of antigen-induced airway inflammation.[68] Khalil and colleagues were the first to report significant improvements in FEV_1 and exercise tolerance in three patients who were receiving infliximab for treatment of their rheumatoid arthritis but also had a diagnosis of asthma or chronic obstructive pulmonary disease (COPD).[69] The findings in animal models, and in the previously described retrospective review, resulted in further investigative clinical trials designed to assess the efficacy of anti-TNF-α in the treatment of asthma (Table 9.2).[70]

In the first open-label, uncontrolled trial of etanercept in severe (Global Initiative for Asthma stage V) asthma, Howarth and colleagues reported a clear improvement in methacholine airway hyperresponsiveness (AHR), asthma quality of life (assessed by ACQ) and a modest improvement in lung function (FEV_1).[71] These positive findings were confirmed by a small randomized, placebo-controlled, crossover trial with etanercept for 10 weeks in chronic severe asthma.[66] In addition to the improvements in FEV_1, methacholine AHR and asthma quality of life (assessed by asthma quality of life questionnaire (AQLQ)), the clinical response to anti-TNF-α treatment was closely correlated with the expression of TNF-α receptor 1 on circulating mononuclear cells.[66] More recently, the results from a randomized, placebo-controlled, parallel group trial in subjects with severe corticosteroid-refractory asthma were reported by Morjaria and colleagues.[72] After 12 weeks of treatment with etanercept, subjects in the treatment group had only a small but significant reduction in asthma control (assessed by ACQ) and, in contrast with the two previous studies, no improvements in lung function, AHR or asthma-related quality of life were found when compared to the placebo group.[72] Several factors may have contributed to these differences compared with the findings of Howarth et al. and Berry et al.. First, Morjaria et al. were not performing methacholine challenges in some of their asthma subjects due to safety reasons as these subjects had severe airflow obstruction (mean percent predicted FEV_1 58–59%). Secondly, there was no TNF-α detected in the sputum of the severe asthma subjects, which supports the concept that only a select subgroup of asthma may respond to anti-TNF-α therapy.

The use of anti-TNF-α therapy in milder forms of asthma has been addressed in two studies. The first study was designed to assess changes in markers of inflammation and AHR.[73] After 2 weeks of treatment in mild-moderate allergic asthma subjects, there was no change in AHR to methacholine and no attenuation of pulmonary eosinophilia.[73] Erin and colleagues conducted a randomized, placebo-controlled, parallel group trial of the use of infliximab in asthma subjects with moderate disease.[7] There was no improvement in the primary endpoint of the study, morning peak flow, but there was a 50% reduction in the number of mild exacerbations in subjects receiving infliximab.

Table 9.2 Summary of clinical trials of anti-TNF-α therapy in asthma.

Authors	No./severity	Design	Treatment	Outcome	Result
Howarth et al.	15/GINA V	Open-label, uncontrolled	Etanercept, 12 wk	1° ACQ	Improvement ACQ
				2° FEV$_1$, AHR	Improvement FEV$_1$, AHR
Berry et al.	10/7 GINA V, 3 GINA IV	Randomized placebo-controlled crossover	Etanercept, 10 wk	1° AHR and AQLQ	Improvement AHR, AQLQ
				2° FEV$_1$, eNO, sputum cell counts	Improvement FEV$_1$, ↓ sputum histamine
Morjaria et al.	39/21 GINA V, 18 GINA IV	Randomized placebo-controlled, parallel group	Etanercept, 12 wk	1° AQLQ	No benefit compared with placebo
				2° ACQ, FEV$_1$, PEF, AHR, exacerbations	Improvement in ACQ, ↓ sputum macrophages, ↓ CRP
Rouhani et al.	21/β-agonist only	Segmental allergen challenge	Etanercept, 2 wk	Markers of inflammation, AHR	Increased TNFR2 in BAL, no change in AHR
Erin et al.	38/ICS only	Randomized placebo-controlled, parallel group	Infliximab, 6 wk	1° morning PEF	No change in morning PEF
				2° FEV$_1$, exacerbations, sputum markers	↓ PEF variability, ↓ exacerbations

GINA, Global Initiative for Asthma; 1°, primary outcomes; 2°, secondary outcomes; ACQ, asthma control questionnaire; AHR, airway hyperresponsiveness; AQLQ, asthma quality-of-life questionnaire; BAL, bronchoalveolar lavage; CRP, C-reactive protein ; eNO, exhaled nitric oxide; FEV$_1$, forced expiratory volume in 1 second;; ICS, inhaled corticosteroids; PEF, peak expiratory flow; TNFR2, TNF receptor 2.

Source: Reprinted from Journal of Allergy and Clinical Immunology, 121, Brightling C, Berry M, and Amrani Y. Targeting TNF-α: A novel therapeutic approach for asthma. 5–10 (2008), with permission from Elsevier.

None of the other studies has found any differences in exacerbation rates thus far, which may reflect therapeutic differences of etanercept and infliximab.

The extensive use of anti-TNF-α therapies in other chronic inflammatory diseases has helped to establish the safety profile for these medications. Both anti-TNF-α drugs are given as infusions and have been well tolerated in both chronic inflammatory disease and asthma patients. Increased risks of infection and malignancy have been identified as possible side effects of the anti-TNF-α drugs, both of which are still being addressed. With the results of larger clinical trials using anti-TNF-α therapies being eagerly awaited, it will still be necessary to consider the 'risk–benefit ratio' of these drugs as they may only be efficacious in a subpopulation of our asthma patients.

9.7   Immunoglobulin E

Asthma

The importance of immunoglobulin E (IgE) as a mediator of allergic airway disease is well established and recognized.[74] Correlations between IgE and clinical manifestations of allergic disease have been previously described and include elevated serum IgE levels associated with airway responsiveness in both children and adults with asthma, emergency room visits for asthma, and skin-test reactivity to allergens.[74–77] The role IgE plays in the biphasic reactions to inhaled antigens that occur in asthma has been studied by Fahy and colleagues. They demonstrated an attenuation of the early- and late-phase reactions to inhaled antigen in mild asthma subjects when IgE was inhibited by anti-IgE.[78]

IgE binds to high-affinity IgE receptor (FcϵRI), which are found on tissue mast cells and circulating basophils. When IgE is bound to the cell surface, an allergen can attach to IgE and cause cross-linking of the IgE to set off a cascade of events that leads to the release of inflammatory mediators such as histamine, leukotrienes and prostaglandins. These mediators are responsible for many of the histological findings seen in asthma that lead to airflow obstruction, including mucosal oedema and smooth muscle contraction.[78]

Until recently, allergen-specific immunotherapy and anti-inflammatory medications, such as inhaled corticosteroids, were mainstays to treat allergic asthma. The clinical efficacy of these treatments has been reported but many asthma patients continue to be symptomatic despite maximum pharmacotherapy.[79] The significance of IgE to allergic disease has made it an obvious target in the development of disease modification therapy.

Omalizumab is a humanized monoclonal IgG1-blocking antibody directed towards the Fc portion of the IgE molecule. This monoclonal antibody acts by forming soluble complexes with free circulating IgE and IgE found on B-cells, which are then cleared by the reticuloendothelial system.[80] Anti-IgE decreases free-IgE as well as reducing FcϵRI expression on mast cells, basophils and dendritic cells. Consequently, reducing circulating IgE inhibits IgE binding to its effector cells, and presumably, leads to

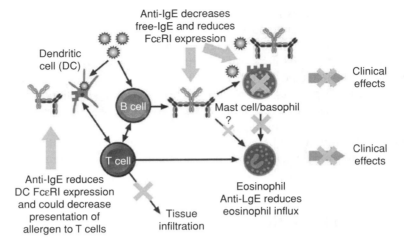

Figure 9.5 Proposed mechanisms of action of omalizumab. Omalizumab decreases free IgE levels and reduces FcεRI receptor expression on mast cells and basophils. This results in decreased mast cell activation and sensitivity, leading to a reduction in eosinophil influx and activation. Anti-IgE treatment with omalizumab might result in decreased mast cell survival. Omalizumab also reduces dendritic cell FcεRI receptor. Reprinted with permission from Journal of Allergy and Clinical Immunology, 115, Holgate S, Casale T, Wenzel S, et al. The anti-inflammatory effects of omalizumab confirm the central role of IgE in allergic inflammation. 459–65 (2005), with permission from Elsevier.

decreased mast cell activation, a reduced eosinophil influx and activation, and finally suppression of airway inflammation (Figure 9.5).[81]

Rapidly after infusion of anti-IgE there is a significant decrease in free IgE levels in the serum and decreased expression of FcεRI on mast cells, basophils and dendritic cells.[82,83] Over time, the amount of cell-bound IgE also declines because of the decrease in free IgE. In addition, allergic asthma subjects treated with anti-IgE have shown a significant decrease in: sputum and peripheral eosinophils; IL-13, IL-5, IL-8, and histamine levels; CD3[+], CD4[+] and CD8[+] T-lymphocytes; and B-lymphocytes (Table 9.3).[23,84]

Several studies have shown omalizumab to be a safe and effective treatment of moderate-to-severe persistent allergic asthma. The use of this treatment in clinical asthma began in 2003 when it was approved by the US FDA, and it was recently included in the Expert Panel Report-3 on Asthma Guidelines for the treatment of asthma in patients whose symptoms are not controlled with standard therapies, Steps 5 and 6.[15]

Milgrom and colleagues were the first to show the efficacy of intravenous anti-IgE antibody in moderate-to-severe allergic asthma.[85] In their cohort, omaluzimab improved asthma control and the quality of life compared to placebo, as well as allowing a significant reduction in the dose of both inhaled and oral corticosteroids.[85] Three additional large, randomized, double-blind, placebo-controlled trials followed evaluating the use of subcutaneous anti-IgE in moderate-to-severe asthma; all showed

Table 9.3 Median (range) change from baseline in cell counts of the epithelial and submucosal compartments of bronchial biopsies after 16 weeks of treatment with omalizumab or placebo.

Cell Type	Epithelium (cells/mm)		Submucosa (cells/mm²)	
	Omalizumab (n = 10)	Placebo (n = 13)	Omalizumab (n = 14)	Placebo (n = 14)
Basophils	0 (−0.77 to 0)	0 (−0.22 to 0)	−1.02 (−8.49 to 3.89)	1.07 (−9.86 to 6.83)
Mast cells	−2.06 (−4.63 to 1.66)	−0.74 (−4.81 to 4.38)	−8.77 (−20.94 to 29.42)	3.24 (−10.76 to 31.28)
Eosinophils	−0.4 (−2.44 to 0.51)	0 (−0.79 to 9.55)	−3.95* (−20.95 to −0.10)	0.35 (−40.80 to 38.47)
T lymphocytes				
CD3$^+$	−4.13* (−17.55 to 7.98)	3.86 (−10.02 to 33.41)	−36.96† (−258.00 to 79.54)	40.52 (−50.00 to 199.09)
CD4$^+$	−0.53 (−1.84 to 1.60)	0.47 (−2.41 to 6.98)	−27.81† (−149.15 to 56.17)	40.90 (−28.02 to 138.89)
CD8$^+$	−0.60 (−10.27 to 4.79)	2.86 (−6.95 to 14.14)	−8.95* (−78.31 to 32.22)	15.71 (−22.07 to 35.92)
B lymphocytes (CD20$^+$)	−0.14 (−0.91 to 0.37)	0 (−0.79 to 0.46)	−0.83* (−20.02 to 6.53)	3.36 (−11.62 to 82.09)
FcεRI	−3.3† (−8.75 to 0)	0 (−0.41 to 7.25)	−21.26‡ (−48.00 to 3.13)	2.44 (−16.15 to 25.65)
FcεRII	0 (0 to 0)	0 (−0.58 to 0)	−0.76 (−5.98 to 0)	−0.73 (−5.02 to 1.55)
IL-4 (cell surface)	−1.0* (−3.64 to 0)	0 (−1.08 to 0.87)	−15.28‡ (−37.74 to 0.29)	0 (−20.21 to 14.67)
IL-4 (cytoplasmic)	0 (−0.14 to 0)	0 (−0.14 to 0.29)	0.47 (−7.61 to 13.96)	0.72 (−8.69 to 15.26)
IL-5	0 (0 to 0)	0 (−0 to 0.45)	−0.44 (−11.06 to 6.33)	1.41 (−12.22 to 18.69)
IgE	−6.22‡ (−13.28 to −0.78)	0 (−3.15 to 10.00)	−31.33‡ (−92.45 to −6.44)	6.16 (−89.39 to 35.24)

Definition of abbreviations: FcεR = Fc receptor specific for IgE; IL = interleukin.
*p ≤ 0.05 versus placebo (Wilcoxon test).
†p ≤ 0.01 versus placebo (Wilcoxon test).
‡p ≤ 0.001 versus placebo (Wilcoxon test).

Source: Reprinted with permission from Effects of treatment with anti-immunoglobulin E antibody omalizumab on airway inflammation in allergic asthma. Djukanović R, Wilson SJ, Kraft M, et al. American Journal of Respiratory and Critical Care Medicine, 170;583–93. (2004) © The American Thoracic Society.

a reduction in asthma exacerbations and a corticosteroid-sparing effect compared to placebo.[86–88] The asthma subjects receiving anti-IgE treatment also had fewer asthma symptoms, less rescue medication use and improved quality-of-life scores. Busse et al. and Solèr et al. both found a small but significant improvement in peak expiratory flow and FEV_1 values in subjects in the treatment group compared with placebo.[86, 88] Subsequent studies have also found that anti-IgE treatment reduces the rates of unscheduled outpatient visits, asthma-related emergency room visits and hospitalizations in patients with moderate-to-severe allergic asthma.[89] In summary, omalizumab therapy in asthma has been shown to positively affect several clinical outcomes such as exacerbations, hospitalizations, symptoms and asthma-specific quality of life but primarily in those with more severe disease.

Allergic rhinitis

Omalizumab has been shown to significantly reduce nasal volume in response to nasal allergen challenge and TNF-α, as well as inhibiting the increase of serum albumin after allergen challenge in allergic rhinitis (Figure 9.6).[90, 91] Early randomized controlled

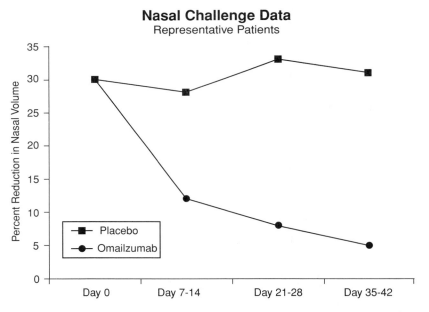

Figure 9.6   Nasal challenge data in placebo-treated and omalizumab-treated subjects. In the omalizumab group there was a gradual blunted response to ragweed challenge, whereas in the placebo group there was a 30% reduction in nasal volume after ragweed nasal challenge. Reprinted with permission from Journal of Allergy and Clinical Immunology, 113, Lin H, Boesel KM, Griffith DT, et al. Omalizumab rapidly decreases nasal allergic response and FcεRI on basophils. 297–302 (2004). Reprinted with permission from Journal of Allergy and Clinical Immunology, 113, Lin H., Boesel K.M., Griffith D.T., et al. Omalizumab rapidly decreases nasal allergic response and FcεRI on basophils 297-302. (2004)

studies to evaluate anti-IgE in seasonal allergic rhinitis found a significant decrease in nasal symptom scores, improved rhinitis quality-of-life scores, and reduced need for rescue antihistamine use.[92,93] Its effectiveness in perennial allergic rhinitis has also been reported by Chervinsky and colleagues, who showed that treatment effectively controlled symptoms, improved rhinitis quality-of-life scores, and decreased reliance on rescue antihistamines.[94] Despite these outcomes, the precise therapeutic role of omalizumab in allergic rhinitis has yet to be defined. The previously mentioned studies showed the benefit of omalizumab over placebo, but none has assessed any benefit over standard therapy for allergic rhinitis. However, Vignola and colleagues did examine the efficacy of omalizumab as add-on therapy in patients with concomitant allergic asthma and persistent allergic rhinitis who were using inhaled corticosteroids and intranasal steroids. In this setting, they found a significant improvement in asthma exacerbations, asthma and rhinitis quality-of-life questionnaires, and composite asthma/rhinitis scores.[95]

When added to specific allergen immunotherapy (IT), omalizumab has shown promising benefits such as better efficacy and reduced acute allergic reactions to immunotherapy. When omalizumab was given with allergen-specific immunotherapy to children who were allergic to birch and grass along, a significant decrease in seasonal allergic rhinitis symptoms and rescue medication scores occurred in the omalizumab + IT group compared to the IT-alone group.[96] The concomitant use of these medications did not confer any increased risk when compared to IT alone. Moreover, Casale and colleagues showed that when omalizumab was used as pretreatment in rush immunotherapy with ragweed, fewer adverse events were noted as compared to those allergic subjects receiving immunotherapy alone.[97] Therefore, in the future clinicians may be able to administer a more effective therapeutic immunotherapy dose in a more rapid fashion confident of a low risk of adverse events. With the great amount of interest in the use of omalizumab for the treatment of allergic diseases, it will be necessary to conduct further trials before we can fully understand its impact in allergic rhinitis.

9.8   DNA vaccines

The first proposed mechanism to explain the 'hygiene hypothesis' and the rise in allergic disease was a current reduction in the stimulation of the Th1 arm of the immune system due to decreased childhood infections, which in turn led to an overactive Th2 immunalogical pathway immunological and greater tendency to develop allergic disease.[98,99] The concept of this immune imbalance as a key factor for the development of allergic disease is still of considerable interest and has, in turn, become the target for new therapeutics in allergic diseases.

Treatments to both upregulate the Th1 arm and downregulate the Th2 phase of the immune system have been developed in the form of DNA vaccines (Figure 9.7). One approach to stimulate Th1-mediated responses and suppress Th2-mediated responses has involved the use of immunostimulatory DNA sequences from bacterial extracts.[100] These immunostimulatory DNA sequences in microbial organisms were identified as

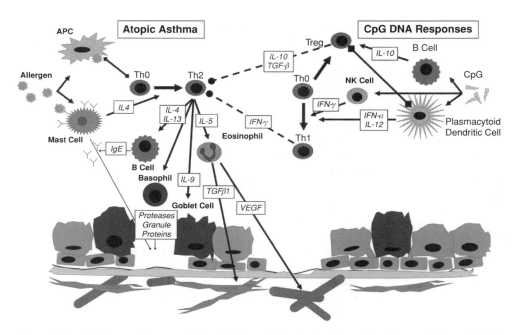

Figure 9.7   Mediators of acute and chronic airway inflammation in atopic asthma and effect of CpG DNA. Environmental exposure of a sensitized individual to aeroallergen induces interleukin-4 (IL-4) release from mast cells; antigen presentation by antigen-presenting cells (APCs) in the setting of IL-4 promotes proliferation and activation of T-helper type 2 (Th2)-committed cells. Th2 cytokine products activate eosinophils, basophils, and B-cells and induce goblet cell hyperplasia/metaplasia. Products of mast cells, basophils and eosinophils promote epithelial denudement, myofibroblast hyperplasia, extracellular matrix/collagen production and organization, and angiogenesis. CpG DNA induces Th1 and T-regulatory (T_{reg}) responses that are primarily (in humans) mediated via plasmacytoid dendritic cells and B-cells. These cells suppress the activation of Th2 cells, preventing (or reversing) acute eosinophilic inflammation and subchronic/chronic remodelling of the airways. IFN, interferon; NK, natural killer; TGF, transforming growth factor; VEGF, vascular endothelial growth factor. Reprinted with permission from Eat Dirt: CpG DNA and Immunomodulation of Asthma. Kline JN. Proceedings of the American Thoracic Society, 4, 283–288. (2007) © The American Thoracic Society.

unmethylated CpG dinucleotides; they exert their effects via Toll-like receptor 9 (TLR-9) binding.[101, 102] In vertebrates, the CpG motifs are heavily suppressed or methylated and thus are not recognized by the innate immune system. With TLR-9 binding, CpG can directly affect B-cells and dendritic cells and indirectly act on T-cells, natural killer (NK) cells and neutrophils.[100] Soon after TLR-9 interaction, B-cells and dendritic cells are activated to release cytokines and chemokines such as IL-10, IFN-α/β, IL-12 and IFN-inducible protein-10, thus leading to an induction of a regulatory/Th1 anti-allergic inflammatory response.[103] One of the downstream effects of CpGs in B-cells is the upregulation of T-cell differentiation transcription factors, such as T-bet.[104] T-bet suppresses the Th2 phenotype by enhancing the production of Th1 cytokines (IFN-γ,

IL-12) while decreasing the production of Th2 cytokines (IL-4, IL-5).[105] Additional downstream effects include an inhibition of IgG1 and IgE class-switching, which is induced by IL-4, inhibition of CD40 signalling in B-cells, and activation of a cascade of cellular responses that promote adaptive immune responses.[105]

To evaluate the immunostimulatory effects of these CpG motifs in both animal and human models, synthetic oligodeoxynucleotides (ODNs) containing unmethylated CpG dinucleotides were developed. Early studies with these CpG ODNs found their efficacy was improved when they were conjugated to an antigen or allergen.[106] Broide and colleagues, along with others, have found the CpG ODNs to be effective in regulating allergic disease in mouse models.[107–111] These studies have shown CpG-ODN treatment decreases eosinophilic airway inflammation, blood and bone marrow eosinophilia, IgE levels, Th2 inflammatory cytokine expression and airway hyperresponsiveness, and increases Th1 inflammatory cytokine expression as well as anti-inflammatory cytokine production.

In humans, thus far, studies are limited and have shown CpG-ODN treatment is well tolerated and safe, yet long-term safety data are not available. Moreover, the majority of the data published have been in ragweed-induced allergic disease using a CpG motif that is conjugated to Ambrosia a 1 allergen (Amb a 1) (Tolamba). Creticos and colleagues conducted a randomized, double-blind, placebo-controlled phase 2 trial with Tolamba in which patients who were allergic to ragweed received six weekly injections of treatment with CpG-ODN or with placebo.[112] Patients received active treatment or placebo before the first ragweed season and were followed for two subsequent ragweed seasons. The subjects who received Tolamba had significantly improved peak-season rhinitis scores and mid-season quality-of-life scores. Furthermore, the clinical benefits of improved rhinitis scores persisted during the following ragweed seasons without additional treatment. Interestingly, the rise in Amb a 1-specific IgE antibody, normally seen during ragweed season, was suppressed during both years of the study, and a transient increase in Amb a 1-specific IgG levels was noted during the first ragweed season. This study showed that CpG-ODN may induce prolonged immune modulation along with benefits in clinical markers. More recently, a large, multicentre, placebo-controlled trial examining the efficacy and tolerability of higher doses of Tolamba found no clinical benefit, though problems in study design and low symptom scores in the placebo groups during peak season have made the interpretation of the results difficult.[113]

Experience in the use of CpG-ODNs in human allergic asthma is limited. Gauvreau and colleagues treated allergic asthma subjects with an inhaled CpG preparation weekly for 4 weeks to study the safety, pharmacological activity and efficacy of this targeted therapy.[114] The treatment was well tolerated, and sputum samples of the subjects showed an increase in IFN-α and -γ and IFN-inducible gene expression. Despite these changes, there was no inhibition of Th2 mRNA expression in the airway of treated subjects and no improvement in allergen-induced bronchoconstriction, post-challenge hyperresponsiveness or sputum-derived eosinophils.[114]

In summary, the current experience with DNA vaccines is limited but thus far they have been shown to be safe, and in the right setting have shown clinical efficacy and prolonged immune modulation in allergic disease. Additional studies will provide further information regarding the value of this class of drugs for allergic disease modification.

9.9   Future directions

The knowledge gained from the use of biological agents in the treatment of allergic disease is significant and continues to grow. Multiple mechanisms, both defined and undefined, have been found to be involved in the pathogenesis of asthma. Consequently, it will likely require the blockage of several cytokines or inflammatory cell types to see a significant change in disease modification. New targets of therapy beyond monoclonal antibodies that block cytokine production and receptor function are being developed and are eagerly awaited to determine if they will have a major impact on the course of allergic disease. In the meantime, other approaches have emerged.

Bronchial thermoplasty

Bronchial thermoplasty is a procedure where controlled thermal energy is applied directly to small- to medium-sized airways, via a bronchoscope device, in the anticipation of a prolonged reduction of airway smooth muscle mass.[115] The success of this treatment is predicated on the concept that a reduction in airway smooth muscle mass by heating will improve airway responsiveness and reduce exacerbations in asthma subjects.[115] This procedure has recently gained interest with the publication of two human studies by Cox and colleagues to illustrate the safety and efficacy of this procedure in subjects with either controlled or uncontrolled asthma.[116, 117]

The first study was a non-randomized, prospective safety design study including subjects with controlled mild-to-moderate asthma.[116] All subjects had a statistically significant reduction in airway hyperresponsiveness associated with clinical improvements in peak expiratory flow and number of symptom-free days. Interestingly, these findings persisted for 2 years after treatment; no severe reactions to treatment occurred. Although, these results provide reassuring data on the safety and feasibility of bronchial thermoplasty in mild-to-moderate controlled asthma, the subjects greatest in need to benefit from this therapy have uncontrolled severe asthma.

Cox and colleagues examined the safety and efficacy of this procedural treatment in moderate-to-severe asthma subjects and, once again, found the treatment to be well tolerated.[117] The most common adverse event related to worsening asthma symptoms during the period immediately after treatment. The primary outcome of this study was the frequency of mild exacerbations, which attained statistical significance in the treatment group when compared to the control population. Twelve months after the initial treatment there was persistence of significantly greater improvement than the control group in morning peak expiratory flow, AQLQ and ACQ scores. Moreover, these improvements occurred in the setting of a reduced requirement for the amount of rescue medication needed in the treatment group. Although still in an experimental phase, bronchial thermoplasty appears to be a unique and promising therapy in difficult-to-treat asthma.

Kinase inhibitors

Interactions between recruited inflammatory cells and resident airway cells can result in the production of multiple cytokines, chemokines, growth factors and inflammatory mediators, all contributing to the pathogenesis of allergic asthma. Protein tyrosine kinases are necessary in the activation and proliferation of inflammatory cells and airway resident cells to aid in the regulation of critical inflammatory and immune processes. Certain tyrosine kinases, such as epidermal growth factor receptor (EGFR), platelet-derived growth factor receptor (PDGFR) and spleen tyrosine kinases (Syk), have been shown to play a role in allergic immune responses. Inhibitors of these tyrosine kinases have been used in the treatment of chronic myeloid leukaemia and epidermal cancers, and are now being considered for use in asthma.

Imatinib (Glivec) is an effective therapy for chronic myeloid leukaemia as well as hypereosinophilic syndrome and blocks c-kit ligand, stem cell factor (SCF) and PDGFR-α protein tyrosine kinase.[118] Al-Muhsen and colleagues reported that significantly increased amounts of SCF and c-kit expression in the airway were associated with greater severity of asthma.[119] These findings suggest that PDGFR inhibitors may be effective by targeting an overactive c-kit pathway. Berlin and Lukacs studied the effects of imatinib in a murine allergic asthma model and found that mice treated with imatinib had a significant decrease in airway hyperreactivity as well as in Th2 cytokines, IL-4 and IL-13.[118] It is unclear, despite these positive findings, what are the exact mechanisms by which imatinib exerts its effects as multiple tyrosine kinase pathways may be affected. Further investigation into these newly discovered inflammatory targets in allergic airway disease is needed and may uncover a new approach to asthma treatment.

The role of epidermal growth factor (EGF) and its receptors (EGFR) in asthma has been evaluated. The findings of increased expression in the airway of asthma subjects suggest a potential role.[120] Activation of EGFR modulates mucin production in the airway epithelium by way of the *MUC5AC* mucin gene.[121] The degree of EGFR expression appears to reflect the intensity of epithelial damage and activation, and has been shown to be enhanced with increasing asthma severity.[122] Gefitinib, an inhibitor of EGFR, has been developed for the treatment of epidermal cancers and has been studied in a murine model of allergic asthma. Hur and colleagues found that pretreatment with gefitinib of OVA-sensitized mice reduced inflammatory cell counts and cytokine concentrations (IL-4 and IL-13) in bronchoalveolar lavage fluid (BALF).[123] Furthermore, a reduction in airway eosinophil recruitment and airway hyperresponsiveness in a dose-dependent manner was also shown in the mice pretreated with gefitinib. These preliminary studies suggest that EGFR inhibition may have a role in the treatment of severe asthma.

Syk kinase may play an essential role in allergic inflammation via multiple mechanisms. This intracellular protein tyrosine kinase is involved in the signalling of high-affinity IgE receptor on mast cells as well as in the survival of eosinophils in response to IL-5 and GM-CSF.[124, 125] By affecting the signalling, Syk kinase has an important role in mast cell activation and the release of its mediators, making it a potential target in the treatment of allergic disease. BAY 61–3606 has been developed and is a potent and selective inhibitor of Syk kinase. Its use *in vitro* in atopic human basophils, eosinophils and monocytes had inhibitory effects.[126] R-112, an intranasal Syk kinase inhibitor, has been studied in allergic rhinitis in phase II clinical trials and been reported to have a rapid onset of action, improvements in symptom scores, and duration of action exceeding 4 hours.[127] In addition, the medication was well tolerated with no significant adverse events reported. Additional studies are under development to further evaluate the effect of Syk kinases in allergic disease including asthma.

Chemokine antagonists

Chemokines are chemotactic cytokines involved in the recruitment of leukocytes. Eotaxin is an eosinophil-specific chemoattractant, and contributes to the early recruitment of eosinophils in the airway during allergen challenge.[128] In addition, mucosal biopsies from the lungs of asthma subjects have shown increased mRNA and protein synthesis of eotaxin and its receptor, CCR3.[129] In CCR3-knockout mouse models, eosinophil infiltration and airway hyperresponsiveness were diminished, suggesting that CCR3 blockade could be of benefit in asthma.[130]

Monoclonal antibodies to eotaxin (CCL-11) and CCR3 antagonists have been developed and are currently being assessed for their efficacy in allergic disease. Bertilimumab (CAT-213), an anti-eotaxin-1 monoclonal antibody, has been studied in phase I/IIa clinical studies in patients with seasonal allergic rhinitis. The results from these studies have shown bertilimumab to be well tolerated and, in addition, to reduce allergen-induced infiltration of submucosal eosinophils and mast cells.[131] CCR3 antagonists are still being tested in the murine model of allergic disease but theoretically are thought to be more efficacious than eotaxin antibodies as they will block other chemokines (RANTES, eotaxin-2, eotaxin-3, MCP-3 and MCP-4) that use CCR3 as their receptor. In a mouse model of allergy, the use of a CCR3 antagonist, YM-344031, prevented both the immediate- and late-phase allergic skin reactions.[132] In addition, Fryer and colleagues showed that the use of GW-701897B, a CCR3 antagonist, prevented antigen-induced clustering of eosinophils along the nerves and also decreased hyperresponsiveness to vagal stimulation in a guinea pig model of asthma.[133] The results from these preliminary studies demonstrate that targeting eotaxin or its receptor (CCR3) may be a novel way to target allergic disease.

9.10   Conclusion

The use of biological agents in the treatment of allergic disease is still in its early stages of development. Despite relatively small number of biologicals approved for the treatment of allergic disease currently, the development of these immunomodulating agents is occurring rapidly as more is learned about the myriad of molecular mechanisms involved in asthma. As with the application of anti-IL-5 in asthma, the use of these biologicals will not only teach us more about the pathophysiology of these diseases but also generate many questions that may lead to additional targets for therapy. As asthma is a heterogeneous disease and redundancy exists in the immune system, it is unlikely that the targeting of one cytokine, chemokine or inflammatory cell will result in the resolution of the disease process. Instead, it is likely that a combination of these immunomodulators in specific phenotypes of asthma will produce the best results. Furthermore, the long-term safety of these medications needs to be assessed with long-term follow-up so clinicians and their patients can address the risk–benefit ratio in the treatment of their allergic disease. In conclusion, this is an extremely exciting time in the field of allergic diseases as we eagerly await the results of many clinical trials assessing the biological targets discussed in this chapter and hope to provide our patients with agents that will change the course of their disease.

References

1. Masoli M, Fabian D, Holt S, Beasley R, for the Global Initiative for Asthma (GINA) Program. The global burden of asthma: executive summary of the GINA Dissemination Committee Report. Allergy 2004;59:469–78.
2. Braman S. The global burden of asthma. Chest 2006;130:4–12.
3. Serra-Batlles J, Plaza V, Morejon E, et al. Costs of asthma according to the degree of severity. Eur Respir J 1998;12:1322–6.
4. Antonicelli L, Bucca C, Neri M, et al. Asthma severity and medical resource utilisation. Eur Respir J 2004;23:723–9.
5. Godard P, Chanez P, Siraudin L, et al. Costs of asthma are correlated with severity: a 1-yr prospective study. Eur Respir J 2002;19:61–7.
6. Drazen JM, Arm JP, Austen KF. Sorting out the cytokines of asthma. J Exp Med 1996;183: 1–5.
7. Erin EM, Leaker BR, Nicholson GC, et al. The effects of a monoclonal antibody directed against tumor necrosis factor-α in asthma. Am J Resp Crit Care Med 2006;174:753–62.
8. Wenzel SE, Szefler SJ, Leung DYM, et al. Bronchoscopic evaluation of severe asthma. Am J Resp Crit Care Med 1997;156:737–43.
9. Jatakanon A, Uasuf C, Maziak W, et al. Neutrophilic inflammation in severe persistent asthma. Am J Resp Crit Care Med 1999;160:1532–9.
10. Wenzel SE, Schwartz LB, Langmack EL, et al. Evidence that severe asthma can be divided pathologically into two inflammatory subtypes with distinct physiologic and clinical characteristics. Am J Resp Crit Care Med 1999;160:1001–8.
11. Wenzel SE, Busse WW. Severe asthma: lessons from the Severe Asthma Research Program (SARP). J Allergy Clin Immun 2007;119:14–21.
12. Sanford AJ, Chagani T, Zhu S, et al. Polymorphisms in the IL4, IL4RA, and FCERIB genes and asthma severity. J Allergy Clin Immun 2000;106:135–40.
13. Burchard EG, Silvermann EK, Rosenwasser LJ, et al. Association between a sequence variant in the IL-4 gene promoter and FEV_1 in asthma. Am J Resp Crit Care Med 1999;160:919–22.
14. Barnes PJ. Therapeutic strategies for allergic diseases. Nature 1999;402:B31–8.
15. National Asthma Education and Prevention Program. Guidelines for the diagnosis and management of asthma: Expert Panel Report 3. Publication no. 08-4051. Bethesda, MD: National Institutes of Health/National Heart, Lung, and Blood Institute, 2007. Available at: http://www.nhlbi.nih.gov/guidelines/asthma/asthgdln.htm.

16. Garrone P, Djossou O, Galizzi JP, Banchereau J. A recombinant extracellular domain of the human interleukin 4 receptor inhibits the biological effects of interleukin 4 on T and B lymphocytes. Eur J Immunol 1991;21:1365–9.

17. Borish LC, Nelson HS, Corren J. Efficacy of soluble IL-4 receptor for the treatment of adults with asthma. J Allergy Clin Immunol 2001;107:963–70.

18. Kotsimbos TC, Ghaffar O, Minshall EM, et al. Expression of the IL-4 receptor α-subunit is increased in bronchial biopsy specimens from atopic and nonatopic asthmatic subjects. J Allergy Clin Immunol 1998;102:859–66.

19. Renz H, Enssle K, Lauffer L, et al. Inhibition of allergen-induced IgE and IgG1 production by soluble IL-4 receptor. Int Arch Allergy Imm 1995;106:46–54.

20. Temann UA, Prasad B, Gallup MW, et al. A novel role for murine IL-4 in vivo: induction of MUC5AC gene expression and mucin hypersecretion. Am J Resp Cell Mol 1997: 16;471–8.

21. Henderson WR Jr, Chi EY, Maliszewski CR. Soluble IL-4 receptor inhibits airway inflammation following allergen challenge in a mouse model of asthma. J Immunol 2000;164:1086–95.

22. Humbert M, Durham SR, Ying S, et al. IL-4 and IL-5 mRNA and protein in bronchial biopsies from patients with atopic and nonatopic asthma: evidence against "intrinsic" asthma being a distinct immunopathologic entity. Am J Resp Crit Care Med 1996;154:1497–504.

23. Djukanović R, Wilson SJ, Kraft M, et al. Effects of treatment with anti-immunoglobulin E antibody omalizumab on airway inflammation in allergic asthma. Am J Resp Crit Care Med 2004;170:583–93.

24. Thyphronitis G, Tsokos GC, June CH, et al. IgE secretion by Epstein-Barr virus-infected purified human B lymphocytes is stimulated by interleukin 4 and suppressed by interferon γ. Proc Natl Acad Sci USA 1989;86:5580–4.

25. Boguniewicz M, Schneider LC, Milgrom H, et al. Treatment of steroid-dependent asthma with recombinant interferon-gamma. Clin Exp Allergy 1993;23:785–90.

26. Andrews AL, Holloway JW, Holgate ST, Davies DE. IL-4 receptor alpha is an important modulator of IL-4 and IL-13 receptor binding: implications for the development of therapeutic targets. J Immunol 2006;176:7456–61.

27. Borish LC, Nelson HS, Lanz MJ, et al. Interleukin-4 receptor in moderate atopic asthma, a phase I/II randomized, placebo-controlled trial. Am J Resp Crit Care Med 1999;160:1816–23.

28. Holtzman MJ. Drug development for asthma. Am J Resp Cell Mol 2003;29:163–71.

29. Bousquet J, Chanez P, Lacoste JY, et al. Eosinophilic inflammation in asthma. New Engl J Med 1990;323:1033–9.

30. Sanderson CJ. Interleukin-5, eosinophils, and disease. Blood 1992;79:3101–9.

31. Flood-Page PT, Menzies-Gow AN, Kay AB, Robinson DS. Eosinophil's role remains uncertain as anti-interleukin-5 only partially depletes numbers in asthmatic airway. Am J Resp Crit Care Med 2003;167:199–204.

32. Hamid Q, Azzawi M, Ying S, et al. Expression of mRNA for interleukin-5 in mucosal bronchial biopsies from asthma. J Clin Invest 1991;87:1541–6.

33. Corrigan CJ, Haczku A, Gemou-Engesaeth V, et al. CD4 T-lymphocyte activation in asthma is accompanied by increased serum concentrations of interleukin-5. Effect of glucocorticoid therapy. Am Rev Respir Dis 1993;147:540–7.

34. van der Veen MJ, Van Neerven RJ, De Jong EC, et al. The late asthmatic response is associated with baseline allergen-specific proliferative responsiveness of peripheral T lymphocytes in vitro and serum interleukin-5. Clin Exp Allergy 1999;29:217–27.

35. Shi HZ, Xiao CQ, Zhong D, et al. Effect of inhaled interleukin-5 on airway hyperreactivity and eosinophilia in asthmatics. Am J Resp Crit Care Med 1998;157:204–9.

36. Leckie MJ, ten Brinke A, Khan J, et al. Effects of an interleukin-5 blocking monoclonal antibody on eosinophils, airway hyper-responsiveness, and the late asthmatic response. Lancet 2000;356:2144–8.

37. Kips JC, O'Connor BJ, Langley SJ, et al. Effect of SCH55700, a humanized anti-human IL-5 antibody, in severe persistent asthma. Am J Resp Crit Care Med 2003;167: 1655–9.

38. Flood-Page P, Swenson C, Faiferman I, et al. (International Mepolizumab Study Group). A study to evaluate safety and efficacy of mepolizumab in patients with moderate persistent asthma. Am J Resp Crit Care Med 2007;176:1062–71.

39. Green RH, Brightling CE, McKenna S, et al. Asthma exacerbations and sputum eosinophil counts: a randomised controlled trial. Lancet 2002;360:1715–21.

40. Jayaram L, Pizzichini MM, Cook RJ, et al. Determining asthma treatment by monitoring sputum cell counts: effect on exacerbations. Eur Respir J 2006;27:483–94.

41. Liu LY, Sedgwick JB, Bates ME, et al. Decreased expression of membrane IL-5 receptor alpha on human eosinophils: I. Loss of membrane IL-5 receptor alpha on airway eosinophils and increased soluble IL-5 receptor alpha in the airway after allergen challenge. J Immunol 2002;169:6452–8.

42. Gregory B, Kirchem A, Phipps S, et al. Differential regulation of human eosinophil IL-3, IL-5, and GM-CSF receptor alpha-chain expression by cytokines: IL-3, IL-5, and GM-CSF down-regulate IL-5 receptor alpha expression with loss of IL-5 responsiveness, but up-regulate IL-3 receptor alpha expression. J Immunol 2003;170:5359–66.

43. Rothenberg ME, Klion AD, Roufosse FE, et al. (Mepolizumab HES Study Group). Treatment of patients with the hypereosinophilic syndrome with mepolizumab. New Engl J Med 2008;358:1215–28.

44. Garrett JK, Jameson SC, Thomson B, et al. Anti-interleukin-5 (mepolizumab) therapy for hypereosinophilic syndromes. J Allergy Clin Immunol 2004;113:115–9.

45. Wynn TA. IL-13 effector functions. Annu Rev Immunol 2003;21:425–56.

46. Wills-Karp M, Luyimbazi J, Xu X, et al. Interleukin-13: central mediator of allergic asthma. Science 1998;282:2258–61.

47. Grünig G, Warnock M, Wakil AE, et al. Requirement for IL-13 independently of IL-4 in experimental asthma. Science 1998;282:2261–3.

48. Zhu Z, Homer RJ, Wang Z, et al. Pulmonary expression of interleukin-13 causes inflammation, mucus hypersecretion, subepithelial fibrosis, physiologic abnormalities, and eotaxin production. J Clin Invest 1999;103:779–88.

49. Huang SK, Xiao HQ, Kleine-Tebbe J, et al. IL-13 expression at the sites of allergen challenge in patients with asthma. J Immunol 1995;155:2688–94.

50. Wills-Karp M. The gene encoding interleukin-13: a susceptibility locus for asthma and related traits. Respir Res 2000;1:19–23.

51. Saha SK, Berry MA, Parker D, et al. Increased sputum and bronchial biopsy IL-13 expression in severe asthma. J Allergy Clin Immunol 2008;121:685–91.

52. Wenzel SE, Wilbraham D, Fuller R, et al. Effect of an interleukin-4 on late phase asthmatic response to allergen challenge in asthmatic patients: results of two phase 2a studies. Lancet 2007;370:1422–31.

53. Bazzoni F, Beutler B. The tumor necrosis factor ligand and receptor families. New Engl J Med 1996;334:1717–25.

54. Medzhitov R, Janeway C. Innate immune recognition: mechanisms and pathways. Immunol Rev 2000;173:89–97.

55. Gosset P, Tsicopoulos A, Wallaert B, et al. Increased secretion of tumor necrosis factor alpha and interleukin-6 by alveolar macrophages consecutive to the development of the late asthmatic reaction. J Allergy Clin Immunol 1991;561:561–71.

56. Ying S, Robinson D, Varney V, et al. TNF alpha mRNA expression in allergic inflammation. Clin Exp Allergy 1991;21:745–50.

57. Bradding P, Roberts JA, Britten KM, et al. Interleukin-4, -5, and -6 and tumor necrosis factor-alpha in normal and asthmatic airways: evidence for the human mast cell as a source of these cytokines. Am J Respir Cell Mol Biol 1994;10:471–80.

58. Ackerman V, Marini M, Vittori E, et al. (1994) Detection of cytokines and their cellular sources in bronchial biopsy specimens from asthmatic patients. Relationship to atopic status, symptoms, and level of airway hyperresponsiveness. Chest. 1994 Mar;105 (3):687–96.

59. Thomas PS, Yates DH, Barnes PJ. Tumor necrosis factor-α increases airway responsiveness and sputum neutrophilia in normal human subjects. Am J Respir Crit Care Med 1995;152:76–80.

60. Huber M, Beutler B, Keppler D. Tumor necrosis factor alpha stimulates leukotriene production in vivo. Eur J Immunol 1988;18:2085–8.

61. Lassalle P, Gosset P, Delneste Y, et al. Modulation of adhesion molecule expression on endothelial cells during the late asthmatic reaction: role of macrophage-derived tumour necrosis factor-alpha. Clin Exp Immunol 1993;94:105–10.

62. Yamamoto H, Sedgwick JB, Busse WW. Differential regulation of eosinophil adhesion and transmigration by pulmonary microvascular endothelial cells. J Immunol 1998;161:971–7.

63. Slungaard A, Vercellotti GM, Walker G, et al. Tumor necrosis factor alpha/cachectin stimulates eosinophil oxidant production and toxicity towards human endothelium. J Exp Med 1990;171:2025–41.

64. Franchimont D, Martens H, Hagelstein MT, et al. Tumor necrosis factor alpha decreases, and interleukin-10 increases, the sensitivity of human monocytes to dexamethasone: potential regulation of the glucocorticoid receptor. J Clin Endocr Metab 1999;84:2834–9.

65. Desmoulière A, Geinoz A, Gabbiani F, Gabbiani G. Transforming growth factor-beta 1 induces alpha-smooth muscle actin expression in granulation tissue myofibroblasts and in quiescent and growing cultured fibroblasts. J Cell Biol 1993;122:103–11.

66. Berry MA, Hargadon B, Shelley M, et al. Evidence of a role of tumor necrosis factor α in refractory asthma. New Engl J Med 2006;354:697–708.

67. Feldmann M, Maini RN. TNF defined as a therapeutic target for rheumatoid arthritis and other autoimmune diseases. Nat Med 2003;9:1245–50.

68. Renzetti LM, Paciorek PM, Tannu SA, et al. Pharmacological evidence for tumor necrosis factor as a mediator of allergic inflammation in the airways. J Pharmacol Exp Ther 1996;278:847–53.

69. Khalil SC, Brown DM, Chumney-Malacara J, Crow J. Infliximab therapy for rheumatoid arthritis (RA) and asthma or asthma/COPD in addition to improving RA status [abstract]. J Allergy Clin Immunol 2002;109:s243.

70. Brightling C, Berry M, Amrani Y. Targeting TNF-α: A novel therapeutic approach for asthma. J Allergy Clin Immunol 2008;121:5–10.

71. Howarth PH, Bau KS, Arshad HS, et al. Tumour necrosis factor (TNFα) as a novel therapeutic target in symptomatic corticosteroid dependent asthma. Thorax 2005;60:1012–8.

72. Morjaria JB, Chauhan AJ, Babu KS, et al. The role of a soluble TNF-α receptor fusion protein (etanercept) in corticosteroid refractory asthma: a double-blind, randomised placebo-controlled trial. Thorax 2008;63:584–91.

73. Rouhani FN, Meitin CA, Kaler M, et al. Effect of tumor necrosis factor antagonism on allergen-mediated asthmatic airway inflammation. Respir Med 2005;99:1175–82.

74. Burrows F, Martinez FD, Halonen RA, et al. Association of asthma with serum IgE levels and skin test reactivity to allergens. New Engl J Med 1989;320:271–7.

75. Sears MR, Burrows B, Flannery EM, et al. Relation between airway responsiveness and serum IgE in children with asthma and in apparently normal children. New Engl J Med 1991;325:1067–71.

76. Pollart SM, Chapman MD, Fiocco GP, et al. Epidemiology of acute asthma: IgE antibodies to common inhalant allergens as a risk factor for emergency room visits. J Allergy Clin Immunol 1989;83:875–82.

77. Sunyer J, Anto JM, Sabria J, et al. Relationship between serum IgE and airway responsiveness in adults with asthma. J Allergy Clin Immunol 1995;95:966–706.

78. Fahy JV, Fleming HE, Wong HH, et al. The effect of an anti-IgE monoclonal antibody on the early- and late-phase responses to allergen inhalation in asthmatic subjects. Am J Resp Crit Care Med 1997;155:1828–34.

79. Cockcroft DW, Swystun VA, Bhagat R. Interaction of inhaled β_2 agonist and inhaled corticosteroid on airway responsiveness to allergen and methacholine. Am J Resp Crit Care Med 1995;152:1485–9.

80. Presta LG, Lahr SJ, Shields RL, et al. Humanization of an antibody directed against IgE. J Immunol 1993: 151;2623–32.

81. Holgate S, Casale T, Wenzel S, et al. The anti-inflammatory effects of omalizumab confirm the central role of IgE in allergic inflammation. J Allergy Clin Immunol 2005;115:459–65.

82. Prussin C, Griffith DT, Boesel KM, et al. Omalizumab treatment downregulates dendritic cell FcεRI expression. J Allergy Clin Immunol 2003;112:1147–54.

83. Beck LA, Marcotte GV, MacGlashan D, et al. Omalizumab-induced reductions in mast cell FcεRI expression and function. J Allergy Clin Immunol 2004;114:527–30.

84. Noga O, Hanf G, Kunkel G. Immunological and clinical changes in allergic asthmatics following treatment with omalizumab. Int Arch Allergy Immunol 2003;131:46–52.

85. Milgrom H, Fick RB, Su JQ (The rhuMAb-E25 study group). Treatment of allergic asthma with monoclonal anti-IgE antibody. New Engl J Med 1999;341:1966–73.

86. Busse WW, Corren J, Lanier BQ, et al. Omalizumab, anti-IgE recombinant humanized monoclonal antibody, for the treatment of severe allergic asthma. J Allergy Clin Immunol 2001;108:184–90.

87. Milgrom H, Berger W, Nayak A. Treatment of childhood asthma with anti-immunoglobulin E antibody (omalizumab). Pediatrics 2001;108:e36.

88. Solèr M, Matz J, Townley R, et al. The anti-IgE antibody omalizumab reduced exacerbations and steroid requirement in allergic asthmatics. Eur Respir J 2001;18:254–61.

89. Corren J, Casale T, Deniz Y, Ashby M. Omalizumab, a recombinant humanized anti-IgE antibody, reduces asthma-related emergency room visits and hospitalizations in patients with allergic asthma. J Allergy Clin Immunol 2003;111:87–90.

90. Lin H, Boesel KM, Griffith DT, et al. Omalizumab rapidly decreases nasal allergic response and FcεRI on basophils. J Allergy Clin Immunol 2004;113:297–302.

91. Hanf G, Noga O, O'Connor A, Kunkel G. Omalizumab inhibits allergen challenge-induced nasal response. Eur Respir J 2004;23:414–18.

92. Casale TB, Condemi J, LaForce C, et al. (Omalizumab Seasonal Allergic Rhinitis Trial Group). Effect of omalizumab on symptoms of seasonal allergic rhinitis, a randomized controlled trial. JAMA 2001;286:2956–67.

93. Ädelroth E, Rak S, Haahtela T, et al. Recombinant humanized mAb-E25, an anti-IgE mAb, in birth pollen-induced seasonal allergic rhinitis. J Allergy Clin Immunol 2000;106:253–9.

94. Chervinsky P, Casale T, Townley R, et al. Omalizumab, an anti-IgE antibody, in the treatment of adults and adolescents with perennial allergic rhinitis. Ann Allerg Asthma Immunol 2003;91:160–7.
95. Vignola AM, Humbert M, Bousquet J, et al. Efficacy and tolerability of anti-immunoglobulin E therapy with omalizumab in patients with concomitant allergic asthma and persistent allergic rhinitis: SOLAR. Allergy 2004;59:709–17.
96. Kuehr J, Brauburger J, Zielen S, et al. Efficacy of combination treatment with anti-IgE plus specific immunotherapy in polysensitized children and adolescents with seasonal allergic rhinitis. J Allergy Clin Immunol 2002;109:274–80.
97. Casale TB, Busse WW, Kline JN, et al. Omalizumab pretreatment decreases acute reaction after rush immunotherapy for ragweed-induced seasonal allergic rhinitis. J Allergy Clin Immunol 2006;117:134–40.
98. Strachan DP. Hay fever, hygiene, and household size. Brit Med J 1989;299:1259–60.
99. Folkerts G, Walzl G, Openshaw PJ. Do common childhood infections "teach" the immune system not to be allergic? Immunol Today 2000;21:118–20.
100. Silverman ES, Drazen JM. Immunostimulatory DNA for asthma: better than eating dirt. Am J Respir Cell Mol Biol 2003;28:645–7.
101. Yamamoto S, Yamamoto T, Kataoka T, et al. Unique palindromic sequences in synthetic oligonucleotides are required to induce IFN and augment IFN-mediated natural killer activity. J Immunol 1992;148:4072–6.
102. Krieg AM. CpG motifs in bacterial DNA and their immune effects. Annu Rev Immunol 2002;20:709–60.
103. Kline JN. Eat dirt: CpG DNA and immunomodulation of asthma. Proc Am Thoracic Soc 2007;4:283–8.
104. Stokes J, Casale TB. Rationale for new treatments aimed at IgE immunomodulation. Ann Allergy Asthma Immunol 2004;93:212–17.
105. Liu N, Ohnishi N, Ni L, et al. CpG directly induces T-bet expression and inhibits IgG1 and IgE switching in B-cells. Nat Immunol 2003;4:687–93.
106. Tighe H, Takabayashi K, Schwartz D, et al. Conjugation of immunostimulatory DNA to the short ragweed allergen Amb a 1 enhances its immunogenicity and reduces its allergenicity. J Allergy Clin Immunol 2000;106:124–34.
107. Broide D, Schwarze J, Tighe H, et al. Immunostimulatory DNA sequences inhibit IL-5, eosinophilic inflammation, and airway hyperresponsiveness in mice. J Immunol 1998;161:7054–62.
108. Sur S, Wild JS, Choudhury BK, et al. Long term prevention of allergic lung inflammation in a mouse model of asthma by CpG oligodeoxynucleotides. J Immunol 1999;162:6284–93.
109. Choudhury BK, Wild JS, Alam R, et al. In vivo role of p38 mitogen activated protein kinase in mediating the anti-inflammatory effects of CpG oligodeoxynucleotide in murine asthma. J Immunol 2002;169:5955–61.
110. Kline JN, Waldschmidt TJ, Businga TR, et al. Modulation of airway inflammation by CpG oligodeoxynucleotides in a murine model of asthma. J Immunol 1998;160:2555–9.
111. Santeliz JV, Van Nest G, Traquina P, et al. Amb a 1-linked CpG oligodeoxynucleotides reverse established airway hyperresponsiveness in a murine model of asthma. J Allergy Clin Immunol 2002;109:455–62.
112. Creticos PS, Schroeder JT, Hamilton RG, et al. Immunotherapy with a ragweed-Toll-like receptor 9 agonist vaccine for allergic rhinitis. New Engl J Med 2006;355:1445–55.
113. Bernstein DI, Segall N, Nayak A, et al. Safety and efficacy of the novel vaccine TOLAMBA in ragweed allergic adults, a dose finding study. J Allergy Clin Immunol 2007;119:s78.

114. Gauvreau GM, Hessel EM, Boulet LP, et al. Immunostimulatory sequences regulate interferon-inducible genes but not allergic airway responses. Am J Resp Crit Care Med 2006;174: 15–20.

115. Cox PG, Miller J, Mitzner W, Leff AR. Radiofrequency ablation of airway smooth muscle for sustained treatment of asthma: preliminary investigations. Eur Respir J 2004;24:659–63.

116. Cox G, Miller JD, McWilliams A, et al. Bronchial thermoplasty for asthma. Am J Resp Crit Care Med 2005;173:965–9.

117. Cox G, Thomson NC, Rubin AS, et al. Asthma control during the year after bronchial thermoplasty. New Engl J Med 2007;356:1327–37.

118. Berlin AA, Lukacs NW. Treatment of cockroach allergen asthma model with imatinib attenuates airway responses. J Allergy Clin Immunol 2004;171:35–9.

119. Al-Muhsen SZ, Shablovsky G, Olivenstein R, et al. The expression of stem cell factor and c-kit receptor in human asthmatic airways. Clin Exp Allergy 2004;34:911–16.

120. Wong WSF, Leong KP. Tyrosine kinase inhibitors: a new approach for asthma. Biochim Biophys Acta 2004;1697:53–69.

121. Takeyama K, Dabbagh K, Lee HM, et al. Epidermal growth factor system regulates mucin production in airways. Proc Natl Acad Sci U S A 1999;96:3081–6.

122. Puddicombe SM, Polosa R, Richter A, et al. Involvement of the epidermal growth factor in epithelial repair in asthma. FASEB J 2000;14:1362–74.

123. Hur GY, Lee SY, Lee SH, et al. Potential use of an anticancer drug gefinitib, an EGFR inhibitor, on allergic airway inflammation. Exp Mol Med 2007;39:367–75.

124. Yousefi S, Hoessli DC, Blaser K, et al. Requirement of Lyn and Syk tyrosine kinases for the prevention of apoptosis by cytokines in human eosinophils. J Exp Med 1996;183:1407–14.

125. Costello PS, Turner M, Walter AE, et al. Critical role for the tyrosine kinase Syk in signaling through the high affinity IgE receptor of mast cells. Oncogene 1996;13:2595–605.

126. Yamamoto N, Takeshita K, Shichijo M, et al. The orally available spleen tyrosine kinase inhibitor 2-[7-(3,4-dimethoxyphenyl)-imidazo[1,2-c]pyrimidin-5-ylamino]nicotinamide dihydrochloride (BAY 61–3606) blocks antigen-induced airway inflammation in rodents. J Pharmacol Exp Ther 2003;306:1174–81.

127. Meltzer EO, Berkowitz RB, Grossbard EB. An intranasal Syk-kinase inhibitor (R112) improves the symptoms of seasonal allergic rhinitis in a park environment. J Allergy Clin Immunol 2005;115:791–6.

128. Rothenberg M, MacLean JA, Pearlman E, et al. Targeted disruption of the chemokine eotaxin partially reduces antigen-induced tissue eosinophilia. J Exp Med 1997;185:785–90.

129. Ying S, Meng Q, Zeibecoglou K, et al. Eosinophil chemotactic chemokines (eotaxin, eotaxin-2, RANTES, monocyte chemoattractant protein-3 (MCP-3), and MCP-4), and C-C chemokine receptor 3 expression in bronchial biopsies from atopic and nonatopic (intrinsic) asthmatics. J Immunol 1999;163:6321–9.

130. Humbles AA, Lu B, Friend DS, et al. The murine CCR3 receptor regulates both the role of eosinophils and mast cells in allergen-induced airway inflammation and hyperresponsiveness. Proc Natl Acad Sci U S A 2002;99:1479–84.

131. Ding C, Li J, Zhang X. Bertilimumab Cambridge Antibody Technology Group. Curr Opin Invest Dr 2004;5:1213–18.

132. Suzuki K, Morokata T, Morihira K, et al. In vitro and in vivo characterization of a novel CCR3 antagonist, YM-344031. Biochem Biophys Res Comm 2006;339:1217–23.

133. Fryer AD, Stein LH, Nie Z, et al. Neuronal eotaxin and the effects of CCR3 antagonist on airway hyperreactivity and M2 receptor dysfunction. J Clin Invest 2006;116;228–36.

10

Anti-infective treatments in asthma and COPD

Jonathan D.R. Macintyre and Sebastian L. Johnston

Department of Respiratory Medicine, National Heart and Lung Institute,
MRC & Asthma UK Centre in Allergic Mechanisms of Asthma,
Imperial College London, UK

10.1   Introduction

Asthma is a multifactorial disease with interactions between genetic susceptibility and environmental agents, such as allergens, pollutants and respiratory tract pathogens; its prevalence is increasing. The major costs of asthma-related morbidity, mortality and healthcare are a result of acute exacerbations. These occur despite optimal use of currently available therapies. There is a wealth of evidence to implicate viruses in acute exacerbations of asthma, and growing evidence that infections with atypical bacteria may also play a role in asthma exacerbations; moreover, both viruses and atypical bacteria may be implicated in persistent asthma. Viruses implicated include rhinoviruses, coronaviruses, respiratory syncytial virus, parainfluenzaviruses, influenzaviruses, adenoviruses, human metapneumovirus and human bocavirus. Bacteria, particularly the atypical bacteria *Mycoplasma pneumoniae* and *Chlamydophila pneumoniae*, have been implicated. It is likely that recurrent infection or chronic infection with these agents plays a role in disease progression.

Chronic obstructive pulmonary disease (COPD) is one of the most prevalent diseases in developed countries, and the number of people affected by the disease is increasing. COPD exacerbations are characterized by increasing dyspnoea, sputum volume and purulence.[1] There is mounting evidence that as well as being the major cause of morbidity, mortality and healthcare costs in COPD, exacerbations accelerate decline in lung function, leading to significantly impaired long-term health status of patients. This makes prevention of exacerbations all the more important. A cardinal feature of exacerbations is an increase in the degree of airway inflammation above that of baseline. Bacteria, viruses or a combination of both are implicated in up to 78% of exacerbations.[2]

Advances in Combination Therapy for Asthma and COPD, First Edition. Edited by Jan Lötvall.
© 2012 John Wiley & Sons, Ltd. Published 2012 by John Wiley & Sons, Ltd.

The same organisms that are implicated in asthma are also implicated in COPD, as well as the common bacteria *Haemophilus influenzae*, *Streptococcus pneumoniae* and *Moraxella catarrhalis*. Bronchoscopic and sputum sampling for studies of infections in COPD have confirmed that many stable patients carry bacteria in the lower respiratory tract, such as non-typable *S. pneumoniae*, *H. influenzae* and *M. catarrhalis*.

Combination inhaler therapy in asthma and COPD has been used for some years. There is a wealth of evidence to support its use, as discussed elsewhere in this volume. A Cochrane review examined the use of a combination of a long-acting β_2-agonist (LABA) and inhaled corticosteroid (ICS) versus high-dose inhaled steroids in asthmatics.[3] It concluded that combination therapy resulted in improved lung function and symptoms and decreased use of reliever therapy. Another Cochrane review comparing combination fluticasone and salmeterol versus fixed-dose budesonide and formoterol concluded that there was no statistically significant difference between the combinations in the need for oral corticosteroids or number of adverse events.[4] This contrasts with the CONCEPT trial, which showed that patients having a stable dose of salmeterol/fluticasone had more symptom-free days and half the exacerbation rate compared to patients having an adjustable dose of formoterol/budesonide.[5] The use of formoterol/budesonide both in maintenance and relief has been investigated. Rabe et al. compared this with high-dose budesonide and as-required terbutaline.[6] They found an improvement in morning peak expiratory flow, fewer hospitalizations, less oral corticosteroid requirement and overall lower steroid load in the combination group. Also formoterol/budesonide maintenance and reliever therapy has been compared to high-dose salmeterol/fluticasone plus a short-acting beta-agonist.[7] This study showed a reduced incidence of exacerbations and hospitalizations in the formoterol/budesonide group. Other agents are also used in combination, particularly the leukotriene antagonists. In a recent systematic review Joos et al. concluded that montelukast as an add-on treatment to ICS was more effective than ICS alone.[8] However, salmeterol/ICS was more effective than montelukast/ICS.

A Cochrane review assessing combination ICS and LABA versus ICS alone in COPD found a significant reduction in morbidity and mortality in the combination group with no significant difference in adverse events.[9] The TORCH study investigated salmeterol/fluticasone as a single inhaler compared to placebo and single-agent inhalers.[10] Although the primary endpoint of death from all causes did not reach statistical significance, there were significant benefits in frequency of exacerbations, health status and spirometric values in the combination group. The use of tiotropium in combination has also been extensively investigated. The UPLIFT study was a randomized, double-blind trial comparing four years of tiotropium versus placebo in COPD patients permitted to use all respiratory medications except inhaled anticholinergics.[11] There was a significant decrease in the risk of exacerbation and number of hospitalizations in the tiotropium arm, along with improvements in lung function and quality of life, though no significant reduction in the rate of decline of forced expiratory volume in 1 second (FEV_1). Vogelmeier et al. recently published a 6-month study of formoterol and tiotropium in combination versus single agents and placebo, concluding that combination therapy was superior in the primary endpoint (FEV_1 2 hours post-dose after

24 weeks) and all groups were better than placebo in the number of bad days, symptoms, use of rescue medication and quality of life.[12] Similarly, Singh et al. discovered greater improvements in bronchodilation in COPD patients having a combination of tiotropium and salmeterol/fluticasone compared to single agents.[13]

These studies highlight the evidence for the use of combination inhaler therapy in asthma and COPD. However, the role of anti-infectives in asthma and COPD has long been a contentious issue and their role in combination therapy has yet to be determined. In this chapter we aim to address their role, by discussing the microbiology of airways disease, examining the evidence for a role for infection in disease pathogenesis, both in stable disease and exacerbations, evaluating the current evidence for the use of antibiotics and antivirals and their mechanisms of action, and commenting on future directions in this field.

10.2   Current guidelines

All the guidelines published thus far discuss the role of anti-infectives in exacerbations of airways disease. Currently there are no recommendations for the use of these agents in stable disease.

Asthma

National Asthma Education and Prevention Program Expert Panel (NAEPP)

The NAEPP report, in 2002, indicates that antibiotics are not currently recommended for the treatment of acute asthma exacerbations except when fever, purulent sputum or clear evidence of infection are present.[14] This advice is based on two rather old trials. They both were randomized, double-blind, placebo-controlled trials testing routine antibiotic administration in addition to standard care in adult[15] and paediatric[16] populations with asthma exacerbations. No association was found between antibiotic treatment and improvement in any asthma outcome, though both studies were small and used penicillin derivatives, to which atypical pathogens such as *M. pneumoniae* and *C. pneumoniae* show poor responses. The 2007 NAEPP guidelines continue not to support the routine use of antibiotics in asthma exacerbations. They do discuss a role for macrolide antibiotics in chronic asthma but conclude that current data are insufficient to support their use.[17]

British Thoracic Society (BTS)

The BTS/SIGN guidelines[18] state that 'when an infection precipitates an exacerbation of asthma it is likely to be viral in type'. These guidelines cite the same trial as NAEPP for saying the role of bacterial infection has been overestimated.[15] They cite a Cochrane review that concludes that there is little evidence to support the use of antibiotics in acute asthma,[19] leading to the recommendation that routine prescription of antibiotics is not indicated for acute asthma in both adults and children. Likewise, antivirals are not recommended.

COPD

European Respiratory Society/American Thoracic Society

These guidelines state that antibiotics may be initiated in COPD exacerbations in patients who have a change in sputum characteristics (purulence and/or volume), that the choice should be based on local bacterial resistance patterns, and that amoxicillin/clavulanate or fluoroquinolones should be used, except where *Pseudomonas* spp. are suspected, when combination therapy should be used.[20]

National Institute for Health and Clinical Excellence (NICE)

The NICE guidelines[21] in the UK comment on the controversy about whether antibiotics have a benefit in exacerbations. They note that a meta-analysis of nine trials found a small, but statistically significant effect favouring antibiotics over placebo in patients with exacerbations of COPD.[22] Anthonisen et al. showed a better outcome with antibiotic compared to placebo based upon the severity of exacerbations. Type I exacerbations (increased amount and purulence of sputum and dyspnoea) benefited the most, with resolution of symptoms in 63% of the antibiotic-treated exacerbations and 43% of the placebo group. Patients with type III exacerbations (who met only one of the three criteria) did not show any benefit.[1] The guidelines therefore recommend that (i) antibiotics should be used to treat exacerbations of COPD associated with a history of more purulent sputum, and (ii) patients with exacerbations without more purulent sputum do not need antibiotic therapy unless there is consolidation on a chest radiograph or clinical signs of pneumonia.

Canadian

The Canadian guidelines for the management of acute exacerbations of COPD state that antimicrobial therapy is warranted for patients in the Anthonisen type I or II categories, but not for type III.[23] An assessment of risk of treatment failure should be made on clinical grounds as well as features such as significant impairment of lung function (FEV_1 ≤50% predicted), frequent exacerbations (≥4 per year), long duration of disease, significant comorbidity (particularly ischaemic heart disease and congestive cardiac failure), use of supplemental oxygen and chronic oral corticosteroid use. Broad-spectrum agents such as fluoroquinolones or amoxicillin/clavulanate are recommended for high-risk groups. Patients presenting with an exacerbation within 3 months of an acute exacerbation should be treated with a different class of antibiotic.

The published guidelines all support a role for antibiotics in acute exacerbations of COPD. None mention any role for antivirals.

Table 10.1   Causes of exacerbations of asthma.

Viral	Bacterial	Other
Rhinoviruses	*Mycoplasma pneumoniae*	Allergens
Respiratory syncytial virus	*Chlamydophila pneumoniae*	Environmental pollutants
Influenzaviruses		Occupational irritants
Human metapneumovirus		Medication: aspirin,
Adenoviruses		beta-blockers
Coronaviruses		Exercise
Parainfluenzavirus		

10.3   Acute exacerbations of asthma

Asthma exacerbations are characterized by an exaggerated lower respiratory tract response to environmental exposures leading to worsening of asthma symptoms and lung function. The causes of exacerbations are illustrated in Table 10.1, with viral infections being the most common cause.

10.4   Increased susceptibility to infection in asthmatics

Asthmatic individuals have increased susceptibility to viral infection. Corne et al. showed that in cohabiting couples, one of whom had asthma, asthmatics were no more likely than controls to develop rhinovirus (RV) infections (10.1% vs 8.5% controls).[24] However, lower respiratory tract symptoms associated with RV infections were significantly more severe ($P = 0.001$) and longer lasting ($P = 0.005$) in asthmatics compared to healthy controls. Kling et al. showed that RV ribonucleic acid (RNA) was detectable in over 40% of asthmatic children 6 weeks after an acute exacerbation.[25] In patients who had persistent RV RNA after 6 weeks, measurements of peak expiratory flow in the emergency room were significantly lower than in patients in whom RV RNA was present in the emergency room but absent after 6 weeks ($P = 0.009$). This suggests that the severity of acute asthma may be linked to prolonged and possibly more severe RV infections.

It has also been reported that asthma is a risk factor for invasive pneumococcal disease. Talbot et al. conducted a nested case-control study to examine the association between asthma and invasive pneumococcal disease.[26] They found that asthma was an independent risk factor for invasive pneumococcal disease, with a risk among asthmatics at least double that of controls. The mechanisms for this increased susceptibility are not known, but interferon production has been found to be deficient in asthmatic bronchoalveolar macrophages following stimulation with lipopolysaccharide.[27] The association of *C. pneumoniae* and *M. pneumoniae* with asthma has prompted further research.

There is some evidence that virus-induced asthma exacerbations may be worsened by concomitant bacterial infection. Ishizuka et al. examined the effects of rhinovirus infection on *S. pneumoniae* adherence to human tracheal epithelial cells.[28] They found that with cells infected with RV-14, the number of *S. pneumoniae* adhering increased and that the use of nuclear factor kappa B (NF-κB) inhibitors decreased adherence. This suggests that RV infection stimulates bacterial adhesion to airway epithelial cells and that this is, at least in part, mediated through activation of transcription factors. Oliver et al. further investigated the possibility of RV infection increasing the risk of bacterial infection.[29] They identified impaired cytokine responses to bacterial lipopolysaccharide and lipoteichoic acid (components of Gram-negative and Gram-positive bacterial cell walls) by alveolar macrophages following infection with both major- and minor-group RVs. This has important implications in the pathogenesis of asthma exacerbations.

10.5 Role of atypical bacteria in asthma

Mycoplasma pneumoniae and *Chlamydophila pneumoniae* are atypical bacteria with very different life cycles. *M. pneumoniae* is an extracellular bacterium. *C. pneumoniae* is an obligate intracellular bacterium that exists in two forms: the elementary body (the infectious form) and the reticulate body (the metabolic form). It has the ability to persist in an inactive state in humans, hence the interest in this pathogen in the development of chronic asthma. Acute and chronic diseases of the respiratory tract are caused by both of these organisms, and subclinical infection is common. There is a high prevalence of humans with antibodies to *M. pneumoniae* and *C. pneumoniae*.[30]

These bacteria are difficult to culture due to their extreme fastidiousness, making studies investigating the association of atypical bacteria and asthma difficult. Studies have mostly relied on serological tests to diagnose infection. The only serological method currently recommended for the routine diagnosis of *C. pneumoniae* is the microimmunofluorescence (MIF) test.[31] The MIF test allows distinction between acute infection (defined by a four-fold rise in IgG between acute and convalescent samples or an acute IgM titre ≥ 1:16) or past exposure (indicated by an IgG titre ≥ 1:16). Laboratory detection of *M. pneumoniae* is largely based on enzyme-linked immunosorbent assay (ELISA). Elevated IgM levels can effectively indicate recent or current infection, particularly in children, but are not always elevated in adults. Hence both IgM and IgG measurement by ELISA allows a more accurate diagnosis. A repeat measurement of IgG 2–3 weeks later would identify an acute infection if there were a four-fold or greater increase in the IgG titre. The polymerase chain reaction (PCR) is widely used for the rapid diagnosis of *M. pneumoniae* and *C. pneumoniae* in the research setting. Unlike *M. pneumoniae*, assays for *C. pneumoniae* are not yet available as standardized commercial tests.

The possible mechanisms by which these atypical bacteria may promote the development and exacerbation of asthma are poorly understood. Both infections cause ciliostasis, increase mucus production in the lung and cause chronic lower airway inflammation.[30] The following discussion will evaluate some of the evidence for the association of these bacteria in stable asthma and exacerbations.

Atypical bacteria in stable asthma

Chlamydophila pneumoniae

Numerous studies have investigated the association of *C. pneumoniae* and stable asthma. As many studies rely on serology they are unable easily to distinguish between acute and chronic infection. In a study, spouse pairs consisting of an atopic asthmatic and a non-atopic non-asthmatic, were investigated with regular nasal aspirate sampling, and actively replicating *C. pneumoniae* infection was detected by reverse transcriptase-PCR (RT-PCR). Spouse pairs were chosen to match exposure to infection as closely as possible. *C. pneumoniae* was positive in 6.4% of samples from atopic asthmatics compared to 2.3% of samples from controls ($P = 0.007$).[32] This study confirmed that *C. pneumoniae* infection is detected more frequently among asthmatics than non-asthmatic participants.

Another study examined the association between IgG and IgA titres to *C. pneumoniae* and the severity of asthma.[33] The authors found that higher titres of antibodies were associated with markers of asthma severity. High-dose inhaled steroid use was associated with a 74.1% increase in IgG titre ($P = 0.04$) and a 70.6% increase in IgA ($P = 0.0001$) compared to low-dose inhaled steroid use. The titre of antibody increased by 0.8% for every 1% decrease in percent predicted FEV_1. An elevation in IgA was associated with a higher daytime symptom score.

In a recent study, investigating the prevalence of *C. pneumoniae* infection in asthmatic patients, the frequency of PCR positivity for *C. pneumoniae* in throat wash samples was higher in stable asthmatics (28.6%) than in healthy controls (11.8%) ($P < 0.01$).[34]

These studies confirm increased detection of *C. pneumoniae* in patients with asthma. The importance of this association requires further study.

Mycoplasma pneumoniae

Although a role for *M. pneumoniae* in exacerbations of asthma has been proposed for some years its role in chronic asthma was not investigated until the late 1990s. Kraft et al. showed that *M. pneumoniae* was detected by PCR in 10 out of 18 subjects with chronic stable asthma compared to 1 out of 11 control subjects ($P = 0.02$). Interestingly all enzyme-linked immunoassays for respiratory viruses were negative.[35]

A further extension of this study, published in 2001, found 25 out of 55 stable asthmatics had a positive PCR result to *M. pneumoniae* compared to 1 out of 11 control subjects.[36] Some patients were in common with the previous study.[35] Both these studies demonstrate the association of stable asthma and *M. pneumoniae*. Further research is needed to determine whether this infection is important for disease development or whether there is increased prevalence of this bacterium due to another as yet unidentified predisposing factor.

Atypical bacteria in asthma exacerbations

Virus infections have been associated with 80–85% of asthma exacerbations in children and 75–80% of adult exacerbations. There is also evidence suggesting a role for atypical bacteria in the aetiology of asthma exacerbations.

Chlamydophila pneumoniae

A longitudinal study of 108 children with asthma symptoms was performed.[37] When respiratory symptoms were reported a nasal aspirate was obtained, the presence of *C. pneumoniae* infection was tested by PCR and *C. pneumoniae*-specific secretory IgA was detected by ELISA. This showed that although *C. pneumoniae* detections were similar between the symptomatic and asymptomatic episodes, those children who reported multiple episodes tended to remain PCR positive, suggesting chronic *C. pneumoniae* infection. IgA antibodies were more than seven times greater in subjects who reported four or more exacerbations compared to those who reported just one ($P < 0.02$). The authors concluded that immune responses to *C. pneumoniae* are positively associated with frequency of asthma exacerbations. Of interest, samples were analysed from a previous study that had detected virus infections in 80–85% of exacerbations,[38] indicating that virus infections interact with *C. pneumoniae* to increase risk/frequency of exacerbations. The mechanisms of this interaction are poorly understood.

Similarly, in an adult asthmatic population presenting to the emergency department who underwent sputum induction and spirometry within 4 hours of presentation and had acute and convalescent serology for *C. pneumoniae*-specific IgA and IgG, 20 (38%) subjects demonstrated an increase in *C. pneumoniae* antibody levels.[39] Fifteen of these had an increase in IgA levels on a background of raised IgG, suggesting reactivation of chronic infection, and five had a rise in IgG having been serologically negative at the first visit, indicating an acute infection. The patients who had serological responses to *C. pneumoniae* also had four times higher sputum neutrophil levels and sputum eosinophilic cationic protein concentrations than those patients who had exacerbation symptoms without serological responses. This may suggest that *C. pneumoniae* reactivation is associated with increased airway inflammation.

Mycoplasma pneumoniae

The clinical association between *M. pneumoniae* and asthma exacerbations has been proposed for many years, but the nature of this association is still unclear. Lieberman et al. showed that in a serologically based prospective study of adults hospitalized with asthma exacerbations, 18% of subjects had evidence of acute infection with *M. pneumoniae* (using immunofluorescence and ELISA) compared to 3% of matched controls ($P = 0.0006$).[40] Of note, in most of these *M. pneumoniae*-infected patients, there was also evidence of infection with a respiratory virus. In another prospective study, in children hospitalized for severe asthma, acute *M. pneumoniae* infection was found in 20% of asthmatics compared to 5.2% of controls – children with stable asthma or rhinitis $(P < 0.005)$.[41]

Proposed pathological mechanisms

Several mechanisms have been proposed to explain the potential role of these atypical bacteria in the pathogenesis of asthma and airway inflammation.[31]

   C. pneumoniae infection induces secretion of cytokines from peripheral blood mononuclear cells and alveolar macrophages. It induces tumor necrosis factor-α (TNF-α) and interleukin (IL)-8, interferon-γ (IFN-γ) and activates NF-κB in airway epithelial cells. NF-κB activates genes encoding a wide range of proinflammatory cytokines. In animal models of asthma, NF-κB activity has been shown to correlate with the degree of lung dysfunction. *C. pneumoniae* infection has been shown to cause both sustained bronchial hyperresponsiveness (BHR) and airway inflammation in a mouse model of asthma.[42] In this study mice were inoculated intranasally with *C. pneumoniae* and chemokines were measured at different time points. IFN-γ and macrophage inflammatory chemokine-2 (MIP-2) levels in bronchoalveolar lavage (BAL) fluid were increased and TNF-α was increased from day 7 post-infection. From day 7 to day 21 epithelial damage and secretory cell hypertrophy was seen. This study suggested that inflammatory mediators, epithelial damage and secretory cell hypertrophy caused by *C. pneumoniae* contributes to BHR, which has clinical implications for asthma and COPD. *In vitro* studies of human bronchial smooth muscle cells have demonstrated that *C. pneumoniae* infection induces production of IL-6, IFN-β and basic fibroblast growth factor (bFGF).[43,44] IFN-β and bFGF mediate smooth muscle cell proliferation, so *C. pneumoniae* infection may lead to airway remodelling by this mechanism. Human airway smooth muscle cells have been shown to express and secrete matrix metalloproteinases (MMPs),[45] which have been linked with airway remodelling in asthma.[46] *C. pneumoniae* increases the production of MMPs in human vascular smooth muscle cells. If this were to occur in bronchial smooth muscle cells it would strengthen the link between *C. pneumoniae* and airway remodelling. It has been suggested that *C. pneumoniae* may inhibit apoptosis of the host cell,[47] enhancing its survival in patients with chronic asthma. The role of this apoptosis inhibition is unclear but asthmatics have impaired apoptotic responses, which increases susceptibility to respiratory virus infection.[48] If *C. pneumoniae*-induced apoptosis inhibition led to increased viral infection this would provide a link between *C. pneumoniae* and the pathogenesis of asthma exacerbations.

   Less work has been done on elucidating the mechanism of action of *M. pneumoniae*, but it has been shown to induce the secretion of IL-8 and TNF-α by human lung epithelial cells *in vitro*.[49] *M. pneumoniae* has been shown to significantly increase BHR and suppress IFN-γ in mice.[50] In another study in a mouse model of allergic asthma, the influence of timing of *M. pneumoniae* infection relative to allergen (ovalbumin) sensitization and challenge on BHR, lung inflammation and BAL cytokines was investigated.[51] The authors found that infection prior to allergen sensitization led to reduced BHR and lung inflammation, but infection after sensitization resulted in an initial reduction but subsequent increase in BHR and lung inflammation, suggesting *M. pneumoniae* can modulate physiological and immunological responses in the mouse asthma model. In a study by Martin et al., asthmatics with positive PCR results to *M. pneumoniae* and *C. pneumoniae* had significantly greater mast cell infiltration and a trend toward greater numbers of T-lymphocytes on airway biopsy than asthmatics with negative PCR results.[36] This highlights a potential interaction between infection and airway inflammation.

Role of macrolide and ketolide antibiotics

Macrolides (clarithromycin, azithromycin, erythromycin and roxithromycin) have activity against *C. pneumoniae* and *M. pneumoniae*. The newer macrolides accumulate intracellularly and have good activity against atypical organisms. Clarithromycin has been shown to reduce the degree of BHR in patients with asthma.[52] In this randomized, double-blind, placebo-controlled study stable adult asthmatic patients undergoing treatment with budesonide 400 μg twice daily and salbutamol 200 μg less than twice weekly were recruited to three arms – clarithromycin 250 mg twice daily for 8 weeks; clarithromycin 250 mg three times a day for 8 weeks; or placebo. BHR was measured by a methacholine provocation test causing a 20% fall in FEV_1. BHR in patients with asthma improved significantly after completion of an 8-week clarithromycin regimen compared to placebo. There was no statistical significance between the two doses of clarithromycin.

Ketolides are a new class of antibacterial agents. They are related to macrolides but have structural modifications that confer a broader range of antibacterial activity. Two ketolides are in clinical use, telithromycin and cethromycin. Telithromycin is known to accumulate in epithelial cells, making it well suited for the treatment of infections caused by intracellular organisms. It has bactericidal effect against *C. pneumoniae* and *M. pneumoniae*.[53] There have been reports of serious hepatotoxicity with telithromycin. Compared with telithromycin, cethromycin has similar tissue penetration, pharmacokinetics, pharmacodynamics and *in vitro* activity against a number of Gram-positive and Gram-negative organisms, including *C. pneumoniae* and *M. pneumoniae*.[54] As yet there are no known hepatotoxic side effects with cethromycin. There are no studies of cethromycin in airways disease, a subject that may become of interest.

As well as their antimicrobial properties, macrolides have various anti-inflammatory actions. Clarithromycin has been shown to act synergistically with dexamethasone in suppressing lymphocyte activation, thereby potentiating glucocorticoid responsiveness in patients with asthma.[55] Macrolides have been shown to inhibit superoxide generation by polymorphonuclear leukocytes. An *in vitro* study of human ciliated respiratory epithelium showed that macrolides may protect the epithelium against oxidative damage inflicted by phospholipid-sensitized phagocytes.[56] Erythromycin has been shown to suppress IL-6 and IL-8 expression in human bronchial epithelial cells.[57,58] These are proinflammatory cytokines important in airway inflammation. One of these studies also showed that erythromycin inhibits the activation of the transcription factor

NF-κB.[58] Erythromycin has been shown to inhibit human airway mucus secretion in culture.[59] Erythromycin, roxithromycin and clarithromycin have also been shown to inhibit neurally mediated contraction of human bronchial smooth muscle.[60] For a review of macrolides as immunomodulatory compounds in chronic lung diseases see Lopez-Boado and Rubin.[61]

Ketolides also have immunomodulatory effects, and Feldman et al. have studied these. They found that HMR 3004 (another ketolide with a carbazate residue) also antagonizes the direct and polymorphonuclear leukocyte-mediated injurious effects of phospholipids on human ciliated epithelium.[62] Telithromycin has been shown to inhibit secretion of IL-1α and TNF-α from human monocytes.[63] It has also been shown to suppress both IL-6 and IL-10 in a mouse model of infection.[64] A recent study has shown that telithromycin reduces the release of inflammatory mediators through NF-κB inhibition and, in the later phase of inflammation, enhances inflammatory cell apoptosis.[65]

The antimicrobial and anti-inflammatory properties of macrolides and ketolides make them of interest both in the context of inflammation in asthma, as well as the influence of atypical bacterial infections in asthma pathogenesis. They are also of potential use in providing further anti-inflammatory effects, perhaps acting synergistically in combination with other anti-inflammatory treatments discussed elsewhere.

Macrolides and ketolides in stable asthma

A 2005 Cochrane review to determine whether macrolides are effective in the management of patients with chronic asthma identified only seven studies, recruiting a total of 416 patients, that met the inclusion criteria (randomized, controlled clinical trials involving children and adult patients treated with macrolides for more than 4 weeks, vs placebo).[66] Four studies showed a positive effect on symptoms with macrolides in different types of asthmatic patients. There were no significant differences in FEV_1, though there were significant differences in eosinophilic inflammation and symptoms. Overall conclusions were that there was insufficient evidence to make recommendations for the use of macrolides in chronic asthma.

One of these studies, the *Chlamydia pneumoniae*, Asthma, Roxithromycin, Multinational (CARM) study, investigated the effect of roxithromycin in subjects with asthma and serological evidence of *C. pneumoniae* infection (IgG antibodies to *C. pneumoniae* $\geq 1:64$, IgA antibodies $\geq 1:16$, or both).[67] The study was randomized, double-blinded and placebo-controlled. Subjects received 6 weeks of roxithromycin or placebo. There were significant differences in evening peak expiratory flow by the end of treatment ($P = 0.02$) but these differences abated within 6 months. There was a trend for improvements in the asthma symptom score, though this was not significant.

More recently, a randomized double-blind study was performed to determine the effect of clarithromycin therapy in patients with chronic stable asthma.[68] Presence of *M. pneumoniae* and *C. pneumoniae* was confirmed by PCR of BAL fluid and was found in 31 of 55 asthmatics. Treatment with clarithromycin 500 mg twice daily for 6 weeks resulted in a significant improvement in FEV_1 ($P = 0.05$) in patients with evidence of atypical infection (PCR-positive). In situ hybridization of inflammatory mediators TNF-α, IL-2, IL-4, IL-5 and IL-12 from airway biopsies and BAL fluid showed no baseline differences between PCR-positive and PCR-negative subjects, but did show reductions in TNF-α ($P = 0.006$), IL-5 ($P = 0.007$) and IL-12 ($P = 0.004$) mRNA in BAL fluid in PCR-positive subjects who received clarithromycin. This study suggested the beneficial effects of clarithromycin in stable asthma through its antimicrobial action. The Asthma Clinical Research Network is currently conducting a PCR-stratified, prospective study (the Macrolides In Asthma trial; ClinicalTrials.gov identifier NCT00318708) to explore the importance of PCR positivity in determining the response to clarithromycin therapy by evaluating the effectiveness of clarithromycin at reducing asthma symptoms. However, Adding clarithromycin to inhaled glucocorticoids alone did not further improve asthma control, although an improvement in airway hyperresponsiveness was observed.

Overall, atypical bacterial infection might have a role in the pathogenesis of stable asthma in subgroups of patients, and further placebo-controlled studies are required to investigate both the antimicrobial and anti-inflammatory actions of macrolides in stable asthma.

Macrolides and ketolides in asthma exacerbations

As discussed earlier, guidelines do not support the routine use of antibiotics in acute exacerbations of asthma, in view of the fact that viral infections appear to be the major cause. And yet there is evidence, as already discussed, that atypical bacterial infection contributes to the aetiology of asthma exacerbations.

In a recent study, the effect of telithromycin in acute exacerbations of asthma was investigated. This Telithromycin, Chlamydophila, and Asthma (TELICAST) study was a multicentre, double-blind, randomized, placebo-controlled trial,[69] in which 278 adults diagnosed with asthma were enrolled within 24 hours of an acute exacerbation requiring acute medical care. The subjects were randomly assigned to receive telithromycin 800 mg daily, or placebo, for 10 days as well as standard care. Primary endpoints were a change from baseline over the treatment period in symptoms (from the subjects' diary cards) and a change in the home morning peak expiratory flow. The mean decrease in symptom scores during the treatment period was 1.3 for telithromycin and 1.0 for placebo (mean difference, -0.3; 95% confidence interval -0.5 to -0.1; $P = 0.004$), showing that there was a greater reduction in asthmatic symptom score in patients receiving telithromycin. There was no significant difference in the home peak expiratory flow between the groups but there was an improvement in clinic-performed lung function tests in the telithromycin group. The proportion of symptom-free days was significantly greater in the telithromycin group than in the placebo group (16% vs 8%, $P = 0.006$). The presence of C. pneumoniae and M. pneumoniae was determined by serological analysis, PCR and culture. Sixty-one percent of subjects met criteria for these atypical infections, mainly from serological data, but there was no relationship between bacteriological status and response to treatment.

This trial is of clinical importance but the mechanisms of action are yet to be determined particularly in view of the fact that there was no clear indication of greater treatment effect in those with evidence of infection compared with that seen in those without. More studies are required to further define patient populations who are most likely to benefit from treatment, to elucidate the mechanisms of action, as well as investigating other antibiotics.

10.6   Role of viruses in asthma exacerbations

Respiratory viruses are implicated in the development of asthma and in exacerbations. For the purposes of this discussion we shall concentrate on virus-induced exacerbations. Viral upper respiratory tract infections are associated with 80–85% of asthma exacerbations in school age children.[38] The most common viruses to be implicated are RVs. Other exacerbation-causing viruses include respiratory syncytial virus (RSV), influenzaviruses, parainfluenzaviruses, adenoviruses, coronaviruses and metapneumoviruses.

Rhinoviruses

Rhinoviruses belong to the Picornaviridae family of viruses. These are small non-enveloped single-stranded RNA viruses, with at least 100 serotypes known. They are divided into major and minor groups depending on receptor binding properties. The major group bind human intercellular adhesion molecule-1 (ICAM-1) and form the majority of RVs. The minor group bind to low-density lipoprotein receptors. Following binding to these receptors intracellular internalization occurs, leading to virus replication and induction of inflammatory mediators.

Epidemiological studies

Rhinovirus is the major virus associated with exacerbations of asthma. Using techniques of RT-PCR and virus culture, studies have shown that, in adults and in children over the age of 2 years, RV is responsible for 60–65% of viral exacerbations. The peak period for RV infection is September in the northern hemisphere, and peaks of asthma exacerbation requiring hospital treatment occur globally after school return. Johnston et al. performed a time trend analysis of upper respiratory infections and hospital admissions for asthma.[70] Strong correlations were found between the seasonal patterns of infection and hospital admissions ($r = 0.72$; $P < 0.0001$). This relationship was stronger for paediatric ($r = 0.68$; $P < 0.0001$) than for adult admissions ($r = 0.53$; $P < 0.01$). RV was the major pathogen implicated in these infections. The authors speculated that it was the children's school attendance that facilitates the spread of virus, leading to an increased number of asthma admissions. Another study showed human picornaviruses were detected in 52% of paediatric asthma admissions and 29% of controls ($P = 0.002$), and these cases were less likely to have been prescribed controller medication (inhaled corticosteroid, 49% vs 85%; $P < 0.0001$; leukotriene receptor antagonist, 9% vs 21%; $P = 0.04$), suggesting that children with asthma prescribed anti-inflammatory medications are less likely to require emergency department treatment during this period of high risk of exacerbation.[71]

Is there a role for antiviral therapy?

The mainstay of treatment of asthma exacerbations is oxygen, inhaled short-acting β_2-adrenoceptor agonists and intravenous or oral corticosteroids. There have been few studies investigating specifically exacerbations of viral aetiology, and few trials have addressed the use of antiviral therapy in virus-induced asthma exacerbations. Of these, only agents targeting influenza have been studied. Johnston et al. studied the effects of oseltamivir amongst asthmatic children infected with influenza.[72] The authors concluded that oseltamivir may reduce symptom duration, improve lung function and lead to fewer asthma exacerbations. Murphy et al. investigated the efficacy of inhaled zanamivir in treating influenza in adults with asthma or COPD.[73] Zanamivir significantly reduced the time to alleviation of influenza symptoms and the incidence of complications and was well tolerated.

There are treatments that have been shown to have efficacy against rhinovirus infections. In this section we discuss various antirhinoviral drugs as potential targets for treatment of asthma exacerbations.

Antirhinoviral compounds

Several anti-RV agents have been investigated, including capsid binders and viral protease inhibitors. The outer capsid of RV consists of four viral proteins, VP1–4. Several compounds have been developed to bind to VP1, thus interfering with viral attachment and uncoating. The viral capsid binder R61837 was found to prevent colds, but not RV infection. In a double-blind, placebo-controlled trial volunteers were challenged with RV-9.[74] R61837 was given by intranasal spray 4 hours before virus challenge and continued for 6 days. There were substantial reductions in clinical score and nasal mucus weight compared to placebo.

More recently the antipicornaviral agent, pleconaril, has been investigated up to phase II clinical trials. Pleconaril has been shown to inhibit *in vitro* replication of most RVs and enteroviruses. It binds into a hydrophobic pocket within VP1, stabilizing the capsid, thus inhibiting cell attachment and RNA uncoating. The efficacy and safety of oral pleconaril in the treatment of naturally occurring colds was studied in two large randomized, double-blind, placebo-controlled, multicentre trials.[75] Those subjects taking pleconaril had reduced symptoms and shorter duration (by 1.5 days) of colds where picornaviruses were detected (65% of subjects). Pleconaril was shown to be safe and well tolerated, with a small excess in frequencies of headache, nausea and diarrhoea in the treatment vs placebo group. However, pleconaril induces CYP3A4, which likely led to menstrual abnormalities and intermenstrual bleeding in women taking pleconaril and oestrogen-based oral contraceptives.[76] A recent double blind, placebo-controlled, multi-centre phase II trial has been completed evaluating the efficacy of pleconaril nasal spray in preventing exacerbations in asthmatics exposed to picornavirus infections. The results are awaited (ClinicalTrials.gov identifier: NCT00394914).

Rhinovirus relies on a viral-encoded 3C protease for replication to occur. Ruprintrivir is a 3C protease inhibitor that has been shown *in vitro* to have potent activity against many RV serotypes. Hayden et al. conducted three double-blind, placebo-controlled trials in healthy volunteers, who randomly received intranasal ruprintrivir or placebo nasal sprays, either as prophylaxis, starting 6 hours before experimental infection, or as treatment, 24 hours after infection.[77] Prophylaxis reduced the proportion of subjects with positive viral cultures but did not decrease the frequency of colds. The treatment group had a reduced daily symptom score, viral titres and nasal mucus weights. Ruprintrivir was well tolerated, with blood-tinged mucus and nasal passage irritation as the most common side effects. Its use in exacerbations of asthma has not been investigated.

ICAM-1 and derivatives

As discussed, the major group of rhinoviruses require the cellular receptor ICAM-1 for attachment to target cells. Thus receptor blockade with a competitive binding inhibitor could be a target for prevention of RV infection, as would soluble ICAM-1 delivered to the site of infection, to saturate binding sites on the virus capsid. Turner et al. performed a randomized, double-blind, placebo-controlled trial to determine the efficacy of intranasal administration of tremacamra, a recombinant soluble ICAM-1, in experimental RV-39 colds in humans.[78] Tremacamra reduced the severity of colds, with significant reductions in symptom scores, proportion of clinical colds and nasal mucus weights. There was also a significant reduction in virus titre in nasal lavage fluid compared to controls. There were no significant adverse effects but medication had to be used six times a day. Tremacamra given both before and after inoculation, but prior to the development of symptoms, was useful in controlling symptoms. No further studies have been carried out and tremacamra has not been tested in the context of asthma exacerbations.

Interferon therapy

Type I interferons (IFNs) include IFN-α (13 subtypes) and IFN-β. They play an important role in the defence against viruses, acting on virally infected cells and inducing a wide range of antiviral proteins. They upregulate and activate IFN-inducible genes, such as antiviral protein kinase (PKR). IFNs induce apoptosis, preventing virus replication, and induce further IFN gene expression in an autocrine and paracrine manner. They activate natural killer (NK) cells and are required for NK cell survival. The study by Wark et al.[48] showed that asthmatic bronchial epithelial cells are more susceptible to infection with RV than non-asthmatics through a deficient IFN-β response that results in reduced apoptosis, increased viral replication and subsequent increases in inflammatory processes; it thus highlights interferons as an important therapeutic target in viral exacerbations of asthma. A novel class of IFNs has recently been discovered and named type III IFNs: IFN-λ1 (IL-29) and IFN-λ2/3 (IL-28A/B). The IFN-λs have similar functions to type I IFNs;[79, 80] however, little is known regarding their role in human diseases. Recently, Contoli et al. identified deficient induction of IFN-λs in response to RV in asthmatic bronchial epithelial cells and alveolar macrophages.[27] The authors also found that, following experimental inoculation with RV of asthmatic and normal volunteers, there were significant inverse correlations between production of IFN-λ and severity of symptoms, BAL virus load, reductions in lung function and airway inflammation.

IFNs-α and -β have been studied in the prevention of the common cold since the 1980s, with conflicting results. Hayden and Gwaltney assessed the therapeutic efficacy of recombinant IFN-α2 in experimental infection with RV-39.[81] They delivered IFN-α2 to adult volunteers by nasal spray or drops three times a day for 5 days beginning 28 hours after RV-39 inoculation. Treatment with drops and to a lesser extent by spray was associated with reduced virus shedding. Use of drops also resulted in a significant but modest reduction in nasal mucus weights, but neither treatment reduced the frequency of clinical colds. A recurrent side effect of this therapy in clinical trials is nasal bleeding and a lymphocytic nasal infiltrate. In a randomized, double-blind study, Farr et al. administered sprays of human IFN-α2 (10^7 IU/day) or placebo once daily to adult volunteers to determine the prophylactic efficacy of IFN in the prevention of natural RV colds.[82] During the 22 days of treatment no IFN-treated volunteers had respiratory illnesses documented secondary to RV infection compared to 13 (8.5%) placebo controls ($P = 0.0002$). There was one episode of tracheobronchitis in the IFN group compared to eight episodes in the control ($P = 0.04$). The authors concluded that intranasal IFN-α2 was efficacious in preventing RV colds under natural conditions but noted some confounding with the increased side effects of nasal obstruction and blood-stained nasal mucus in the IFN group.

Studies have also addressed the use of prophylactic intranasal IFN-α2 and viral exacerbations of chronic respiratory disease.[83] Patients with asthma or chronic bronchitis who had been in close contact with someone with symptoms of upper respiratory tract infection were randomly allocated to receive recombinant IFN-α2 nasal spray (3×10^6 IU) or placebo twice daily for 5 days. The use of prophylactic IFN-α2 was not associated with a significant reduction in upper or lower respiratory tract symptoms (23% of IFN group vs 27% placebo group, $P = 0.58$). Of note and unusually, coronavirus was the most common viral diagnosis and the incidence of adverse effects was similar in the two groups. A more recent study, by Simon et al., investigated 10 patients with corticosteroid-resistant asthma (with and without Churg–Strauss syndrome) with low-dose IFN-α treatment.[84] Treatment resulted in improved lung function and a reduction in oral corticosteroid use. Immunological changes included decreased blood leukocyte numbers, increased number of T-helper (Th) 1 cells and increased expression of IL-10 in peripheral blood mononuclear cells. IL-10 is an anti-inflammatory cytokine, and corticosteroids mediate their effects in part by inducing the IL-10 gene. It has been observed that patients with corticosteroid-resistant asthma have a defect in IL-10 production. These observations make this study particularly interesting in that the IFN-α may break the corticosteroid resistance in this group of patients by increasing the expression of IL-10. There were significant side effects in this study, particularly flu-like symptoms, nausea and headache and one episode of leukopenia severe enough to warrant temporary cessation of treatment.

Several studies have investigated the use of IFN-β in the treatment of and prophylaxis against clinical colds. Higgins et al. administered intranasal recombinant human IFN-β serine (IFN-β ser) or placebo to volunteers and challenged them with experimental RV-9 and RV-14 infection.[85] There were significant reductions in clinical scores, quantity of nasal secretions and virus release in the IFN-β group compared to controls. Sperber et al. investigated the tolerance and efficacy of intranasal recombinant IFN-β ser in healthy adults.[86] The tolerance study identified side effects of nasal mucosal bleeding particularly in the high-dose IFN-β group compared to placebo. The efficacy study, where volunteers received nasal drops of IFN-β ser or placebo 36 hours before RV challenge and for 3 days afterwards, reported significant reductions in incidence of clinical colds and nasal mucus weights, particularly in the high-dose group, but no difference in viral release, suggesting some role for IFN-β in the prevention of clinical colds. A subsequent study by the same group, investigating the use of recombinant IFN-β ser nasal drops for prophylaxis against natural colds, showed illness frequency and number of days with subjective colds did not differ between the IFN-β group and placebo.[87]

These studies provide a background for the investigation of the use of interferons in exacerbations of asthma. In all studies the mode of delivery and dose of interferons have been contentious issues. Side effects have been problematic with most studies, and this is pertinent in asthmatics where increased airway inflammation would be likely to be troublesome. More investigation is required into the effectiveness of interferons in RV-induced asthma exacerbations, particularly in light of the finding that asthmatics have deficient production of IFN-β[48] and IFN-λ.[27]

Inhaled corticosteroids (ICS)

Inhaled corticosteroids are the mainstay of asthma treatment. Papi et al. investigated the *in vitro* effect of corticosteroids on RV-induced ICAM-1 upregulation.[88] They showed that this upregulation was inhibited by corticosteroid pretreatment of cultured primary bronchial cells and in A549 respiratory epithelial cells. Despite *in vitro* studies showing the effect of corticosteroids on RV-induced inflammatory responses, several *in vivo* studies of experimental RV infection have reported poor efficacy of corticosteroids.

Farr et al. carried out a placebo-controlled study into the effects of combined intranasal and systemic corticosteroids, given 4 days before experimental RV infection in adult volunteers.[89] For up to 48 hours after viral inoculation, nasal obstruction, nasal mucus weights and nasal lavage kinin concentrations were lower in the steroid recipients. After 48 hours, increases in these measurements in the steroid group resulted in no overall differences between treatment groups.

Grunberg et al. investigated the possible effects of inhaled budesonide in mild asthmatics following experimental RV infection.[90] In this double blind, placebo-controlled study treatment was started 2 weeks prior to RV challenge. The investigators examined inflammatory cell numbers in bronchial biopsies 2 days before and 6 days after RV infection. Budesonide treatment reduced BHR and eosinophil numbers but did not reduce the total number of inflammatory cells following infection. The authors concluded that RV infection by itself induces subtle worsening of inflammation in the asthmatic airway, on which ICS have no effect.

Studies therefore show that there is evidence that ICS alone are only partially protective in viral-induced exacerbations of asthma. It has been shown that ICS in combination with a LABA, if used early in worsening asthma, may prevent deterioration leading to severe exacerbations.[91] This study did not identify the cause of asthma exacerbations, but viral triggers are likely to be a major component. It has thus been postulated that ICS/LABA combination therapy may improve treatment/prevention of viral exacerbations. Edwards et al. found that combination therapy can synergistically and additively suppress RV-induced bronchial epithelial cell chemokine production thus reducing the inflammatory effects of RV.[92] It remains unclear what, if any, effect combination therapy of ICS and LABA will have in the treatment or prevention of viral-induced asthma exacerbations. Indeed, if an effect is shown, the combination of ICS/LABA and antiviral therapies could have an important therapeutic role in asthma exacerbations.

NF-κB inhibitors

NF-κB is a transcription factor that is involved in induction of proinflammatory mediators in RV infection. This signalling pathway represents a target for anti-inflammatory intervention. For a review of the development of drugs that inhibit NF-κB activation and what the potential applications of these drugs will be in airway diseases see Edwards et al.[93] NF-κB inhibitors have not yet been tested in human models of asthma. In the mouse model of allergic asthma, MOL 294, a small molecule inhibitor of redox-regulated NF-κB, was shown to reduce eosinophils, IL-13 and eotaxin in BAL fluid and decrease BHR *in vivo*.[94] IκB kinase (IKK) is required for activation of NF-κB. In a more recent study, IKK inhibitors were used in A549 cells stimulated with IL-1β and TNF-α.[95] Following stimulation the induction of NF-κB-dependent transcription was subsequently repressed by IKK-selective inhibitors. Epithelial production of chemokines was also significantly repressed in a concentration-dependent manner. This study suggests a role for IKK inhibitors on the bronchial epithelium and possibly in the development of therapeutic agents for asthma.

Macrolides and ketolides

As discussed above macrolides and ketolides have anti-inflammatory as well as antimicrobial properties. Macrolides have been shown to inhibit the production of ICAM-1, IL-6 and IL-8. RV induces the expression of ICAM-1 through upregulation of NF-κB-mediated transcription.[96] Suzuki et al. studied the effects of erythromycin on RV infection of human tracheal epithelial cells.[97] They showed that erythromycin inhibited RV-induced expression of ICAM-1, the major group RV receptor, although the inhibitory effects of erythromycin on the expression of the LDL receptor, the minor group RV receptor, were small. Jang et al. went on to investigate the effect of clarithromycin on RV infection in epithelial cells (A549 cells).[98] They showed that treating RV-infected cells with clarithromycin resulted in inhibition of the RV-induced increase in ICAM-1 mRNA and protein and the RV-induced secretion of IL-1β, IL-6 and IL-8. The authors suggested, therefore, that clarithromycin might have the potential to treat airway inflammation caused by RV.

Despite this, clinical studies have shown that the use of clarithromycin following experimental RV infection in healthy volunteers has little effect on the development of cold symptoms or nasal inflammation.[99] Further studies on the role of macrolides and ketolides in asthma exacerbations are needed.

Antiviral treatments have thus been investigated in the context of the common cold and the only studies investigating their use in asthma exacerbations have been with anti-influenza treatments. The clear link between RV and asthma exacerbations should prompt more interest in the antirhinoviral agents pleconaril and tremacamra as potential therapeutic options. With the described deficiency in IFN-β in asthmatics,[48] type I interferon treatment remains a potential option, particularly if the issues of safety, adverse effects and drug delivery can be addressed. The recent study by Wark et al. found release of IFN-γ-induced protein 10 (IP-10) was relatively specific to acute virus-induced asthma (median of 604 pg/mL in virus-induced asthma, compared to 167 pg/mL in non-virus induced asthma; $P < 0.01$).[100] Increased serum IP-10 levels were strongly associated with more severe airflow obstruction ($r = -0.8$, $P < 0.01$). This finding should allow more causal relationships between virus and asthma to be investigated, potentially allowing the development of specific viral-induced exacerbation treatments. Also, the recent development of the mouse model of RV infection[101] should prove invaluable in investigating therapeutic targets in future.

10.7   Anti-infectives in COPD exacerbations

Exacerbations of COPD are characterized by an acute worsening of respiratory symptoms. They are of major health and economic importance, with long-lasting effects on patients. It is well recognized that exacerbations are an important part of the natural history of the disease. There is evidence that patients with a higher frequency of exacerbations (greater than three per year) have a faster decline in lung function.[102] As will be discussed, bacterial and viral infections are the main cause of exacerbation.

Anthonisen et al. defined a COPD exacerbation based on the presence of three specific symptoms: increased shortness of breath, increased sputum volume and increased sputum purulence.[1] In this study three subtypes (I, II and III) were proposed depending on the occurrence of all or some of the symptoms:

- type I with all three symptoms;
- type II with two of three symptoms;
- type III with one of three symptoms, with evidence of fever of upper respiratory tract infection.

Table 10.2 Causes of exacerbations of COPD. Viral and/or bacterial infections are the commonest causes.

Viral	Bacterial	Other
Rhinoviruses	*Haemophilus influenzae*	Air pollution
Respiratory syncytial virus	*Streptococcus pneumoniae*	Congestive cardiac failure
Influenzavirus A and B	*Moraxella catarrhalis*	Pulmonary embolus
Parainfluenzavirus	*Streptococcus aureus*	Cold temperatures
Adenoviruses		Sulphur dioxide
Coronaviruses		Particulates
		Ozone

A second definition, proposed by a working group in 2000, is 'a sustained worsening of the patient's condition, from the stable state and beyond normal day-to-day variations, that is acute in onset and necessitates a change in regular medication in a patient with underlying COPD.'[103]

Causes of COPD exacerbations

The causal agents for COPD exacerbations are shown in Table 10.2. Papi et al. investigated the relationship between infections and exacerbation severity in COPD exacerbations requiring hospitalization.[2] They found that viral and/or bacterial infections were detected in 78% of exacerbations. The frequency of infections is shown in Figure 10.1. Patients with infectious exacerbations had longer hospitalizations ($P < 0.02$) and greater impairment of lung function ($P < 0.05$) than those with non-infectious exacerbations.

Bronchoscopic specimens have shown the presence of bacteria in 50% of exacerbations. Groenewegen et al. performed a prospective study to investigate the frequency

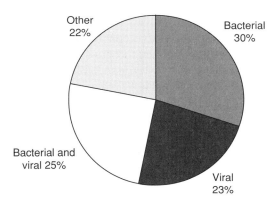

Figure 10.1 Triggers for exacerbations of COPD. Viral and bacterial infections account for up to 78% of causes of COPD exacerbations. Data from Papi et al.[2]

of bacterial infections in patients admitted to hospital with an acute exacerbation of COPD.[104] Fifty percent of patients had positive sputum culture results. Patients with lower FEV_1 had a higher incidence of bacterial infections ($P = 0.026$), but no differences were seen in clinical outcomes between those patients with and those without bacteria isolated. It was previously thought that bacteria do not cause exacerbations and that their presence in sputum was due to chronic colonization. However, Sethi et al. performed a study from 81 patients with COPD in the stable state and during exacerbations.[105] An exacerbation was diagnosed at 33% of clinic visits involving a new strain of bacteria, compared to 15.4% of visits not involving a new strain ($P < 0.001$). The authors concluded that isolation of new strains of *H. influenzae*, *M. catarrhalis* and *S. pneumoniae* was associated with a significantly increased risk of exacerbations, and that this supports a role for bacteria in causing COPD exacerbations. In a recent study, Sethi et al. went on to determine if systemic and airway inflammation was distinct in new strain acquisition exacerbations.[106] They found that new strain exacerbations were associated with significantly more intense inflammation than those with pre-existing strains and non-bacterial episodes. Also, the clinical severity was well correlated with levels of inflammatory markers.

Upper respiratory tract virus infections are detected in approximately 50% of exacerbations. Seemungal et al. evaluated the effects of viral infection in COPD exacerbations.[107] Patients were sampled during the exacerbation and when stable. Using culture, PCR and serology, respiratory viruses were identified. Sixty-four percent of exacerbations were associated with a cold occurring up to 18 days prior to the exacerbation. Forty percent of exacerbations had viruses detected, of which 58% were rhinoviruses. Similarly, Rohde et al. found that viruses were detected in induced sputum and nasal lavage in 56% of exacerbations requiring hospitalization.[108] Exacerbations associated with viral infections have a longer median symptom recovery time (13 days vs 6 days) and higher levels of airway inflammatory markers compared to non-viral exacerbations.[107] Prevention of viral infections may lead to reductions in frequency and severity of exacerbations, thus having important health and economic consequences.

As discussed above, exacerbations can be associated with bacteria, viruses or both.[2] There is evidence that bacteria and viruses interact to worsen exacerbation severity. Wilkinson et al. performed a prospective cohort study of 56 COPD exacerbations in 39 patients to investigate the interaction between bacterial and RV infection,[109] and found that 69.6% of exacerbations were associated with a bacterial pathogen, most commonly *H. influenzaei*; RV was found in 19.6% of exacerbations. Exacerbations with both pathogens had higher bacterial loads and serum IL-6 than exacerbations without both pathogens. Also, exacerbations with cold symptoms and a bacterial pathogen had a greater decline in lung function and a higher symptom count than those exacerbations associated with bacteria alone. The authors concluded that airway bacteria and viruses interact, worsening inflammation and the severity of exacerbation.

Atypical bacteria have also been implicated in exacerbations of COPD. As discussed, due to the poor sensitivity of atypical bacterial culture there are difficulties in diagnosing acute atypical bacterial infection. Studies rely on PCR and serology. *C. pneumoniae* has been implicated in 4–16% of exacerbations. Blasi et al. studied IgG and IgM to

C. pneumoniae by microimmunofluorescence in outpatient exacerbations of COPD and compared them to healthy controls.[110] The mean titre of IgG was significantly higher in COPD than controls. At least 4% of exacerbations were associated with *C. pneumoniae*, diagnosed from specific IgM or a four-fold increase in IgG titre. Similarly, Mogulkoc et al. identified *C. pneumoniae* as a sole causative agent in 16% of exacerbations.[111] There is debate as to whether chronic infection with *C. pneumoniae* leads to more frequent exacerbation rates. Blasi et al. performed PCR to detect *C. pneumoniae* DNA in sputum from subjects with chronic bronchitis.[112] They reported that chronic colonization was significantly associated with a lower FEV_1 and a higher rate of exacerbations. Seemungal et al. found no relationship between *C. pneumoniae* detection in the airway at exacerbation and exacerbation frequency.[113] Also, unlike RV-triggered exacerbations, they found no relationship between *C. pneumoniae* detection and inflammatory markers (IL-6, IL-8 and total and differential cell counts in induced sputum), suggesting that *C. pneumoniae* exacerbations do not differ from exacerbations not associated with *C. pneumoniae*.

Non-infective causes include air pollution, low temperatures, pulmonary embolus and heart failure. Particulate matter is known to induce oxidative stress, leading to a pro-inflammatory response. This has been shown to be enhanced by adenoviral early region 1A protein,[114] suggesting a possible interaction between air pollution and latent viral infection in triggering COPD exacerbations.

Antibiotic use

Antibiotics are widely used in exacerbations of COPD. As discussed there are compelling data to show that bacteria are causative agents in a significant proportion of exacerbations. The study by Anthonisen et al. remains one of the most influential in addressing the use of antibiotics in acute exacerbations of COPD.[1] Over 3.5 years, 362 exacerbations were treated, with a success rate of 55% placebo vs 68% antibiotic, and a failure rate of 19% with placebo vs 10% with antibiotic. These differences were statistically significant, demonstrating the benefit of antibiotics in exacerbations of COPD.

A meta-analysis performed in 1995 of randomized trials of antibiotics in exacerbations of COPD, reviewed nine trials and showed a small but significant improvement in the antibiotic groups.[22] More recently, Puhan et al. performed a systematic review of antibiotic use in exacerbations of COPD.[115] They concluded that antibiotics reduce treatment failure and mortality in patients with severe exacerbations requiring hospitalization and not in patients with mild-moderate exacerbations treated as outpatients. This highlights the need for further studies to be carried out in the mild-moderate group to guide antibiotic prescription. The most recent Cochrane review reports that in exacerbations with increased cough and sputum purulence, antibiotics reduce the short-term mortality by 77% and the risk of treatment failure by 53%, supporting the view that antibiotics for COPD exacerbation patients with increased cough and sputum purulence have a mortality benefit.[116]

The question of which antibiotic class to use remains a debate. Ram et al. concluded that antibiotic therapy reduced mortality regardless of type.[116] A recent meta-analysis by Siempos et al. concluded that macrolides, quinolones and amoxicillin/clavulanate were equivalent in the short term, that quinolones had better microbiological success and fewer recurrences than macrolides, and that amoxicillin/clavulanate was associated with more adverse effects.[117] Wilson et al. showed that in an Anthonisen type I exacerbation, 5 days of gemifloxacin (an enhanced affinity quinolone) was at least as effective as 7 days of clarithromycin, and significantly more patients were exacerbation-free after 6 months in the gemifloxacin group.[118]

The MOSAIC study (Moxifloxacin Oral tablets to Standard oral antibiotic regimen given as first-line therapy in out patients with Acute Infective exacerbations of Chronic bronchitis) aimed to compare a 5-day course of moxifloxacin with 7 days of standard antibiotic therapy.[119] Patients were identified during a stable phase of illness. During an Anthonisen type I exacerbation, patients returned to the clinic with a sputum sample and were randomized to receive 5 days of moxifloxacin (with 2 extra days of placebo) or 7 days standard antibiotic treatment (amoxicillin, clarithromycin or cefuroxime, depending on therapeutic habits, local pathogen epidemiology, *in vitro* susceptibilities and clinical presentation of the patient). Patients were followed for up to 9 months after treatment. Moxifloxacin was equal to standard treatment in clinical success and achieved significantly superior bacteriological eradication, greater cure rate and improved long-term outcomes (twice the number of antibiotics were prescribed in the weeks following the exacerbation in the standard therapy group, and the time to the next exacerbation was longer in the moxifloxacin group). An important feature of this study was that the subjects were identified during a stable phase so that a baseline assessment could be made to judge recovery.

Other studies have examined the use of fluoroquinolones in COPD exacerbations. Nouira et al. assessed the effects of ofloxacin in exacerbation patients requiring mechanical ventilation.[120] Patients were eligible if they were admitted with an acute exacerbation of COPD and acute respiratory failure. They were excluded if they had had recent antimicrobial treatment or had pneumonic infiltrates on chest radiograph. In a randomized, double-blind, placebo-controlled trial, the frequency of in-hospital death, need for additional antibiotics, duration of mechanical ventilation and hospital stay was significantly lower in the ofloxacin versus placebo group, concluding that ofloxacin is beneficial in COPD exacerbations requiring mechanical ventilation. Recently, Ruiz-Gonzales et al. investigated the long-term outcome of COPD exacerbation patients treated with 10 days of levofloxacin vs standard antibiotic therapy (clarithromycin, cefuroxime or amoxicillin/clavulanate).[121] Use of levofloxacin significantly reduced hospitalizations compared to the standard group, though there were no other differences in outcome variables.

Guidelines discuss the class of antibiotics used in exacerbations, but do not discuss the duration of antibiotic therapy. El Moussaoui et al. performed a recent systematic review of randomized double-blind studies of short-course (≤5 days) antibiotic treatment versus conventional longer treatment in COPD exacerbations.[122] Of the 21 studies included, short-course therapy was as effective as longer courses in the treatment of mild-moderate exacerbations, of Anthonisen type I and II. Eradication of bacteria from sputum was also comparable for both treatment regimes. Similar results were found when antibiotics were grouped by class. The authors felt that their study should be interpreted with caution in patients with severe exacerbations. The benefits of shorter antibiotic courses are numerous – better compliance, fewer side effects, less financial cost and, importantly, reduced risk of the development of resistant organisms.

Is there a biomarker for bacterial exacerbations of COPD?

The fact that not all groups of patients benefit from antibiotic therapy prompted research into the discovery of a biomarker that would specify which exacerbations warrant antibiotic therapy. There is an evolving role for the measurement of serum procalcitonin in exacerbations of COPD. Procalcitonin is a small protein, normally undetectable, whose serum levels increase rapidly in the presence of bacterial infection. Christ-Crain et al. performed a study that showed procalcitonin guidance markedly reduces antibiotic prescriptions and length of antibiotic treatment in patients with community-acquired pneumonia.[123] This prompted the same group to perform a prospective, single-blinded, randomized, controlled, single-centre trial comparing patients with exacerbations of COPD treated according to internationally accepted guidelines or to procalcitonin levels.[124] Patients were followed up during the hospitalization, at a short-term follow-up visit and at 6 months. In the procalcitonin group, patients with a procalcitonin level below 0.1 µg/mL (measured by a time-resolved amplified cryptate emission technology assay) were considered non-bacterial and antibiotics were discouraged; those with a level greater than 0.25 µg/mL were considered bacterial and antibiotics were encouraged; whereas for those with a level in the range 0.1–0.25 µg/mL antibiotics were used 'based on the stability of the patient's clinical condition'. Procalcitonin guidance reduced antibiotic prescribing compared to standard therapy (40% vs 72%, $P < 0.0001$). There was also a significant sustained reduction in total antibiotic exposure for up to 6 months, suggesting that procalcitonin guidance for exacerbations of COPD has advantages over standard therapy in reducing use of antibiotics for up to 6 months. An important question, raised by Martinez and Curtis,[125] is whether patients with low serum procalcitonin levels derive any benefit from antimicrobials? This was not answered by this study. Also, as this was a single-centre study, it is not known whether similar results could be achieved from a multicentre trial. Another recent study by Nseir et al. addressed the use of procalcitonin in COPD exacerbations, particularly by investigating factors predicting bacterial isolation in severe acute exacerbations of COPD requiring intubation and mechanical ventilation.[126] A positive Gram stain of endotracheal aspirates and procalcitonin level less than 0.5 ng/mL (measured using the monoclonal immunoluminometric quantitative method) were independently associated with bacterial isolation, with a negative predictive value of more than 95%.

Antiviral use

As discussed above there are a number of antiviral agents targeting RV that are in development and, as yet, have not been applied to viral exacerbations of asthma or COPD. Indeed, some of the deficiencies discovered in asthma, such as the interferon deficiencies, have not yet been identified in COPD. Some of the antiviral treatments described above may not be as relevant to COPD. More work needs to be done in this area. As will be discussed later, vaccination has an important role in the prevention of viral infection, particularly influenza. Indeed vaccination is the mainstay for prevention of influenza. There are other treatment options, however, with amantadine and the neuraminidase inhibitors, zanamivir and oseltamivir. Amantadine has not gained wide acceptance due to its poor adverse events profile, the rapid emergence of resistant strains and its ineffectiveness against influenza B. The neuraminidase (NA) inhibitors have the advantage of action against both influenza A and B.[127] They block influenza neuraminidase, preventing the cleavage of sialic residues, thus interfering with virus release and reducing infectivity. Few studies have been performed into the use of NA inhibitors in COPD. Murphy et al. investigated the clinical efficacy of inhaled zanamivir for the treatment of influenza in patients with asthma and COPD.[73] Zanamivir significantly reduced the median time to alleviation of influenza symptoms by 1.5 days ($P = 0.009$), and the incidence of complications (requiring antibiotics and a change in respiratory medication) by 58% compared to placebo ($P = 0.064$).

10.8   Use of antibiotics in stable COPD

The latest Cochrane review of prophylactic antibiotic therapy for chronic bronchitis in 2003 evaluated nine randomized controlled trials all performed before 1970.[128] The authors concluded that prophylactic antibiotics in chronic bronchitis/COPD have a small effect in reducing the length of illness due to exacerbations, though they acknowledged that the available data were over 30 years old.

A study by Suzuki et al., published in 2001, was a prospective, randomized, controlled, but not blinded, trial of 109 patients with COPD to investigate whether the use of erythromycin lowers the frequency of the common cold and exacerbations of COPD.[129] The mean number of colds per person over 12 months was significantly lower in the erythromycin group compared to control (1.24 ± 0.07 vs 4.54 ± 0.02, $P = 0.0002$). The relative risk of an exacerbation in the control group compared to the erythromycin group was 4.71 (95% CI, $P = 0.007$). The authors concluded that erythromycin therapy is of benefit in the prevention of exacerbations of COPD.

Recently, Seemungal et al. went on to perform a single-centre randomized, double-blind, placebo-controlled trial to test the hypothesis that long-term low-dose treatment with the macrolide erythromycin reduces exacerbation frequency in patients with moderate to severe COPD.[130] One hundred and nine patients were randomized to receive erythromycin 250 mg or placebo twice daily over 12 months. The primary outcome variable was the number of moderate and/or severe exacerbations – moderate being defined as a worsening of baseline symptoms for at least 2 days requiring oral corticosteroid and/or antibiotic treatment, severe being defined as an exacerbation requiring hospitalization. The study showed that the rate ratio for exacerbations in the erythromycin group compared to the placebo group was 0.648 (95% CI: 0.489–0.859; $P = 0.003$). These patients also had a shorter length of exacerbation. No differences were noticed in stable FEV_1, sputum IL-6, IL-8, myeloperoxidase and bacterial flora, serum CRP or IL-6. The drug was well tolerated with adverse event frequency being equal in both groups. The data suggested that the effect of the macrolide occurred in addition to any effect that inhaled steroids have on reducing exacerbation frequency. It is of interest that no difference in stable FEV_1 was seen, especially in view of previous studies showing that a higher exacerbation frequency is associated with an increased rate of FEV_1 decline.[102] Indeed, if the exacerbations decreased in the macrolide arm it could be hypothesized that there would be a corresponding decrease in the rate of FEV_1 decline. The authors explain this by stating that the study was not powered to detect such a difference. The fear that resistance can develop with long-term antibiotics could at least in part be allayed by the finding that the sputum microbiological profile was not influenced by the use of erythromycin. The authors therefore conclude that macrolide therapy was associated with a significant reduction in exacerbations compared to placebo, and suggest that macrolides may have a role in moderate to severe COPD to augment therapy and decrease the disease burden of this patient group. They could therefore be of use in combination therapy in COPD.

10.9 Role of vaccination

The notion that viral and bacterial infections are the cause of the majority of exacerbations of asthma and COPD is well accepted. It follows that if there were an effective vaccine for the various infective agents then the rate of exacerbation should fall. The theory of viral infection being a causative agent in the development of asthma in childhood again makes development of effective antiviral vaccines important. The currently available vaccines are against influenza and pneumococcus. It is generally accepted in routine clinical practice to offer these vaccines to patients with asthma and COPD.

Asthma

There are two Cochrane reviews of vaccines for asthma. The earlier review addressed the efficacy of pneumococcal vaccine in reducing mortality or morbidity from pneumococcal disease in asthmatics.[131] The review found very limited evidence to support the routine use of a pneumococcal vaccine in asthma. Indeed, there was only one study that satisfied the inclusion criteria and this had low methodological quality.[132] This study investigated the use of pneumococcal vaccine in the prophylaxis of otitis media in asthmatic children. In children receiving vaccine and daily sulfisoxazole there was a 90% mean yearly reduction in otitis media and a 56% reduction in frequency of acute asthma attacks. The second Cochrane review's objective was to assess the efficacy of influenza vaccination in children and adults with asthma.[133] The authors concluded that there was no evidence of a significant increase in asthma exacerbations immediately after vaccination and that there is uncertainty about vaccination affording protection from asthma exacerbations. Both live and inactivated vaccines are used. There is concern, however, in infants given live intranasal vaccine, that there is an

increased incidence of wheeze and hospital admissions. A review into the benefits
of influenza vaccination found there was no evidence of vaccines provoking asthma
exacerbations but there was no unequivocal beneficial effect of influenza vaccines, and
more long-term randomized, placebo-controlled studies are required.[134]

The gold standard for prophylaxis against influenza is vaccination. The neuraminidase inhibitors zanamivir and oseltamivir are useful adjuncts to vaccination.
There had been concerns that zanamivir may reduce lung function and induce bronchospasm in asthmatic patients. However, Cass et al. performed a placebo-controlled
trial in mild or moderate asthmatics who were otherwise healthy, and found that inhaled
zanamivir did not significantly affect pulmonary function or BHR.[135]

The viruses most implicated in asthma are RVs and RSV, for which no human vaccines are currently available. More research is needed to develop effective antiviral
strategies, particularly antiviral monoclonal antibodies (mAb), passive immunization
and vaccines.[136] The mAb palivizumab is effective in preventing RSV infection. In the
IMPACT study, in 1998, the use of palivizumab was associated with a 55% reduction
in RSV hospitalization.[137] One problem is that escape mutants have been detected both
in vivo and *in vitro*, hence motavizumab, a derivative of palivizumab, is now in clinical
trials. Passive immunization with RSV immunoglobulin reduced hospitalizations from
lower respiratory tract infections.[138] Much work has been carried out into the development of a vaccine against RSV, but this has been hampered by the confounding effects
of poor neonatal immune responses, the presence of maternal antibodies and the risk of
vaccine-induced disease. Subunit vaccines have the advantage of not inducing disease
and are in development. Likewise, experimental live attenuated viruses for RSV are
being developed for intranasal administration. These are currently the most promising
approached for RSV vaccine development. There are over 100 RV serotypes, and this
antigenic diversity has led to obvious difficulties with vaccine development.

COPD

There is more evidence to support the use of vaccination in patients with COPD. Three
Cochrane reviews have addressed influenza, *Haemophilus influenzae* and pneumococcal vaccines. The review by Poole et al. concluded that use of inactivated influenza
virus reduces COPD exacerbations.[139] There was a mild increase in transient local
adverse events, but no evidence of an increase in early exacerbations. The importance
of an effective influenza prevention programme is highlighted by the study by Smith
et al., which reported that in patients with COPD, influenza infections resulted in the
greatest decreases in pulmonary function compared to other respiratory viruses.[140]
Nichol et al. performed a study into the benefits of influenza vaccination in the elderly
with chronic lung disease.[141] They showed that hospitalization rates for pneumonia
and influenza were twice as high in the influenza seasons in unvaccinated people as in
the non-influenza seasons, suggesting the importance of influenza infections in people
with chronic lung disease and that influenza vaccination is associated with significant
health benefits.

Foxwell et al. assessed the effects of an oral, whole cell, non-typable *H. influenzae* vaccine in protecting against recurrent episodes of chronic bronchitis.[142] They concluded that vaccination in the autumn may reduce the number and severity of exacerbations over the following winter, though a larger clinical trial is still needed to confirm these findings.

Granger et al. assessed the efficacy of pneumococcal vaccines in COPD.[143] They concluded that, from randomized controlled trials, there is no evidence that injectable pneumococcal vaccination has any effect on morbidity or mortality in patients with COPD. However, a study by Alfageme et al. in 2006 investigated the efficacy of the 23-valent pneumococcal polysaccharide vaccine in COPD patients.[144] They concluded that this vaccine was effective in preventing community-acquired pneumonia (radiographically proven) in COPD patients under 65 years and those with severe airflow obstruction (FEV_1 <40% predicted). In a recent review of the current practice of pneumococcal vaccination the authors discuss the evidence in support of vaccination and the challenges in the development of improved vaccines.[145]

As discussed above many challenges exist in the development of other viral vaccines. RSV is an increasingly recognized cause of illness in elderly and high-risk adults – those with chronic heart or lung disease. Indeed, the study by Falsey et al. showed a disease burden similar to non-pandemic influenza A.[146] This stresses the potential role an effective RSV vaccine may have not only in children but also in the adult population.

10.10   Conclusion

In this discussion we have aimed to delineate the role of antibiotics and antiviral agents in asthma and COPD, both in stable disease and exacerbations, and have highlighted the current evidence for their use. Exacerbations of asthma are strongly associated with infection, particularly viral infection, mostly RV. Asthmatics have been shown to have an increased susceptibility to viral infection, and are at increased risk of pneumococcal disease. There is some *in vitro* evidence that virus-induced exacerbations may be worsened by bacterial infection. There is an increasing amount of evidence that atypical bacteria play a role in the pathogenesis of both stable disease and exacerbations and this has generated interest in the role of macrolide and ketolide antibiotics as treatment options. Their actions, particularly the anti-inflammatory ones, could, in future, lead to their use in combination therapy. The large number of exacerbations associated with viral infection has generated much interest in the pathogenesis of viral-induced exacerbations. More targeted treatments against respiratory viruses such as interferons, NF-κB inhibitors, and even macrolides and ketolides, and development of specific treatments against rhinoviruses, namely capsid binders, protease inhibitors and soluble ICAM-1 derivatives, could have a great impact on the outcome of asthma exacerbations. These studies are currently lacking. With bacteria and viruses playing such an important role in the aetiology of asthma, there could be a greater role for the use of vaccination. Difficulties have been encountered in the development of an effective vaccine for both RSV and RV.

Bacterial and/or viral infections account for up to 78% of the causes of COPD exacerbations. Antibiotics are widely used in exacerbations and there is good evidence to support this, particularly in the Anthonisen type I and II exacerbations. The class of antibiotic still remains a debate, with equivalence seen in macrolides, quinolones and amoxicillin/clavulanate. The development of a potential marker for bacterial exacerbations, possibly procalcitonin, should target antibiotic therapy more appropriately. There is little evidence for the use of antiviral agents, other than anti-influenza drugs, particularly the neuraminidase inhibitors. More work needs to be done in this area. There is evidence emerging that antibiotics, particularly the macrolides, may be of use in stable COPD, and this could have profound implications for combination therapy. Vaccination plays a role in COPD arguably more than in asthma. Use of pneumococcal and *H. influenzae* vaccines can reduce the number and severity of exacerbations and prevent pneumonia in this group of patients. Other than the influenza vaccine, development of other viral vaccines has been hampered, so their role in COPD has yet to be determined.

Without doubt, anti-infectives play a role in therapy of airways disease, particularly in the exacerbation state, but evidence is suggesting a role for them in the stable state as well. We wait to see what impact they will have on these diseases, with the identification of further pathogenic processes, the development of alternative therapeutic agents, and trial of these agents in populations of patients with different severities of disease.

References

1. Anthonisen NR, Manfreda J, Warren CP, Hershfield ES, Harding GK, Nelson NA. Antibiotic therapy in exacerbations of chronic obstructive pulmonary disease. Ann Intern Med 1987;106:196–204.
2. Papi A, Bellettato CM, Braccioni F, et al. Infections and airway inflammation in chronic obstructive pulmonary disease severe exacerbations. Am J Respir Crit Care Med 2006;173:1114–21.
3. Greenstone IR, Ni Chroinin MN, et al. Combination of inhaled long-acting beta2-agonists and inhaled steroids versus higher dose of inhaled steroids in children and adults with persistent asthma. Cochrane Database Syst Rev 2005;(4):CD005533.
4. Lasserson TJ, Cates CJ, Ferrara G, Casali L. Combination fluticasone and salmeterol versus fixed dose combination budesonide and formoterol for chronic asthma in adults and children. Cochrane Database Syst Rev 2008;(3):CD004106.
5. FitzGerald JM, Boulet LP, Follows RM. The CONCEPT trial: a 1-year, multicenter, randomized, double-blind, double-dummy comparison of a stable dosing regimen of salmeterol/fluticasone propionate with an adjustable maintenance dosing regimen of formoterol/budesonide in adults with persistent asthma. Clin Ther 2005;27:393–406.
6. Rabe KF, Pizzichini E, Stallberg B, et al. Budesonide/formoterol in a single inhaler for maintenance and relief in mild-to-moderate asthma: a randomized, double-blind trial. Chest 2006;129:246–56.
7. Bousquet J, Boulet LP, Peters MJ, et al. Budesonide/formoterol for maintenance and relief in uncontrolled asthma vs. high-dose salmeterol/fluticasone. Respir Med 2007;101:2437–46.
8. Joos S, Miksch A, Szecsenyi J, et al. Montelukast as add-on therapy to inhaled corticosteroids in the treatment of mild to moderate asthma: a systematic review. Thorax 2008;63:453–62.

9. Nannini LJ, Cates CJ, Lasserson TJ, Poole P. Combined corticosteroid and long-acting beta-agonist in one inhaler versus inhaled steroids for chronic obstructive pulmonary disease. Cochrane Database Syst Rev 2007;(4):CD006826.

10. Calverley PM, Anderson JA, Celli B, et al. Salmeterol and fluticasone propionate and survival in chronic obstructive pulmonary disease. N Engl J Med 2007;356:775–89.

11. Tashkin DP, Celli B, Senn S, et al. A 4-year trial of tiotropium in chronic obstructive pulmonary disease. N Engl J Med 2008;359:1543–54.

12. Vogelmeier C, Kardos P, Harari S, Gans SJ, Stenglein S, Thirlwell J. Formoterol mono- and combination therapy with tiotropium in patients with COPD: A 6-month study. Respir Med 2008;102:1511–20.

13. Singh D, Brooks J, Hagan G, Cahn A, O'Connor BJ. Superiority of "triple" therapy with salmeterol/fluticasone propionate and tiotropium bromide versus individual components in moderate to severe COPD. Thorax 2008;63:592–8.

14. Use of antibiotics to treat asthma exacerbations. J Allergy Clin Immunol 2002;110(5, Suppl. 1):S180–S183.

15. Graham VA, Milton AF, Knowles GK, Davies RJ. Routine antibiotics in hospital management of acute asthma. Lancet 1982;i:418–20.

16. Shapiro GG, Eggleston PA, Pierson WE, Ray CG, Bierman CW. Double-blind study of the effectiveness of a broad spectrum antibiotic in status asthmaticus. Pediatrics 1974;53:867–72.

17. National Asthma Education and Prevention Program. Expert Panel Report 3: Guidelines for the Diagnosis and Management of Asthma. National Heart, Lung and Blood Institute, 2007; available at: www.nhlbi.nih.gov/guidelines/asthma/asthgdln.pdf

18. British Guideline on the Management of Asthma. Thorax 2008;63(Suppl. 4):iv1–121.

19. Graham V, Lasserson T, Rowe BH. Antibiotics for acute asthma. Cochrane Database Syst Rev 2001;(3):CD002741.

20. Celli BR, MacNee W, Agusti A, et al. Standards for the diagnosis and treatment of patients with COPD: a summary of the ATS/ERS position paper. Eur Respir J 2004;23:932–46.

21. Management of exacerbations of COPD. Thorax 2004;59:i131–i156.

22. Saint S, Bent S, Vittinghoff E, Grady D. Antibiotics in chronic obstructive pulmonary disease exacerbations. A meta-analysis. JAMA 1995;273:957–60.

23. Balter MS, La FJ, Low DE, Mandell L, Grossman RF. Canadian guidelines for the management of acute exacerbations of chronic bronchitis. Can Respir J 2003;10(Suppl. B):3B–32B.

24. Corne JM, Marshall C, Smith S, et al. Frequency, severity, and duration of rhinovirus infections in asthmatic and non-asthmatic individuals: a longitudinal cohort study. Lancet 2002;359:831–4.

25. Kling S, Donninger H, Williams Z, et al. Persistence of rhinovirus RNA after asthma exacerbation in children. Clin Exp Allergy 2005;35:672–8.

26. Talbot TR, Hartert TV, Mitchel E, et al. Asthma as a risk factor for invasive pneumococcal disease. N Engl J Med 2005;352:2082–90.

27. Contoli M, Message SD, Laza-Stanca V, et al. Role of deficient type III interferon-lambda production in asthma exacerbations. Nat Med 2006;12:1023–6.

28. Ishizuka S, Yamaya M, Suzuki T, et al. Effects of rhinovirus infection on the adherence of Streptococcus pneumoniae to cultured human airway epithelial cells. J Infect Dis 2003;188:1928–39.

29. Oliver BG, Lim S, Wark P, et al. Rhinovirus exposure impairs immune responses to bacterial products in human alveolar macrophages. Thorax 2008;63:519–25.

30. Hansbro PM, Beagley KW, Horvat JC, Gibson PG. Role of atypical bacterial infection of the lung in predisposition/protection of asthma. Pharmacol Ther 2004;101:193–210.

31. Johnston SL, Martin RJ. Chlamydophila pneumoniae and Mycoplasma pneumoniae: a role in asthma pathogenesis? Am J Respir Crit Care Med 2005;172:1078–89.

32. Biscione GL, Corne J, Chauhan AJ, Johnston SL. Increased frequency of detection of Chlamy-dophila pneumoniae in asthma. Eur Respir J 2004;24:745–9.
33. Black PN, Scicchitano R, Jenkins CR, et al. Serological evidence of infection with Chlamydia pneumoniae is related to the severity of asthma. Eur Respir J 2000;15:254–9.
34. Kocabas A, Avsar M, Hanta I, Koksal F, Kuleci S. Chlamydophila pneumoniae infection in adult asthmatics patients. J Asthma 2008;45:39–43.
35. Kraft M, Cassell GH, Henson JE, et al. Detection of Mycoplasma pneumoniae in the airways of adults with chronic asthma. Am J Respir Crit Care Med 1998;158:998–1001.
36. Martin RJ, Kraft M, Chu HW, Berns EA, Cassell GH. A link between chronic asthma and chronic infection. J Allergy Clin Immunol 2001;107:595–601.
37. Cunningham AF, Johnston SL, Julious SA, Lampe FC, Ward ME. Chronic Chlamydia pneu-moniae infection and asthma exacerbations in children. Eur Respir J 1998;11:345–9.
38. Johnston SL, Pattemore PK, Sanderson G, et al. Community study of role of viral infections in exacerbations of asthma in 9–11 year old children. Brit Med J 1995;310:1225–9.
39. Wark PA, Johnston SL, Simpson JL, Hensley MJ, Gibson PG. Chlamydia pneumoniae immunoglobulin A reactivation and airway inflammation in acute asthma. Eur Respir J 2002;20:834–40.
40. Lieberman D, Lieberman D, Printz S, et al. Atypical pathogen infection in adults with acute exacerbation of bronchial asthma. Am J Respir Crit Care Med 2003;167:406–10.
41. Biscardi S, Lorrot M, Marc E, et al. Mycoplasma pneumoniae and asthma in children. Clin Infect Dis 2004;38:1341–6.
42. Blasi F, Aliberti S, Allegra L, et al. Chlamydophila pneumoniae induces a sustained airway hyperresponsiveness and inflammation in mice. Respir Res 2007;8:83.
43. Rodel J, Woytas M, Groh A, et al. Production of basic fibroblast growth factor and interleukin 6 by human smooth muscle cells following infection with Chlamydia pneumoniae. Infect Immun 2000;68:3635–41.
44. Rodel J, Assefa S, Prochnau D, et al. Interferon-beta induction by Chlamydia pneumoniae in human smooth muscle cells. FEMS Immunol Med Microbiol 2001;32:9–15.
45. Xie S, Issa R, Sukkar MB, et al. Induction and regulation of matrix metalloproteinase-12 in human airway smooth muscle cells. Respir Res 2005;6:148.
46. Suzuki R, Miyazaki Y, Takagi K, Torii K, Taniguchi H. Matrix metalloproteinases in the pathogenesis of asthma and COPD: implications for therapy. Treat Respir Med 2004;3:17–27.
47. Byrne GI, Ojcius DM. Chlamydia and apoptosis: life and death decisions of an intracellular pathogen. Nat Rev Microbiol 2004;2:802–8.
48. Wark PA, Johnston SL, Bucchieri F, et al. Asthmatic bronchial epithelial cells have a deficient innate immune response to infection with rhinovirus. J Exp Med 2005;201:937–47.
49. Yang J, Hooper WC, Phillips DJ, Talkington DF. Regulation of proinflammatory cy-tokines in human lung epithelial cells infected with Mycoplasma pneumoniae. Infect Immun 2002;70:3649–55.
50. Martin RJ, Chu HW, Honour JM, Harbeck RJ. Airway inflammation and bronchial hyperre-sponsiveness after Mycoplasma pneumoniae infection in a murine model. Am J Respir Cell Mol Biol 2001;24:577–82.
51. Chu HW, Honour JM, Rawlinson CA, Harbeck RJ, Martin RJ. Effects of respiratory My-coplasma pneumoniae infection on allergen-induced bronchial hyperresponsiveness and lung inflammation in mice. Infect Immun 2003;71:1520–6.
52. Kostadima E, Tsiodras S, Alexopoulos EI, et al. Clarithromycin reduces the severity of bronchial hyperresponsiveness in patients with asthma. Eur Respir J 2004;23:714–7.

53. Hammerschlag MR, Roblin PM, Bebear CM. Activity of telithromycin, a new ketolide antibacterial, against atypical and intracellular respiratory tract pathogens. J Antimicrob Chemother 2001;48(Suppl. T1):25–31.

54. Hammerschlag MR, Sharma R. Use of cethromycin, a new ketolide, for treatment of community-acquired respiratory infections. Expert Opin Investig Drugs 2008;17:387–400.

55. Spahn JD, Fost DA, Covar R, et al. Clarithromycin potentiates glucocorticoid responsiveness in patients with asthma: results of a pilot study. Ann Allergy Asthma Immunol 2001;87: 501–5.

56. Feldman C, Anderson R, Theron AJ, Ramafi G, Cole PJ, Wilson R. Roxithromycin, clarithromycin, and azithromycin attenuate the injurious effects of bioactive phospholipids on human respiratory epithelium in vitro. Inflammation 1997;21:655–65.

57. Takizawa H, Desaki M, Ohtoshi T, et al. Erythromycin suppresses interleukin 6 expression by human bronchial epithelial cells: a potential mechanism of its anti-inflammatory action. Biochem Biophys Res Commun 1995;210:781–6.

58. Desaki M, Takizawa H, Ohtoshi T, et al. Erythromycin suppresses nuclear factor-kappaB and activator protein-1 activation in human bronchial epithelial cells. Biochem Biophys Res Commun 2000;267:124–8.

59. Goswami SK, Kivity S, Marom Z. Erythromycin inhibits respiratory glycoconjugate secretion from human airways in vitro. Am Rev Respir Dis 1990;141:72–8.

60. Tamaoki J, Tagaya E, Sakai A, Konno K. Effects of macrolide antibiotics on neurally mediated contraction of human isolated bronchus. J Allergy Clin Immunol 1995;95:853–9.

61. Lopez-Boado YS, Rubin BK. Macrolides as immunomodulatory medications for the therapy of chronic lung diseases. Curr Opin Pharmacol 2008;8:286–91.

62. Feldman C, Anderson R, Theron A, Mokgobu I, Cole PJ, Wilson R. The effects of ketolides on bioactive phospholipid-induced injury to human respiratory epithelium in vitro. Eur Respir J 1999;13:1022–8.

63. Araujo FG, Slifer TL, Remington JS. Inhibition of secretion of interleukin-1alpha and tumor necrosis factor alpha by the ketolide antibiotic telithromycin. Antimicrob Agents Chemother 2002;46:3327–30.

64. Niclau DP, Tessier R, Rubinstein I, Nightingale CH. In vivo immunomodulatory profile of telithromycin in a murine pneumococcal infection model. Pharmazie 2006;61:343–7.

65. Leiva M, Ruiz-Bravo A, Jimenez-Valera M. Effects of Telithromycin in in vitro and in vivo models of lipopolysaccharide-induced airway inflammation. Chest 2008;134:20–9.

66. Richeldi L, Ferrara G, Fabbri LM, Lasserson TJ, Gibson PG. Macrolides for chronic asthma. Cochrane Database Syst Rev 2005;(4):CD002997.

67. Black PN, Blasi F, Jenkins CR, et al. Trial of roxithromycin in subjects with asthma and serological evidence of infection with Chlamydia pneumoniae. Am J Respir Crit Care Med 2001;164:536–41.

68. Kraft M, Cassell GH, Pak J, Martin RJ. Mycoplasma pneumoniae and Chlamydia pneumoniae in asthma: effect of clarithromycin. Chest 2002;121:1782–8.

69. Johnston SL, Blasi F, Black PN, Martin RJ, Farrell DJ, Nieman RB. The effect of telithromycin in acute exacerbations of asthma. N Engl J Med 2006;354:1589–600.

70. Johnston SL, Pattemore PK, Sanderson G, et al. The relationship between upper respiratory infections and hospital admissions for asthma: a time-trend analysis. Am J Respir Crit Care Med 1996;154:654–60.

71. Johnston NW, Johnston SL, Duncan JM, et al. The September epidemic of asthma exacerbations in children: a search for etiology. J Allergy Clin Immunol 2005;115:132–8.

72. Johnston SL, Ferrero F, Garcia ML, Dutkowski R. Oral oseltamivir improves pulmonary function and reduces exacerbation frequency for influenza-infected children with asthma. Pediatr Infect Dis J 2005;24:225–32.

73. Murphy KR, Eivindson A, Pauksens K, et al. Efficacy and safety of inhaled zanamivir for the treatment of influenza in patients with asthma or chronic obstructive pulmonary disease: A double-blind, randomised, placebo-controlled, multicentre study. Clin Drug Invest 2000;20:337–49.

74. Al-Nakib W, Higgins PG, Barrow GI, et al. Suppression of colds in human volunteers challenged with rhinovirus by a new synthetic drug (R61837). Antimicrob Agents Chemother 1989;33:522–5.

75. Hayden FG, Herrington DT, Coats TL, et al. Efficacy and safety of oral pleconaril for treatment of colds due to picornaviruses in adults: results of 2 double-blind, randomized, placebo-controlled trials. Clin Infect Dis 2003;36:1523–32.

76. Fleischer R, Laessig K. Safety and efficacy evaluation of pleconaril for treatment of the common cold. Clin Infect Dis 2003;37:1722.

77. Hayden FG, Turner RB, Gwaltney JM, et al. Phase II, randomized, double-blind, placebo-controlled studies of ruprintrivir nasal spray 2-percent suspension for prevention and treatment of experimentally induced rhinovirus colds in healthy volunteers. Antimicrob Agents Chemother 2003;47:3907–16.

78. Turner RB, Wecker MT, Pohl G, et al. Efficacy of tremacamra, a soluble intercellular adhesion molecule 1, for experimental rhinovirus infection: a randomized clinical trial. JAMA 1999;281:1797–804.

79. Kotenko SV, Gallagher G, Baurin VV, et al. IFN-lambdas mediate antiviral protection through a distinct class II cytokine receptor complex. Nat Immunol 2003;4:69–77.

80. Sheppard P, Kindsvogel W, Xu W, et al. IL-28, IL-29 and their class II cytokine receptor IL-28R. Nat Immunol 2003;4:63–8.

81. Hayden FG, Gwaltney JM Jr. Intranasal interferon-alpha 2 treatment of experimental rhinoviral colds. J Infect Dis 1984;150:174–80.

82. Farr BM, Gwaltney JM Jr, Adams KF, Hayden FG. Intranasal interferon-alpha 2 for prevention of natural rhinovirus colds. Antimicrob Agents Chemother 1984;26:31–4.

83. Wiselka MJ, Nicholson KG, Kent J, Cookson JB, Tyrrell DA. Prophylactic intranasal alpha 2 interferon and viral exacerbations of chronic respiratory disease. Thorax 1991;46:706–11.

84. Simon HU, Seelbach H, Ehmann R, Schmitz M. Clinical and immunological effects of low-dose IFN-alpha treatment in patients with corticosteroid-resistant asthma. Allergy 2003;58:1250–5.

85. Higgins PG, Al-Nakib W, Willman J, Tyrrell DA. Interferon-beta ser as prophylaxis against experimental rhinovirus infection in volunteers. J Interferon Res 1986;6:153–9.

86. Sperber SJ, Levine PA, Innes DJ, Mills SE, Hayden FG. Tolerance and efficacy of intranasal administration of recombinant beta serine interferon in healthy adults. J Infect Dis 1988;158:166–75.

87. Sperber SJ, Levine PA, Sorrentino JV, Riker DK, Hayden FG. Ineffectiveness of recombinant interferon-beta serine nasal drops for prophylaxis of natural colds. J Infect Dis 1989;160:700–5.

88. Papi A, Papadopoulos NG, Degitz K, Holgate ST, Johnston SL. Corticosteroids inhibit rhinovirus-induced intercellular adhesion molecule-1 up-regulation and promoter activation on respiratory epithelial cells. J Allergy Clin Immunol 2000;105:318–26.

89. Farr BM, Gwaltney JM Jr, Hendley JO, et al. A randomized controlled trial of glucocorticoid prophylaxis against experimental rhinovirus infection. J Infect Dis 1990;162:1173–7.

90. Grunberg K, Sharon RF, Sont JK, et al. Rhinovirus-induced airway inflammation in asthma: effect of treatment with inhaled corticosteroids before and during experimental infection. Am J Respir Crit Care Med 2001;164:1816–22.

91. O'Byrne PM, Bisgaard H, Godard PP, et al. Budesonide/formoterol combination therapy as both maintenance and reliever medication in asthma. Am J Respir Crit Care Med 2005;171: 129–36.

92. Edwards MR, Johnson MW, Johnston SL. Combination therapy: Synergistic suppression of virus-induced chemokines in airway epithelial cells. Am J Respir Cell Mol Biol 2006;34: 616–24.

93. Edwards MR, Bartlett NW, Clarke D, Birrell M, Belvisi M, Johnston SL. Targeting the NF-kappaB pathway in asthma and chronic obstructive pulmonary disease. Pharmacol Ther 2009;121:1–13.

94. Henderson WR Jr, Chi EY, Teo JL, Nguyen C, Kahn M. A small molecule inhibitor of redox-regulated NF-kappa B and activator protein-1 transcription blocks allergic airway inflammation in a mouse asthma model. J Immunol 2002;169:5294–9.

95. Newton R, Holden NS, Catley MC, et al. Repression of inflammatory gene expression in human pulmonary epithelial cells by small-molecule IkappaB kinase inhibitors. J Pharmacol Exp Ther 2007;321:734–42.

96. Papi A, Johnston SL. Rhinovirus infection induces expression of its own receptor intercellular adhesion molecule 1 (ICAM-1) via increased NF-kappaB-mediated transcription. J Biol Chem 1999;274:9707–20.

97. Suzuki T, Yamaya M, Sekizawa K, et al. Erythromycin inhibits rhinovirus infection in cultured human tracheal epithelial cells. Am J Respir Crit Care Med 2002;165:1113–8.

98. Jang YJ, Kwon HJ, Lee BJ. Effect of clarithromycin on rhinovirus-16 infection in A549 cells. Eur Respir J 2006;27:12–9.

99. Abisheganaden JA, Avila PC, Kishiyama JL, et al. Effect of clarithromycin on experimental rhinovirus-16 colds: a randomized, double-blind, controlled trial. Am J Med 2000;108:453–9.

100. Wark PA, Bucchieri F, Johnston SL, et al. IFN-gamma-induced protein 10 is a novel biomarker of rhinovirus-induced asthma exacerbations. J Allergy Clin Immunol 2007;120:586–93.

101. Bartlett NW, Walton RP, Edwards MR, et al. Mouse models of rhinovirus-induced disease and exacerbation of allergic airway inflammation. Nat Med 2008;14:199–204.

102. Donaldson GC, Seemungal TA, Bhowmik A, Wedzicha JA. Relationship between exacerbation frequency and lung function decline in chronic obstructive pulmonary disease. Thorax 2002;57:847–52.

103. Rodriguez-Roisin R. Toward a consensus definition for COPD exacerbations. Chest 2000;117(5 Suppl. 2):398S–401S.

104. Groenewegen KH, Wouters EF. Bacterial infections in patients requiring admission for an acute exacerbation of COPD; a 1-year prospective study. Respir Med 2003;97:770–7.

105. Sethi S, Evans N, Grant BJ, Murphy TF. New strains of bacteria and exacerbations of chronic obstructive pulmonary disease. N Engl J Med 2002;347:465–71.

106. Sethi S, Wrona C, Eschberger K, Lobbins P, Cai X, Murphy TF. Inflammatory profile of new bacterial strain exacerbations of chronic obstructive pulmonary disease. Am J Respir Crit Care Med 2008;177:491–7.

107. Seemungal T, Harper-Owen R, Bhowmik A, et al. Respiratory viruses, symptoms, and inflammatory markers in acute exacerbations and stable chronic obstructive pulmonary disease. Am J Respir Crit Care Med 2001;164:1618–23.

108. Rohde G, Wiethege A, Borg I, et al. Respiratory viruses in exacerbations of chronic obstructive pulmonary disease requiring hospitalisation: a case-control study. Thorax 2003;58:37–42.

109. Wilkinson TM, Hurst JR, Perera WR, Wilks M, Donaldson GC, Wedzicha JA. Effect of interactions between lower airway bacterial and rhinoviral infection in exacerbations of COPD. Chest 2006;129:317–24.

110. Blasi F, Legnani D, Lombardo VM, et al. Chlamydia pneumoniae infection in acute exacerbations of COPD. Eur Respir J 1993;6:19–22.

111. Mogulkoc N, Karakurt S, Isalska B, et al. Acute purulent exacerbation of chronic obstructive pulmonary disease and Chlamydia pneumoniae infection. Am J Respir Crit Care Med 1999;160:349–53.

112. Blasi F, Damato S, Cosentini R, et al. Chlamydia pneumoniae and chronic bronchitis: association with severity and bacterial clearance following treatment. Thorax 2002;57:672–6.

113. Seemungal TA, Wedzicha JA, MacCallum PK, Johnston SL, Lambert PA. Chlamydia pneumoniae and COPD exacerbation. Thorax 2002;57:1087–8.

114. Gilmour PS, Rahman I, Hayashi S, Hogg JC, Donaldson K, MacNee W. Adenoviral E1A primes alveolar epithelial cells to PM(10)-induced transcription of interleukin-8. Am J Physiol Lung Cell Mol Physiol 2001;281:L598–L606.

115. Puhan MA, Vollenweider D, Latshang T, Steurer J, Steurer-Stey C. Exacerbations of chronic obstructive pulmonary disease: when are antibiotics indicated? A systematic review. Respir Res 2007;8:30.

116. Ram FS, Rodriguez-Roisin R, Granados-Navarrete A, Garcia-Aymerich J, Barnes NC. Antibiotics for exacerbations of chronic obstructive pulmonary disease. Cochrane Database Syst Rev 2006;(2):CD004403.

117. Siempos II, Dimopoulos G, Korbila IP, Manta K, Falagas ME. Macrolides, quinolones and amoxicillin/clavulanate for chronic bronchitis: a meta-analysis. Eur Respir J 2007;29:1127–37.

118. Wilson R, Schentag JJ, Ball P, Mandell L. A comparison of gemifloxacin and clarithromycin in acute exacerbations of chronic bronchitis and long-term clinical outcomes. Clin Ther 2002;24:639–52.

119. Wilson R, Allegra L, Huchon G, et al. Short-term and long-term outcomes of moxifloxacin compared to standard antibiotic treatment in acute exacerbations of chronic bronchitis. Chest 2004;125:953–64.

120. Nouira S, Marghli S, Belghith M, Besbes L, Elatrous S, Abroug F. Once daily oral ofloxacin in chronic obstructive pulmonary disease exacerbation requiring mechanical ventilation: a randomised placebo-controlled trial. Lancet 2001;358:2020–5.

121. Ruiz-Gonzalez A, Gimenez A, Gomez-Arbones X, et al. Open-label, randomized comparison trial of long-term outcomes of levofloxacin versus standard antibiotic therapy in acute exacerbations of chronic obstructive pulmonary disease. Respirology 2007;12:117–21.

122. El Moussaoui R, Roede BM, Speelman P, Bresser P, Prins JM, Bossuyt PM. Short-course antibiotic treatment in acute exacerbations of chronic bronchitis and COPD: a meta-analysis of double-blind studies. Thorax 2008;63:415–22.

123. Christ-Crain M, Stolz D, Bingisser R, et al. Procalcitonin guidance of antibiotic therapy in community-acquired pneumonia: a randomized trial. Am J Respir Crit Care Med 2006;174:84–93.

124. Stolz D, Christ-Crain M, Bingisser R, et al. Antibiotic treatment of exacerbations of COPD: a randomized, controlled trial comparing procalcitonin-guidance with standard therapy. Chest 2007;131:9–19.

125. Martinez FJ, Curtis JL. Procalcitonin-guided antibiotic therapy in COPD exacerbations: closer but not quite there. Chest 2007;131:1–2.

126. Nseir S, Cavestri B, Di Pompeo C, et al. Factors predicting bacterial involvement in severe acute exacerbations of chronic obstructive pulmonary disease. Respiration 2008;76:253–60.

127. Nathan RA, Geddes D, Woodhead M. Management of influenza in patients with asthma or chronic obstructive pulmonary disease. Ann Allergy Asthma Immunol 2001;87:447–54, 487.

128. Black P, Staykova T, Chacko E, Ram FS, Poole P. Prophylactic antibiotic therapy for chronic bronchitis. Cochrane Database Syst Rev 2003;(1):CD004105.

129. Suzuki T, Yanai M, Yamaya M, et al. Erythromycin and common cold in COPD. Chest 2001;120:730–3.

130. Seemungal TA, Wilkinson TM, Hurst JR, Perera WR, Sapsford RJ, Wedzicha JA. Long term erythromycin therapy is associated with decreased COPD exacerbations. Am J Respir Crit Care Med 2008;178:1139–47.

131. Sheikh A, Alves B, Dhami S. Pneumococcal vaccine for asthma. Cochrane Database Syst Rev 2002;(1):CD002165.

132. Schuller DE. Prophylaxis of otitis media in asthmatic children. Pediatr Infect Dis 1983;2:280–3.

133. Cates CJ, Jefferson TO, Rowe BH. Vaccines for preventing influenza in people with asthma. Cochrane Database Syst Rev 2008;(2):CD000364.

134. Bueving HJ, Thomas S, Wouden JC. Is influenza vaccination in asthma helpful? Curr Opin Allergy Clin Immunol 2005;5:65–70.

135. Cass LM, Gunawardena KA, Macmahon MM, Bye A. Pulmonary function and airway responsiveness in mild to moderate asthmatics given repeated inhaled doses of zanamivir. Respir Med 2000;94:166–73.

136. Hansbro NG, Horvat JC, Wark PA, Hansbro PM. Understanding the mechanisms of viral induced asthma: new therapeutic directions. Pharmacol Ther 2008;117:313–53.

137. The IMpact-RSV Study Group. Palivizumab, a humanized respiratory syncytial virus monoclonal antibody, reduces hospitalization from respiratory syncytial virus infection in high-risk infants. Pediatrics 1998;102:531–7.

138. Reduction of respiratory syncytial virus hospitalization among premature infants and infants with bronchopulmonary dysplasia using respiratory syncytial virus immune globulin prophylaxis. The PREVENT Study Group. Pediatrics 1997;99:93–9.

139. Poole PJ, Chacko E, Wood-Baker RW, Cates CJ. Influenza vaccine for patients with chronic obstructive pulmonary disease. Cochrane Database Syst Rev 2006;(1):CD002733.

140. Smith CB, Kanner RE, Golden CA, Klauber MR, Renzetti AD Jr. Effect of viral infections on pulmonary function in patients with chronic obstructive pulmonary diseases. J Infect Dis 1980;141:271–80.

141. Nichol KL, Baken L, Nelson A. Relation between influenza vaccination and outpatient visits, hospitalization, and mortality in elderly persons with chronic lung disease. Ann Intern Med 1999;130:397–403.

142. Foxwell AR, Cripps AW, Dear KB. Haemophilus influenzae oral whole cell vaccination for preventing acute exacerbations of chronic bronchitis. Cochrane Database Syst Rev 2006;(4):CD001958.

143. Granger R, Walters J, Poole PJ, et al. Injectable vaccines for preventing pneumococcal infection in patients with chronic obstructive pulmonary disease. Cochrane Database Syst Rev 2006;(4):CD001390.

144. Alfageme I, Vazquez R, Reyes N, Munoz J, Fernandez A, Hernandez M, et al. Clinical efficacy of anti-pneumococcal vaccination in patients with COPD. Thorax 2006;61:189–95.

145. Schenkein JG, Nahm MH, Dransfield MT. Pneumococcal vaccination for patients with COPD: current practice and future directions. Chest 2008;133:767–74.

146. Falsey AR, Hennessey PA, Formica MA, Cox C, Walsh EE. Respiratory syncytial virus infection in elderly and high-risk adults. N Engl J Med 2005;352:1749–59.

11

Long-acting muscarinic antagonists in asthma and COPD

M. Diane Lougheed, Josuel Ora and Denis E. O'Donnell

Department of Medicine, Queen's University, Ontario, Canada

11.1   Introduction

Asthma and chronic obstructive pulmonary disease (COPD) are two of the most prevalent chronic respiratory diseases in the world.[1,2] Although the pathogenesis of these two conditions is fundamentally different, both are characterized by chronic airway inflammation and airflow obstruction. In the absence of a cure for either disease, management necessarily focuses on effective prevention, self-management education and bronchodilator pharmacotherapy to relieve respiratory symptoms. For asthma, effective anti-inflammatory therapy is available and has been shown to impact favourably on the natural history of the disease. However, therapeutic suppression of the airway inflammation that characterizes COPD remains an elusive goal. Short-acting anticholinergic bronchodilators have played a prominent therapeutic role for many years in obstructive lung diseases. Recent development of long-acting and selective muscarinic antagonists such as tiotropium bromide[3,4] presents novel therapeutic options for the management of COPD and asthma.

This review summarizes current understanding of human airway innervation, focusing on muscarinic receptor function in health and in obstructive lung diseases. This provides the foundation for overviews of the physiological rationale for the use of long-acting anticholinergic bronchodilators in COPD and asthma. Finally, the role of long-acting muscarinic antagonists in COPD and asthma is discussed, based upon a detailed appraisal of the available literature.

11.2   Innervation of the airways

Airway smooth muscles, mucous glands, and the bronchial circulation are regulated by the autonomic nervous system.[5] The human airways are innervated by parasympathetic (cholinergic) and sympathetic (adrenergic) nerves, and the non-adrenergic

Advances in Combination Therapy for Asthma and COPD, First Edition. Edited by Jan Lötvall.
© 2012 John Wiley & Sons, Ltd. Published 2012 by John Wiley & Sons, Ltd.

non-cholinergic (NANC) system.[6,7] The structure and function of cholinergic pathways and their role in the pathophysiology of asthma and COPD have recently been extensively reviewed,[6,8] and are summarized below.

Parasympathetic innervation

Parasympathetic innervation, via the vagus nerve, is the dominant autonomic neural pathway regulating airway smooth muscle tone, airway secretions, bronchial circulation, vascular permeability, and recruitment and activation of inflammatory cells.[5,6,9] The efferent nerves synapse in parasympathetic ganglia, which are situated in the airway walls. This innervation is present along the length of the bronchial tree, but is concentrated in large and medium-sized airways.[10] Postganglionic nerves innervate the target organs, which include airway smooth muscle, submucosal glands and blood vessels. The major neurotransmitter of cholinergic nerves is acetylcholine (ACh), which acts by binding to nicotinic and muscarinic receptors located on these target organs, causing airway smooth muscle contraction and mucous secretion. In addition, ACh feeds back onto prejunctional muscarinic receptors to inhibit further ACh release.

Five muscarinic receptor subtypes have been identified, three of which are known to be present in human airways (M_1, M_2 and M_3) and have different physiological effects.[9,11] Table 11.1 summarizes their location and function in humans. Elegant animal models have clearly elucidated the function of muscarinic receptor subtypes. M_2 receptor knockout mice ($M_2^{-/-}$ genotype) develop greater bronchoconstriction when stimulated than $M_2^{+/+}$ or $M_3^{+/+}$ mice.[12] The M_2 subtype predominates on airway smooth muscle and has an autoinhibitory function, providing a 'physiological brake' to bronchoconstriction. In contrast, since $M_3^{-/-}$ mice do not bronchoconstrict in response to methacholine or vagal stimulation, M_3 receptors are considered to be the primary receptors that mediate bronchoconstriction.

Table 11.1 Location and effects of muscarinic receptors in the airways.

Receptor type	Location	Airway smooth muscle	Submucosal gland	Blood vessel
M_1	Parasympathetic ganglia, submucosal glands, alveolar walls	Facilitation of neurotransmission	Stimulation of mucus secretion	–
M_2	Postganglionic nerve terminals, airway smooth muscle, sympathetic nerves	Inhibition of ACh release (negative feedback); bronchodilation	–	–
M_3	Smooth muscle, submucosal glands, epithelial cells, endothelial cells	Bronchoconstriction	Stimulation of mucus secretion	Vasodilation
M_4		Unknown	Unknown	Unknown

The observation that atropine causes bronchodilation in humans without lung disease indicates that there is resting 'cholinergic' tone.[8] In animals and humans, muscarinic receptors appear to be predominantly located in the central airways and diminish in density towards the smaller peripheral airways.[13] Nonetheless, M_3 receptors are expressed in the airway smooth muscle of smaller airways that lack cholinergic nerve innervation.[10,14] Some studies have provided evidence that inhaled anticholinergics preferentially reduce airway resistance in the central airways of patients with COPD.[15–19] Others, however, have confirmed that the site of action of short-acting anticholinergic agents is at the level of both the central and peripheral airways.[20–22] Currently, cholinergic pathways are generally believed to have relatively less impact on smaller airways, while adrenergic pathways have equal impact on large and small airways. These differences may have important therapeutic implications.

11.3   Cholinergic mechanisms in asthma and COPD

Cholinergic mechanisms have long been recognized to contribute to obstructive lung diseases. Extracts of roots, seeds and leaves of belladonna plants have anticholinergic properties and have been used to treat bronchospasm for thousands of years. Atropine, the primary alkaloid in belladonna, was isolated in the mid-1800s and soon thereafter was recognized to block the cardiac effects of vagal stimulation and effectively treat acute asthma.[23] For decades, inhaled and systemic forms of atropine became the treatment of choice for bronchospasm. But, limited in clinical utility by systemic side effects, they were displaced from this position by ephedrine and epinephrine (adrenaline) in the twentieth century.

The parasympathetic nervous system contributes to the pathophysiology of both asthma and COPD. Whether or not cholinergic tone is increased in these conditions is somewhat controversial.[8] In COPD, normal resting cholinergic tone has a greater effect on airway calibre due to structural narrowing of the airways. Cholinergic tone may be increased in asthma due to: increased afferent stimulation by inflammatory mediators, increased release of ACh from cholinergic nerve terminals, altered muscarinic receptor expression (either increased M_3 or reduced M_2 receptors), and/or a reduction in inhibitory neurotransmitters.[8] Studies have shown that M_1 and M_3 receptor function is normal in both asthma and COPD. Jacoby et al.[24] have shown that inhibitory M_2 receptor function is abnormal in three different animal models of asthma and hyperresponsiveness (viral infections, antigen challenge and exposure to ozone). Experimental blockade of the feedback inhibition of ACh release can increase vagally mediated bronchoconstriction as much as 10-fold.[24] Thus, the increased parasympathetic activity seen in asthma is likely in part attributable to loss of the inhibitory M_2 receptor function, and resultant increase in ACh release.

In COPD, cholinergic tone is an important reversible factor contributing to airway resistance, making anticholinergics a logical therapeutic option. In asthma, however, anticholinergics only counteract the cholinergic reflex component of bronchoconstriction. β_2-agonists are more potent bronchodilators in asthma, presumably because they are functional antagonists and reverse bronchoconstriction regardless of the mechanism.[8] Furthermore, non-selective anticholinergics may block the inhibitory M_2 muscarinic receptors, increase ACh release, and cause so-called paradoxical bronchoconstriction. Thus, there is sound physiological rationale for anticholinergic bronchodilators in the treatment of obstructive pulmonary diseases, particularly more selective cholinergic antagonists.

11.4   Role of long-acting anticholinergic bronchodilators in obstructive lung disease

The advent of selective, long-acting tertiary and quaternary atropine-like derivatives in the past few decades has renewed interest in anticholinergic therapy for obstructive lung diseases, particularly for COPD.[26,27] Several long-acting anticholinergic (LAAC) bronchodilators have been evaluated for use in asthma and COPD, including tiotropium bromide, glycopyrrolate and aclidinium bromide.[28] To date, tiotropium bromide has been evaluated most extensively and is the only LAAC in widespread use for these conditions. Novel ultra-long-acting bronchodilators are on the horizon, as are devices with various combinations of LAAC, long-acting β_2-agonists (LABAs) and inhaled corticosteroids (ICS).

Tiotropium bromide

The quaternary ammonium compound tiotropium bromide binds to all three muscarinic receptor subtypes in humans, but is functionally a selective M_1, M_3 receptor antagonist.

It is approximately 10 times as potent as ipratropium bromide.[3] Delivered by inhalation, at a recommended once-daily dose of 18 µg, it has a rapid onset of action (within minutes), which lasts for over 24 hours. A steady state is achieved within 48 hours, after only two doses.[4,29] It has kinetic selectivity and dissociates slowly from M_1 and M_3 receptors but more rapidly from M_2 receptors. In contrast to ipratropium bromide, tiotropium is therefore linked to relatively less blockade of M_2-mediated inhibition of ACh release from cholinergic nerves.[3,30,31] This attribute may result in pharmacological and clinical advantages for tiotropium over the less selective anticholinergic agents. Indeed a number of comparative studies have confirmed that tiotropium is superior to ipratropium with respect to effects on respiratory physiology and patient-centred outcomes in patients with COPD.[32,33] Some studies have included patients with COPD and coexistent asthma. Fewer studies have been conducted in individuals with asthma alone. The role of LAAC bronchodilators in each of these conditions will be discussed separately.

COPD

COPD is characterized by extensive inflammatory bronchiolitis with varying degrees of emphysematous destruction of the lung parenchyma and its vasculature. The pathophysiological hallmark of COPD is expiratory flow limitation.[34] Its presence indicates that the expired flows generated during spontaneous tidal breathing represent the maximal possible flows that can be generated at that operating lung volume. Increases in lung compliance and airway resistance in heterogeneously distributed alveolar units in the lungs of the COPD patient lead to delays in the time constant for emptying (i.e. the product of compliance and resistance).[35] Thus, in many instances the time available for expiration during resting breathing (dictated by the central brainstem rhythm generator) is insufficient to allow lung volume to decline to its natural relaxation volume: air trapping and dynamic pulmonary hyperinflation is the result. Therefore, in flow-limited patients with COPD end-expiratory lung volume (EELV) is, in part, *dynamically* determined and it is this component that can be successfully manipulated by bronchodilator therapy.

Resting cholinergic tone is the most reversible component of the airway obstruction in COPD that can be targeted for treatment. There is inconclusive evidence that resting vagal cholinergic tone is increased in the airways of patients with COPD compared with health.[36–38] Even normal cholinergic tone in the airway smooth muscle of the COPD patient will result in greater increases in airway resistance than in the normal healthy airway, given the relatively reduced baseline airway diameter in the former.[38] Some studies have provided evidence that inhaled anticholinergics preferentially reduce airway resistance in the central airways of patients with COPD.[15–19] Others, however, have confirmed that the site of action of short-acting anticholinergic agents is at the level of both the central and peripheral airways.[20–22]

The clinical efficacy of tiotropium has been rigorously evaluated over several years in numerous randomized, placebo-controlled clinical trials. In this brief review we will summarize the available information on the impact of tiotropium therapy on several key outcome parameters. Broadly speaking, we will examine the evidence that this medication favourably reduces respiratory impairment and its negative clinical consequences in patients with moderate-to-severe COPD.

Airway function

Several randomized, placebo-controlled trials have confirmed that tiotropium treatment is associated with consistent short-term and longer-term (1–4 years) improvements in peak forced expiratory volume in 1 second (FEV_1) in the range of 0.16–0.36 L (16–29% of the basal FEV_1) in patients with moderate-to-severe COPD.[32,39–42] Improvements in the trough FEV_1 in the range 0.10–0.17 L (10–14% of the basal FEV_1, Table 11.2) have confirmed that tiotropium is an effective once-daily bronchodilator. The UPLIFT study, the largest clinical trial undertaken on the effects of long-acting anticholinergics, has provided evidence that tachyphylaxis does not develop during tiotropium treatment over a 4-year period.[42]

No consensus exists as to what degree of improvement in FEV_1 constitutes a minimal clinically important difference, but most would agree that modest but consistent spirometric improvements of this order (see above) indicate clinical benefit for patients with more advanced disease. Most randomized clinical trials on the efficacy of tiotropium were conducted in patients with more advanced COPD (average

Table 11.2 Summary of 12 published studies evaluating inhaled tiotropium bromide in patients with chronic obstructive pulmonary disease (COPD).

Trial design and duration (months)	Drug	Dosage (μg) and frequency of administration	No. of patients	Baseline FEV$_1$, L (% predicted)	Δ Trough FEV$_1$, L (% basal)	Δ Peak FEV$_1$, L (% basal)	Reference
r, db, pg (1)	TIO	18 o.d.	40	1.23 (45.7)	0.16 (13)***	0.22 (18)	Celli et al. (2003)[50]
	PL		41	1.01 (40.7)			
r, db, pg (1.5)	TIO	18 o.d.	131	1.20 (43.1)	0.17 (14)**	0.26 (22)**	Maltais et al. (2005)[41]
	PL		117	1.22 (42.8)			
r, db, pg (1.5)	TIO	18 o.d.	96	1.25 (42)	0.12 (10)**	0.22 (18)***	O'Donnell et al. (2004)[40]
	PL		91	1.29 (42)			
r, db, (1.5)	TIO	18 o.d.	70	1.04 (37.2)	0.10 (9.6) #	0.22 (21)	Van Noord et al. (2005)[57]
	FORM	12 b.i.d.	69		0.06 (5.7)	0.22 (21)	
	TIO/FORM	18/12 o.d.	71		0.14 (14) ##	0.35 (34) ##	
r, db, pg (1.5)	TIO	18 o.d.	46	1.05 (34.7)	0.12 (11)*	0.24 (23)**	Verkindre et al. (2006)[53]
	PL		54	1.08 (35.8)			
r, db, pg (3)	TIO	18 o.d.	107	2.15 (73.6)	0.074 (3.4)**		Johansson et al. (2008)[43]
	PL		111	2.01 (73.2)			
r, db, pg (6)	TIO	18 o.d.	402	1.12 (39.2)	0.12 (11)*		Brusasco et al. (2003)[61]
	SAL	50 b.i.d.	405	1.07 (37.7)	0.09 (8)*		
	PL		400	1.09 (38.7)			

(continued)

Table 11.2 (Continued)

Trial design and duration (months)	Drug	Dosage (μg) and frequency of administration	No. of patients	Baseline FEV$_1$, L (% predicted)	Δ Trough FEV$_1$, L (% basal)	Δ Peak FEV$_1$, L (% basal)	Reference
r, db, pg (6)	TIO	18 o.d.	209	1.11 (~40)	0.14 (12)***,##	0.24 (22)***,##	Donohue et al. (2002)[51]
	SAL	50 b.i.d.	213	1.07 (~40)	0.09 (8)***	0.16 (15)***	
	PL		201	1.06 (~40)			
r, db, pg (6)	TIO	18 o.d.	915	1.04 (35.6)	0.10 (10)**	0.17 (16)**	Niewoehner et al. (2005)[68]
	PL		914	1.04 (35.6)			
Pooled data (12)	TIO	18 o.d.	550	1.04 (39.1)	0.12 (12)*	0.21 (20)*	Casaburi et al. (2002)[39]
	PL		371	1.00 (38.1)			
r, db, pg (12)	TIO	18 o.d.	191	1.24 (42)	0.16 (13) #	0.36 (29) #	Van Noord et al. (2000)[52]
	IPR	40 q.i.d.	97	1.19 (40)	0.03 (3)	0.31 (26)	
Pooled data (12)	TIO	18 o.d.	356	1.25 (41.9)	0.12 (10) #		Vincken et al. (2002)[32]
	IPR	40 q.i.d.	179	1.18 (39.4)	−0.03 (−3)		

Abbreviations: b.i.d., twice a day; db, double blind; IPR, ipratropium bromide; o.d., once daily; pg, parallel group; PL, placebo; q.i.d., four times daily; r, randomized; SAL, salmeterol; FORM, formoterol; TIO, tiotropium bromide.

Significance levels: *$P < 0.01$, **$P < 0.001$, ***$P < 0.0001$, comparison with placebo. #$P < 0.05$, ##$P < 0.01$, comparison with salmeterol.

$FEV_1 = 40\%$ predicted); minimal information is available on the clinical efficacy of this medication in milder COPD.[43] One study ($n = 227$) in more moderate COPD ($FEV_1 = 73\%$ predicted) showed consistent increases in spirometry compared with placebo.[43] Although the FEV_1 is historically favoured by regulatory authorities for the purpose of drug registration, this physiological parameter has limitations with respect to evaluation of improved airway function after bronchodilator (BD) therapy.[44–46] It is well known, for example, that as disease severity advances the FEV_1 is often poorly responsive to change following bronchodilator therapy.[44–46] Thus, following acute β_2-agonist inhalation, consistent reductions in lung hyperinflation have been reported in the presence of minimal or no change in FEV_1 in patients with severe COPD.[44–46] It is now clear that exclusive reliance on FEV_1 as the sole outcome measure of interest for the purpose of evaluating bronchodilator efficacy may underestimate important physiological improvement in airway function and respiratory mechanics.

The forced vital capacity (FVC) gives complementary information about airway function in COPD although it is less reproducible than the FEV_1. This reflects measurement artifacts related to volume history, thoracic gas compression effects and expiratory time duration during the forced expiratory manoeuvre in patients with more advanced COPD.[47,48] After bronchodilator (BD) therapy the FEV_1/FVC ratio is either unchanged or sometimes decreases: improvement in FEV_1 therefore reflects lung volume recruitment secondary to more effective lung emptying.[49] Tiotropium therapy was associated with increases in FVC in the range of 0.42–0.84 L (17–30% change),[41,50–52] and in slow vital capacity in the range of 0.38–0.41 L.[41,50,53]

The resting inspiratory capacity (IC) is diminished in patients with more advanced COPD who have expiratory flow limitation and lung hyperinflation during spontaneous resting breathing. Studies have confirmed that resting IC was diminished (to less than 80% of the predicted value) in patients with demonstrable expiratory flow limitation at rest.[54,55] Improvement of resting IC following BD treatment in flow-limited COPD patients with lung hyperinflation reflects a more rapid time constant for lung emptying because of reduced airway resistance. Increased IC would *not* be expected following BD treatment in patients with early COPD, who have a preserved resting IC.[56] Tiotropium treatment was associated with consistent increases in resting IC in the range 0.22–0.35 L: the average increase was ~11.5% (predicted). The change in IC following BD therapy may underestimate the true reduction in end expiratory lung volume (EELV) by the amount by which total lung capacity (TLC) falls (i.e. ~0.12 L).[40,41,50]

Lung volume deflation

Only three studies have measured changes in plethysmographic lung volume components following long-acting anticholinergic treatment in patients with moderate-to-severe COPD[40,41,50] (Figure 11.1). The reduction of residual volume (RV) associated with tiotropium treatment (compared with placebo) was on average 0.44 L, or 10% of predicted (0.35–0.56 L). This improvement indicates more effective lung emptying and reduced airway closure during the forced manoeuvre. Reductions in functional residual capacity (FRC) average 0.38 L, or 7.2% of predicted FRC (0.35–0.56 L)

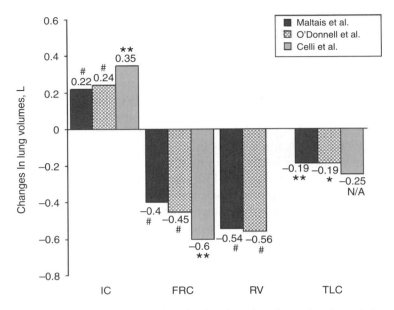

Figure 11.1   Mean difference (tiotropium – placebo) from baseline values in peak lung volumes. $*P < 0.05$; $**P < 0.01$; $\#P < 0.001$; N/A not available. IC, inspiratory capacity; FRC, functional residual capacity; RV, residual volume; TLC, total lung capacity. Data from Maltais et al.,[41] O'Donnell et al.[40] and Celli et al.[50]

confirming reductions in dynamically determined EELV.[40,41,50] Modest but consistent reductions in TLC (by ∼0.12 L) have been reported following tiotropium.[45] Sustained 24-hour pharmacological lung volume reduction during tiotropium therapy was confirmed by showing reductions in the trough (pre-BD) FRC by an average of 0.28 L (range 0.26–0.30 L).

Improvement in airway function and respiratory mechanics following tiotropium monotherapy does not represent the maximal possible bronchodilation that can be achieved in moderate-to-severe COPD. The addition of long-acting β_2-agonists has been shown to be associated with significant *additive* effects with respect to lung volume deflation.[33,57]

Alleviation of chronic activity-related dyspnoea

Currently, the main indication for initiation of therapy with long-acting inhaled anticholinergics is for symptom alleviation in patients who are troubled by persistent dyspnoea. The origins of activity-related dyspnoea are multifactorial but respiratory mechanical abnormalities are undoubtedly important.[58,59] Mechanistic studies have shown that dyspnoea relief following tiotropium therapy is closely associated with the reduction of EELV (and increased IC) during rest and exercise. This reflects the improved time constant for lung emptying as a result of decreased airway resistance

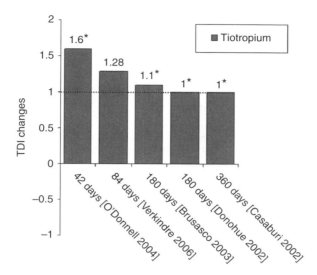

Figure 11.2 Mean difference (tiotropium – placebo) from baseline values in Transition Dyspnoea Index (TDI). TDI of 1 was considered a clinically meaningful difference. *$P < 0.05$ vs placebo. Data from O'Donnell et al.,[40] Verkindre et al.,[53] Brusasco et al.,[61] Donohue et al.[51] and Casaburi et al.[39]

secondary to release of cholinergic bronchomotor tone.[40,60] The increased resting IC allows greater tidal volume expansion capability, and improvement in the ratio of contractile respiratory muscle effort to tidal volume displacement throughout exercise.[60] This improvement in the effort:displacement ratio correlated with reduced dyspnoea ratings and reflects enhanced neuromechanical coupling of the respiratory system on account of the reduced operating lung volumes. A number of placebo-controlled studies have shown that tiotropium therapy is associated with consistent improvements in measures of chronic activity-related dyspnoea such as the Transition Dyspnoea Index (TDI).[39,40,51,53,61] Average improvements in the order of 1.4 units (range: 1–1.6 units) have been reported, which exceeds the threshold value thought to represent the minimal clinically important difference (Figure 11.2).

Improvement of exercise endurance

Two large replicate randomized controlled trials were undertaken to examine the effects of tiotropium on exercise endurance as measured during constant work cycle exercise set at 75% of each patient's peak work capacity.[40,41] After 42 days of treatment there were significant increases in exercise endurance, by 105 and 236 seconds, or 21% and 42% over placebo, respectively (Figure 11.3). These studies therefore confirmed that while receiving tiotropium, patients could consistently undertake a demanding physical task for a longer duration while experiencing less respiratory discomfort. The main mechanism of improved exercise capacity is reduced exertional dyspnoea, which in turn reflects improved dynamic ventilatory mechanics and respiratory muscle

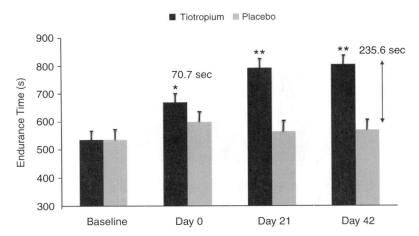

Figure 11.3   Endurance time during constant work rate cycle ergometry to symptom limitation at 75%Wmax. Baseline (day −5) and 2.25 h after dosing on days 0, 21 and 42. Reprinted with permission from O'Donnell DE, Flüge T, Gerken F, et al.[41] (2004). Effects of tiotropium on lung hyperinflation, dyspnoea and exercise tolerance in COPD. The European Respiratory Journal, 23, 832–840, © European Respiratory Society.

function[60] (Figures 11.4 and 11.5). One study reported consistent increases in walking distance measured during the shuttle endurance test in patients receiving tiotropium compared with placebo.[53] Tiotropium treatment was also associated with improved indices of cardio-pulmonary interaction during exercise compared with placebo.[62]

The desired long-term goal of treatment with long-acting anticholinergics is to increase activity levels and to improve functional *status*. Initiation of BD therapy merely improves the patient's functional *capacity*. In other words, this therapy provides patients with the physiological potential to increase daily activity levels. To successfully transform increased functional capacity into habitual increases in daily activity, sustained cognitive-behavioural modification and individualized self-management plans are generally required.[63] Patients receiving optimal bronchodilator therapy should ideally be encouraged to exercise regularly and if possible to enrol in formal pulmonary rehabilitation programmes. The combination of regular tiotropium therapy and participation in a structured exercise training programme has been shown to have additive effects on exercise endurance.[64, 65]

Effect on acute exacerbations of COPD (AECOPD)

The natural history of COPD is punctuated by symptomatic exacerbations, which increase in frequency and severity as the disease advances. AECOPD is associated with increased and often prolonged morbidity and possibly an accelerated progression of respiratory impairment.[66] Exacerbations that require hospitalization carry significant risks for both short-term and long-term mortality. Tiotropium treatment is associated with reduction in the frequency and severity of AECOPD by an average of 20% (range

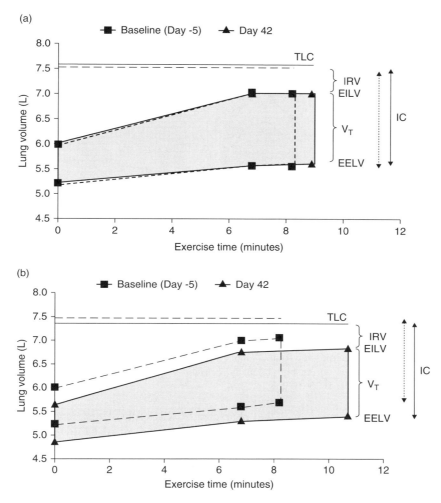

Figure 11.4   Operating lung volumes at rest and during exercise at baseline (■ - - -) and after 42 days (▲ —) of treatment with (a) placebo ($n = 91$) and (b) tiotropium ($n = 96$). TLC, total lung capacity; IRV, inspiratory reserve volume; EILV, end-inspiratory lung volume; V_T, tidal volume; EELV, end-expiratory lung volume; IC, inspiratory capacity. Reprinted with permission from Maltais F, Hamilton A, Marciniuk D, et al.[40] (2005). Improvements in symptom-limited exercise performance over 8 h with once-daily tiotropium in patients with COPD. Chest, 128, 1168–1178.

6–35%) with consequent reduced healthcare utilization and financial costs.[39,42,61,67,68] One study conducted in a total of 1323 patients with severe COPD, compared the effect of tiotropium therapy with that of fluticasone/salmeterol therapy on exacerbation rate (measures by healthcare utilization) and found no difference between the groups.[69]

The mechanisms of reduction of AECOPD in patients receiving long-acting anti-cholinergic therapy are unknown. It is reasonable to speculate that sustained bron-chodilation and lung volume reduction might alter sensory perception thresholds to the

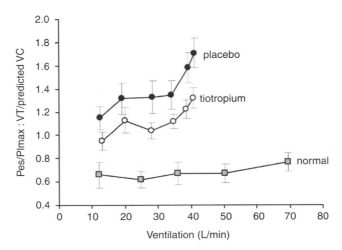

Figure 11.5 Ratio between pressure in eosophagus/peak inspiratory mouth pressure (Pes/PImax) and tidal volume (V_T) displacement (V_T standardized as a fraction of predicted vital capacity, VC), an index of neuromechanical dissociation, is shown during exercise after tiotropium and placebo in chronic obstructive pulmonary disease (COPD; $n = 11$) compared with a group of age-matched normal subjects ($n = 12$). The effort:displacement ratio is increased in COPD compared with normal throughout exercise, with an upward trend after a ventilation of 30 L/min that did not occur in the normal subjects. Compared with placebo, tiotropium reduced this ratio throughout exercise in COPD. Reprinted with permission from O'Donnell DE, Hamilton AL and Webb KA (2006). Sensory-mechanical relationships during high-intensity, constant-work-rate exercise in COPD. Journal of Applied Physiology, 101, 1025–1035.

disrupted respiratory mechanics that characterize AECOPD. Thus, perceived respiratory discomfort during the acute mechanical perturbations of AECOPD (i.e. increased expiratory flow limitation and lung hyperinflation) is diminished because baseline mechanics are favourably altered by long-term tiotropium treatment.[70] Given this scenario, the reporting of AECOPD in RCTs may become diagnostically 'downgraded' from *severe* (requiring oral steroids and antibiotic treatment) to *moderate* or *mild*. Improved and sustained airway patency with enhanced clearance of secretions may be linked to a reduced propensity for developing bacterial AECOPD. An anti-inflammatory action of anticholinergic therapy has also been purported to explain prevention of AECOPD, but this too remains speculative.[71]

Disease progression

The main purpose of the UPLIFT study was to examine the effect of longer-term treatment with tiotropium on the rate of decline of FEV_1 (trough and peak), a surrogate of disease progression, over 4 years.[42] This carefully conducted study enrolled 5993 patients with moderate to severe COPD (mean FEV_1 1.32 ± 0.44) and showed no effect on this primary outcome compared with placebo. While the rate of decline of FEV_1 appears to be a robust and responsive indicator (at least to smoking cessation) of disease progression in younger patients with early COPD, its utility as a marker of progressive respiratory impairment in population studies of advanced COPD is questionable.[72] In the UPLIFT study many of those randomized to placebo received treatment with inhaled long-acting β_2-agonist, corticosteroids or both, making it very difficult to evaluate the relative impact of tiotropium. In this regard, the annual rate of loss of FEV_1 in those randomized to placebo in the UPLIFT study was only 0.03 L/year, a value that is considerably lower than that reported in several previous studies (0.04–0.06 L/year) in patients with similar baseline FEV_1 at study entry who received only short-acting bronchodilators in addition to placebo.[73, 74] These considerations make it impossible to answer the question of whether long-term tiotropium treatment can, *by itself*, attenuate the progressive respiratory impairment of COPD and its clinical sequelae.

Mortality

No study has examined the effect of long-acting anticholinergics on survival as the *primary* outcome variable in COPD. Tiotropium treatment was associated with consistent improvement of a number of recognized independent predictors of survival (FEV_1, IC, activity-related dyspnoea, exercise capacity, frequency of AECOPD).[75–83] Improved dyspnoea and reduced activity limitation should reduce the risk for the development of several systemic consequences of COPD, including: osteoporosis, insulin resistance, skeletal muscle deconditioning/wasting and increased risk factors for the development of cardiovascular disease.[84] Moreover, sustained improvements in respiratory mechanics following surgical lung volume reduction, of similar magnitude to that achieved pharmacologically with tiotropium, have been linked to improved survival in selected patients with advanced COPD.[85] Collectively, these data provide a compelling rationale for potential positive effects on survival in those receiving long-term anticholinergic therapy. A Canadian population study in 7218 patients with COPD, who were discharged from hospital, examined the risk of mortality (within 6 months) in patients receiving a prescription for tiotropium compared with those who were prescribed a long-acting beta-agonist (LABA).[86] All-cause mortality was significantly reduced by 20% (95% confidence ratio = 0.70–0.93) in those receiving tiotropium compared with those in whom a LABA was prescribed after discharge. By contrast, another study compared the effects of treatment with fluticasone/salmeterol combination with tiotropium in 1323 patients with severe COPD (FEV_1 = mean 39% predicted) on mortality as a *secondary* outcome measure over a 1-year period.[69] Mortality rates were significantly higher in those randomized to tiotropium (6%) than those receiving fluticasone/salmeterol (3%). A number of methodological concerns have been raised about the design of this study, including the lack of a placebo arm, and this together with the lack of a convincing biological rationale for the increased death rates make the findings of this study inconclusive.[87] In the UPLIFT study, all-cause and respiratory mortality (as *secondary* outcome measures) were shown to be reduced in those randomized to tiotropium during the 4-year period of active drug treatment.[42] However, these survival improvements in favour of tiotropium did not persist following the washout period

(4 years + 30 days of washout), which was the prespecified survival indicator of interest for this study.

Safety of long-acting anticholinergics in COPD

Kesten et al.[88] conducted a pooled analysis of 19 placebo-controlled, randomized, double-blind clinical trials in order to evaluate the safety of tiotropium (4435 tiotropium patients vs 3384 placebo patients). The most common side effect reported in the pooled trial population was dry mouth (5%) (relative risk (RR) 3.6; 95% CI 2.56–5.05), while urinary retention occurred in 0.4% (RR 10.9; 95% CI 1.26–94.88). The prevalence of dry mouth in the pivotal tiotropium studies was reported to be 9–17 % but tolerance usually developed quickly. Some side effects that were potentially related to mucosal dryness (e.g. epistaxis, hoarseness, laryngitis and pharyngitis) were more frequent in those randomized to tiotropium compared with those randomized to placebo, but this did not reach statistical significance. Conversely, COPD exacerbations, dyspnoea and productive cough were significantly less frequent in those randomized to tiotropium. Some adverse events were reported exclusively in the tiotropium group (dehydration, urinary frequency) but absolute numbers were small (seven participants). In the Lung Health Study (LHS) there was an unexpected tendency for coronary and cardiovascular disease in patients receiving short-acting anticholinergic therapy compared with the placebo group.[75] In a recent meta-analysis of 17 trials, Singh et al.[89] reported an increased risk of cardiovascular death, myocardial infarction and stroke in the triotropium group compared with the placebo group. In the pooled analysis, Kesten et al.[88] reported small increases in 'other arrhythmias' including bradycardia, irregular heartbeat and extrasystoles (0.6%) (RR 2.71; 95% CI 1.10–6.65) but did not find any increase in the total mortality, including cardiovascular and respiratory mortality, in the tiotropium group. Moreover, the risks of tachycardia and fibrillation were similar in both tiotropium and placebo groups. Furthermore, no compelling biological or pharmacological rationale currently exists for the potential arrhythmogenic action of newer kinetically selective anticholinergic agents such as tiotropium. Other studies did not find any association between tiotropium and ambulatory-monitored electrocardiographic changes.[90,91] In the UPLIFT study the overall mortality tended to be lower in the tiotropium group, with a reduction in a range of cardiovascular adverse events (lower congestive heart failure, RR 0.59, 95% CI 0.37–0.96; lower myocardial infarction, RR 0.71, 95% CI 0.52–0.99). The incidence of stroke was not increased in the tiotropium group compared with placebo. These findings of a lack of increased risk for cardiovascular events and cardiac death in a large cohort of elderly patients with moderate-to-severe COPD, followed carefully over a four year, are reassuring.

Asthma

Asthma is a chronic inflammatory condition of the airways that manifests clinically as intermittent or persistent dyspnoea, chest tightness, wheezing, cough and sputum production, associated with variable airflow obstruction and hyperresponsiveness to endogenous or exogenous stimuli.[92,93] Inhaled corticosteroids are universally recommended as the treatment of choice to control airway inflammation in asthma,[92,93] with fast-acting bronchodilators reserved for as-needed use to relieve acute symptoms of bronchospasm.

Inhaled short-acting beta-agonists (SABAs) are the recommended first-line bronchodilators in stable asthma on an as-needed basis and to relieve bronchospasm in acute exacerbations asthma,[92–95] because SABAs have a faster onset of action and produce greater bronchodilation than ipratropium or oxitropium.[25]

Systematic reviews have concluded that *short-acting* anticholinergics are not routinely indicated in stable asthma, but a trial of therapy may be warranted in individual patients since subgroups may benefit.[96] As such, short-acting anticholinergics are second-line bronchodilators for chronic asthma and are typically reserved for specific clinical situations, for example when SABAs are contraindicated due to side effects and to treat bronchospasm cause by beta-blockers.[92–94]

Tiotropium prevents methacholine-induced bronchoconstriction in asthma.[97,98] This effect is seen within 30 minutes,[98] and lasts for at least 48 hours.[97] However, clinical response to anticholinergic therapy seems to vary among patients with asthma, presumably due to inter-individual variation in cholinergic control of bronchomotor tone. The published literature on long-acting anticholinergics in asthma is much less extensive than that on COPD. Subgroups of asthma patients have been identified in whom cholinergic mechanisms are thought to play an important role and, at least theoretically, are most likely to benefit from anticholinergic agents; these subgroups include the elderly, those with nocturnal or allergic (intrinsic) asthma, patients with coexistent COPD, or chronic asthma with fixed obstruction.[27] Additionally, they should be considered in individuals intolerant of β_2-adrenergic agents, to treat bronchospasm caused by beta-blockers, and/or in individuals at real or theoretically increased risk of side effects from other bronchodilators, as may be the case in individuals who are homozygous for arginine (Arg/Arg) rather than glycine (Gly/Gly) at amino acid residue 16 of the β_2-adrenergic receptor.[99–102]

The elderly

A number of physiological changes occur in the respiratory system with age.[103] Structurally, age-related degeneration of elastin fibres, particularly around alveolar ducts, leads to dilation and enlargement of the small airways. In some individuals, loss of supporting tissues can cause alveolar fenestrations and airspace dilation so severe as to resemble emphysema and predispose to small airway collapse and gas trapping. Compliance of the lung decreases with age, while closing volume and residual volume increase. Increased static lung compliance (and reduced driving pressure for expiratory flow) and the resultant reduced alveolar tethering of the airways, predisposes the elderly to expiratory flow limitation and air-trapping, particularly during activity.[104,105] When the airway inflammation of asthma is superimposed on the airway dysfunction that arises as a consequence of natural aging there is the potential for compounded respiratory impairment. Moreover, normal cholinergic bronchomotor tone in the elderly may cause relatively increased airway resistance (compared to youth), which can potentially be reversed by anticholinergic therapy.

There is some evidence that cholinergic tone increases in the elderly,[103, 106] and age-related decline in the bronchodilator effect of beta-agonists exceeds that of anticholinergics.[107] As such, LAAC may be of particular benefit in older individuals with asthma.[26, 28, 103, 106, 108, 109]

Combined COPD/asthma

Clinical trials examining the effects of LAAC in obstructive lung disease have almost universally been done in COPD patients. Patients with coexistent asthma have been excluded. Only one study has been published to date specifically examining the efficacy and safety of tiotropium in patients with COPD and a concomitant diagnosis of asthma.[110] This was a multicentre, 12-week, randomized, double-blind, placebo-controlled, parallel group study of 472 patients over 39 years of age (mean age 59.6 years) with physician-diagnosed asthma before the age of 30 years, plus a physician-diagnosis of COPD and a smoking history exceeding 10 pack-years. Pulmonary function criteria included a post-bronchodilator FEV_1 of less than 80% predicted, a post-bronchodilator FEV_1/FVC ratio less than 70%, and an acute bronchodilator response (≥ 200 mL and $\geq 12\%$ increase in FEV_1). Patients were treated with either 18 µg/day of tiotropium dry powder capsules via the HandiHaler® or placebo inhaler. The primary outcome was FEV_1 area-under-the-curve (AUC). There were small but statistically significant improvements in FEV_1 AUC (from 0 to 6 hours, of 186 ± 24 mL, $P < 0.001$) and pre-dose morning FEV_1 (98 ± 23 mL, $P < 0.001$). Use of salbutamol p.r.n. decreased by 0.5 ± 0.12 puffs/day in the intervention group at week 12, which was also statistically significantly different from that of the placebo group (0.05 ± 0.12 puffs/day; $P < 0.05$). However, clinical relevance of these minor changes in FEV_1 and reliever use is questionable at best. Worth noting is that there were no significant differences in adverse events between groups overall. The frequency of COPD exacerbations was lower in the tiotropium group (5.7%) than in the placebo group (10.7%), but the proportions of subjects who developed asthma exacerbations were similar. This study did not examine resting or dynamic lung volumes, or patient-centred outcomes such as dyspnoea, quality of life or exercise capacity. Thus, additional studies are required in order to determine both the efficacy and safety of tiotropium in this patient population.

Severe/persistent asthma

Similarly, there is only one 'proof of concept' study published that examined the efficacy of reducing the dose of fluticasone in combination with salmeterol and tiotropium in severe persistent asthma.[111] Patients had severe volume-dependent airway closure on an expiratory flow volume loop and a FEV_1 ≤65% predicted, FVC <80% predicted, forced expiratory flow over the middle half of FVC (FEF 25–75) <50% predicted, and at least 15% improvement with ipratropium bromide and salbutamol. In a double-blind, randomized, placebo-controlled crossover study, 18 non-smoking severe asthma patients received either HFA fluticasone propionate 500 µg b.i.d./salmeterol 100 µg b.i.d./hydrofluoroalkane HFA tiotropium bromide 18 µg once daily or fluticasone propionate 500 µg b.i.d./salmeterol 100 µg b.i.d. placebo for 4 weeks. The addition of tiotropium resulted in statistically significant improvements in spirometric measures (FEV_1 improved by 0.17 L (95% CI 0.01–0.32; $P<0.05$); FVC increased by 0.24 L (0.05–0.43; $P<0.05$)). Once again, the magnitude of effect was small and therefore the clinical relevance is uncertain.

Airway remodelling

Airway remodelling is seen as a consequence of longstanding asthma, particularly if airway inflammation has been suboptimally treated. A number of recent studies suggest that many of the features of airway remodelling, such as airway smooth muscle thickening, may be the result of the action of acetylcholine on muscarinic receptors.[112] Tiotropium has been shown to inhibit airway smooth-muscle hypertrophy and contractility in a guinea pig model of allergic asthma.[113] It remains to be seen whether SAAC or LAAC help prevent airway remodelling in humans with asthma.[27]

Nocturnal asthma

Circadian variation in bronchomotor tone is present in normal humans and is exaggerated in individuals with asthma.[114, 115] Increased parasympathetic tone accounts for some, but not all of this variation in airway calibre. In asthma, blockade of parasympathetic efferent activity by atropine[116] or ipratropium[117] diminishes but does not eliminate nocturnal bronchoconstriction. Inhibition of NANC nervous system function, which normally has a bronchodilating effect, likely contributes to overnight bronchoconstriction in healthy individuals and asthmatics.[118] LAAC such as tiotropium have not been specifically evaluated in nocturnal asthma.

Asthma and gastro-oesophageal reflux disease (GERD)

Gastro-oesophageal reflux disease (GERD) is common in individuals with asthma, and is associated with difficult or therapy-resistant asthma.[119–121] One of the postulated mechanisms is bronchoconstriction from an oesophagobronchial vagal reflex.[122] On formal testing, autonomic dysfunction is apparent in individuals with asthma and GERD.[122] Atropine inhibits bronchoconstriction induced by acid present in the oesophagus of individuals with asthma.[123] The role of LAAC such as tiotropium in asthma and GERD has not been specifically evaluated.

Exercise-induced asthma (EIA)

The pathophysiology of airway hyperresponsiveness in exercise-induced asthma is complex, but cholinergic mechanisms may play a role.[124] Athletes have been shown to have greater parasympathetic tone (based upon heart-rate variability on 24-hour ECG recordings) than healthy sedentary individuals[125] and the respiratory sinus arrhythmia method.[126] Some postulate that bronchomotor tone may increase to compensate for prolonged sympathetic stimulation from repeated intense exercise training.[124] However, the role of LAAC in EIA also remains to be determined.

Acute exacerbations/viral infections

During acute attacks of asthma, increased airway resistance contributes to expiratory flow limitation during spontaneous resting breathing and results in air-trapping and dynamic lung hyperinflation. We have shown that during methacholine challenge testing, EELV increases by as much as 0.6 L at PC_{20}.[127] When FEV_1 declined by approximately 50% of the baseline value dynamic, EELV increased by more than 1 L.[128,129] The intensity of dyspnoea and chest tightness correlated well with the extent of dynamic hyperinflation during cholinergic bronchoconstriction.[128–130] SAAC treatment is recommended during acute exacerbations in addition to β_2-agonists to maximize bronchodilation. The role of LAAC agents has not been studied in this setting, but conceivably these could achieve more sustained bronchodilation and lung deflation than SAACs.

Viral infections are known to increase vagally mediated reflex bronchoconstriction in individuals without asthma.[131,132] Animal studies have shown that this is largely due to virus-induced dysfunction of the M_2 receptors, related to release of major basic protein (MBP) from eosinophils.[24,133,134] MBP binds to the M_2 receptors, blocking their function.[135] This may be the mechanism by which viral respiratory tract infections (RTIs) lead to transient airway hyperresponsiveness to histamine, methacholine, exercise and cold air exposure in individuals without underlying asthma, and contribute to increasing bronchospasm in virus-induced acute exacerbations of asthma. Eosinophil activation, eosinophil recruitment to airway nerves and release of MBP is also seen after antigen challenges, exposure to air pollutants such as ozone, and in fatal asthma,[136] suggesting similar mechanisms may be relevant in human airway hyperresponsiveness.[24]

Safety of long-acting anticholinergics in asthma

Due to the paucity of published clinical trials of LAAC in asthma, less is known of the side-effect profile specifically in asthma patients who do not also have COPD. No adverse events were reported in studies assessing the effects of tiotropium bromide on methacholine-induced bronchoconstriction.[97,98] The pooled analysis by Kesten et al.[88] of clinical trial data from pre-approval and post-approval clinical trials indicates that a limited number of trials were included in patients with asthma, but these data are not reported separately. There were no significant differences in the relative risk of asthma exacerbations (RR 1.17; 95% CI 0.30–4.61) or bronchospasm (RR 1.66; 95% CI 0.65–4.24) between tiotropium and placebo groups. The RR of asthma as a serious adverse event was increased in tiotropium compared to placebo (RR 2.52; 95% CI 0.23–27.220), based upon three events in the 2171 tiotropium-treated subjects compared to one event in 1672 patients on placebo.

The largest reported summary of the safety of LAAC used clinically, which includes a substantial proportion of individuals with a combination of COPD and asthma, is an analysis of the UK THIN (The Health Information Network) primary care database.[137] The THIN database is an electronic medical record from over 3 million individuals registered in 220 general practices in the UK. Jara et al. compared the safety of tiotropium bromide with single-ingredient LABAs (salmeterol or formoterol) in patients over 40 years of age who received at least one prescription for one of these medications between November 2002 and the last date of data collection, which ranged from February 2003 to June 2004. They identified 1061 patients prescribed tiotropium and 1801 prescribed a LABA. This study excluded patients whose sole respiratory diagnosis was asthma, to avoid confounding by indication (since beta-agonists are used more widely than anticholinergics in asthma; but morbidity and mortality are higher in COPD patients, who are typically older than asthma patients). Coexistent COPD and asthma diagnoses were present in 30% of those prescribed tiotropium, and 37% of those prescribed LABAs. Risks of total mortality and most cardiac events such as angina, atrial fibrillation or flutter, and myocardial infarction were similar in tiotropium and LABA users. The adjusted hazard ratio (HR) for an asthma exacerbation was decreased in individuals prescribed tiotropium compared to a LABA (HR 0.41; 95% CI 0.26–0.64). Residual confounding by indication was likely, however, in that this risk reduction was less when the analysis was restricted to COPD patients without asthma (HR 0.77; 95% CI 0.31–1.91).

11.5   Summary

Cholinergic mechanisms play an important role in the regulation of bronchomotor tone in humans, forming the physiological rationale for muscarinic antagonist bronchodilator therapy in obstructive lung diseases. In COPD, the long-acting muscarinic receptor antagonist tiotropium bromide has been rigorously scrutinized in clinical trials and shown to consistently provide effective, sustained bronchodilation and lung volume deflation in patients with moderate-to-severe disease. These improvements in respiratory impairment translate into clinically important amelioration of dyspnoea and exercise intolerance, together with reduced exacerbations and enhanced perceived health status. Consequently, evidence-based guidelines have universally advocated the use of long-acting anticholinergics as maintenance therapy for patients with moderate-to-severe COPD who experience persistent dyspnoea.

Although animal and human studies have demonstrated that M_2 receptor dysfunction is unequivocally important in the pathophysiology of asthma, the clinical role of long-acting anticholinergic bronchodilators in asthma remains to be determined. Additional research will help clarify the role in specific subgroups of asthma patients in whom selective long-acting muscarinic antagonists are of greatest theoretical benefit, such as the elderly, individuals with expiratory flow limitation and hyperinflation from fixed predominantly small airways obstruction (similar to moderate-to-severe COPD), individuals with coexistent asthma and COPD, nocturnal asthma, viral-induced asthma exacerbations, and difficult therapy-resistant chronic asthma.

References

1. Bousquet J, Dahl R, Khaltaev N. Global alliance against chronic respiratory diseases. Allergy 2007;62(3):216–23.
2. Masoli M, Fabian D, Holt S, Beasley R. Global Initiative for Asthma (GINA) Program. The global burden of asthma: executive summary of the GINA Dissemination Committee report Allergy. 2004;59(5):469–78.
3. Barnes PJ, Belvisi MG, Mak JC, Haddad EB, O'Connor B. Tiotropium bromide (Ba 679 BR), a novel long-acting muscarinic antagonist for the treatment of obstructive airways disease. Life Sci 1995;56:853–9.
4. Hansel TT, Barnes PJ. Tiotropium bromide: a novel once-daily anticholinergic bronchodilator for the treatment of COPD. Drugs Today (Barc.) 2002;38:585–600.
5. Barnes PJ. Neural control of human airways in health and disease. Am Rev Respir Dis 1986;134:1289–314.
6. van der Velden VHJ, Hulsmann AR. Autonomic innervation of human airways: structure, function, and pathophysiology in asthma. Neuroimmunomodulation 1999;6:145–59.
7. Joos GF. Potential usefulness of inhibiting neural mechanisms in asthma. Monaldi Arch Chest Dis 2000;55:411–14.
8. Barnes PJ, Thomson NC. Neural and humoral control of the airways. In: Barnes PJ et al. (eds), Asthma and COPD: Basic Mechanisms and Clinical Management, 2nd edn. Elsevier Ltd, San Diego, 2008; pp. 381–98.
9. Coulson FR, Fryer AD. Muscarinic acetylcholine receptors and airway diseases. Pharmacol Therapeut 2003;98:59–69.
10. Mak JC, Barnes PJ. Autoradiographic visualization of muscarinic receptor subtypes in human and guinea pig lung. Am Rev Respir Dis 1990;141:1559–68.
11. Barnes PJ. Muscarinic receptor subtypes in airways. Life Sci 1993;52:521–7.
12. Fisher JT, Vincent SG, Gomeza J, Yamada M, Wess J. Loss of vagally mediated bradycardia and bronchoconstriction in mice lacking M2 or M3 muscarinic acetylcholine receptors. FASEB J 2004;18:711–13.
13. Barnes PJ, Basbaum CB, Nadel JA. Autoradiographic localization of autonomic receptors in airway smooth muscle. Marked differences between large and small airways. Am Rev Respir Dis 1983;127:758–62.
14. Mak JC, Baraniuk JN, Barnes PJ. Localization of muscarinic receptor subtype mRNAs in human lung. Am J Respir Cell Mol Biol 1992;7:344–8.
15. Ingram RH, Wellman JJ, McFadden ER, Mead J. Relative contributions of large and small airways to flow limitation in normal subjects before and after atropine and isoproterenol. J Clin Invest 1977;59:696–703.
16. Hensley MJ, O'Cain CF, McFadden ER, Ingram RH. Distribution of bronchodilatation in normal subjects: beta agonist versus atropine. J App Physiol 1978;778–82.

17. Ashutosh K, Mead G, Dickey JC, Berman P, Kuppinger M. Density dependence of expiratory flow and bronchodilator response in asthma. Chest 1980;77:68–75.

18. Yanai M, Ohrui T, Sekizawa K, et al. Effective site of bronchodilation by antiasthma drugs in subjects with asthma. J Allergy Clin Immunol 1991;87:1080–7.

19. Sekizawa K, Yanai M, Shimizu Y, Sasaki H, Takishima T. Serial distribution of bronchoconstriction in normal subjects. Methacholine versus histamine. Am Rev Respir Dis 1988;137: 1312–16.

20. Partridge MR, Saunders KB. Site of action of ipratropium bromide and clinical and physiological determinants of response in patients with asthma. Thorax 1981;36:530–3.

21. Douglas NJ, Davidson I, Sudlow MF, Flenley DC. Bronchodilatation and the site of airway resistance in severe chronic bronchitis. Thorax 1979;34:51–6.

22. Douglas NJ, Sudlow MF, Flenley DC. Effect of an inhaled atropine-like agent on normal airway function. J Appl Physiol 1979;46:256–62.

23. Courty MA. Treatment of asthma. Edin Med J 1859;5:665.

24. Jacoby DB, Costello RM, Fryer AD. Eosinophil recruitment to the airway nerves. J Allergy Clin Immunol 2001;107:211–18.

25. Gross NJ. Anticholinergic agents in asthma and COPD. Eur J Pharmacol 2006;533:36–9.

26. Restrepo RD. Inhaled adrenergics and anticholinergics in obstructive lung disease: do they enhance mucociliary clearance? Respir Care 2007;52:1159–73.

27. Restrepo RD. Use of inhaled anticholinergic agents in obstructive airway disease. Respir Care 2007;52:833–51.

28. Cazzola M, Matera MG. Novel long-acting bronchodilators for COPD and asthma. Brit J Pharmacol 2008;155:291–9.

29. Hansel TT, Tan AJ, Barnes PJ, Kon OM. Anticholinergic bronchodilators. In: Barnes PJ, et al. (eds) Asthma and COPD: Basic Mechanisms and Clinical Management. Elsevier Ltd, San Diego, 2008.

30. Barnes PJ. The pharmacological properties of tiotropium. Chest 2000;117:63S–66S.

31. Disse B, Speck GA, Rominger KL, Witek TJ, Hammer R. Tiotropium (Spiriva): mechanistical considerations and clinical profile in obstructive lung disease. Life Sci 1999;64: 457–64.

32. Vincken W, van Noord JA, Greefhorst AP, et al. Dutch/Belgian Tiotropium Study Group. Improved health outcomes in patients with COPD during 1 yr's treatment with tiotropium. Eur Respir J 2002;19:209–16.

33. van Noord JA, Aumann JL, Janssens E, et al. Effects of tiotropium with and without formoterol on airflow obstruction and resting hyperinflation in patients with COPD. Chest 2006;129: 509–17.

34. Hyatt RE. Expiratory flow limitation. J Appl Physiol 1983;55:1–7.

35. Vinegar A, Sinnett EE, Leith DE. Dynamic mechanisms determine functional residual capacity in mice, Mus musculus. J Appl Physiol 1979;46:867–71.

36. Gross NJ, Skorodin MS. Role of the parasympathetic system in airway obstruction due to emphysema. New Engl J Med 1984;311:421–5.

37. Gross NJ, Co E, Skorodin MS. Cholinergic bronchomotor tone in COPD. Estimates of its amount in comparison with that in normal subjects. Chest 1989;96:984–7.

38. Nisar M, Earis JE, Pearson MG, Calverley PM. Acute bronchodilator trials in chronic obstructive pulmonary disease. Am Rev Respir Dis 1992;146:555–9.

39. Casaburi R, Mahler DA, Jones PW, et al. A long-term evaluation of once-daily inhaled tiotropium in chronic obstructive pulmonary disease. Eur Respir J 2002;19:217–24.

40. O'Donnell DE, Flüge T, Gerken F, et al. Effects of tiotropium on lung hyperinflation, dyspnoea and exercise tolerance in COPD. Eur Respir J 2004;23:832–40.

41. Maltais F, Hamilton A, Marciniuk D, et al. Improvements in symptom-limited exercise performance over 8 h with once-daily tiotropium in patients with COPD. Chest 2005;128:1168–78.

42. Tashkin DP, Celli B, Senn S, et al. UPLIFT Study Investigators. A 4-year trial of tiotropium in chronic obstructive pulmonary disease. New Engl J Med 2008;359:1543–54.

43. Johansson G, Lindberg A, Romberg K, Nordström L, Gerken F, Roquet A. Bronchodilator efficacy of tiotropium in patients with mild to moderate COPD. Primary Care Respir J 2008;17:169–75.

44. Newton MF, O'Donnell DE, Forkert L. Response of lung volumes to inhaled salbutamol in a large population of patients with severe hyperinflation. Chest 2002;121:1042–50.

45. O'Donnell DE, Forkert L, Webb KA. Evaluation of bronchodilator responses in patients with "irreversible" emphysema. Eur Respir J 2001;18:914–20.

46. Walker PP, Calverley PM. The volumetric response to bronchodilators in stable chronic obstructive pulmonary disease. COPD 2008;5:147–52.

47. D'Angelo E, Prandi E, Marazzini L, Milic-Emili J. Dependence of maximal flow-volume curves on time course of preceding inspiration in patients with chronic obstruction pulmonary disease. Am J Respir Crit Care Med 1994;150:1581–6.

48. Pennock BE, Rogers RM, McCaffree DR. Changes in measured spirometric indices. What is significant? Chest 1981;80:97–9.

49. Pennock BE, Rogers RM. An evaluation of tests used to measure bronchodilator drug responses. Chest 1978;73:988–9.

50. Celli BR, ZuWallack R, Wang S, Kesten S. Improvement in resting inspiratory capacity and hyperinflation with tiotropium in COPD patients with increased static lung volumes. Chest 2003;124:1743–8.

51. Donohue JF, van Noord JA, Bateman ED, et al. A 6-month, placebo-controlled study comparing lung function and health status changes in COPD patients treated with tiotropium or salmeterol. Chest 2002;122:47–55.

52. van Noord JA, Bantje TA, Eland ME, Korducki L, Cornelissen PJ. A randomised controlled comparison of tiotropium and ipratropium in the treatment of chronic obstructive pulmonary disease. The Dutch Tiotropium Study Group. Thorax 2000;55:289–94.

53. Verkindre C, Bart F, Aguilaniu B, et al. The effect of tiotropium on hyperinflation and exercise capacity in chronic obstructive pulmonary disease. Respiration 2006;73:420–7.

54. Pellegrino R, Brusasco V. Lung hyperinflation and flow limitation in chronic airway obstruction. Eur Respir J 1997;10:543–9.

55. Tantucci C, Duguet A, Similowski T, et al. Effect of salbutamol on dynamic hyperinflation in chronic obstructive pulmonary disease patients. Eur Respir J 1998;12:799–804.

56. O'Donnell DE, Laveneziana P, Ora J, et al. Evaluation of acute bronchodilator reversibility in symptomatic GOLD stage I COPD. Thorax 2008; doi:10.1136/thx.2008.103598.

57. van Noord JA, Aumann JL, Janssens E, et al. Comparison of tiotropium once daily, formoterol twice daily and both combined once daily in patients with COPD. Eur Respir J 2005;26:214–22.

58. O'Donnell DE, Banzett RB, Carrieri-Kohlman V, et al. Pathophysiology of dyspnea in chronic obstructive pulmonary disease: a roundtable. Proc Am Thorac Soc 2007;4:145–68.

59. O'Donnell DE, Webb KA. The major limitation to exercise performance in COPD is dynamic hyperinflation. J Appl Physiol 2008;105:753–5.

60. O'Donnell DE, Hamilton AL, Webb KA. Sensory-mechanical relationships during high-intensity, constant-work-rate exercise in COPD. J Appl Physiol 2006;101:1025–35.

61. Brusasco V, Hodder R, Miravitlles M, et al. Health outcomes following treatment for six months with once daily tiotropium compared with twice daily salmeterol in patients with COPD. Thorax 2003;58:399–404.
62. Travers J, Laveneziana P, Webb KA, Kesten S, O'Donnell DE. Effect of tiotropium bromide on the cardiovascular response to exercise in COPD. Respir Med 2007;101:2017–24.
63. Pitta F, Troosters T, Probst VS, et al. Are patients with COPD more active after pulmonary rehabilitation? Chest 2008;134:273–80.
64. Casaburi R, Kukafka D, Cooper CB, Witek TJ, Kesten S. Improvement in exercise tolerance with the combination of tiotropium and pulmonary rehabilitation in patients with COPD. Chest 2005;127:809–17.
65. Kesten S, Casaburi R, Kukafka D, Cooper CB. Improvement in self-reported exercise participation with the combination of tiotropium and rehabilitative exercise training in COPD patients. Int J COPD 2008;3:127–36.
66. Donaldson GC, Seemungal TA, Bhowmik A, Wedzicha JA. Relationship between exacerbation frequency and lung function decline in chronic obstructive pulmonary disease. Thorax 2002;57:847–52.
67. Dusser D, Bravo ML, Iacono P. The effect of tiotropium on exacerbations and airflow in patients with COPD. Eur Respir J 2006;27:547–55.
68. Niewoehner DE, Rice K, Cote C, et al. Prevention of exacerbations of chronic obstructive pulmonary disease with tiotropium, a once-daily inhaled anticholinergic bronchodilator: a randomized trial. Ann Intern Med 2005;143:317–26.
69. Wedzicha JA, Calverley PM, Seemungal TA, et al. INSPIRE Investigators. The prevention of chronic obstructive pulmonary disease exacerbations by salmeterol/fluticasone propionate or tiotropium bromide. Am J Respir Crit Care Med 2008;177:19–26.
70. Parker CM, Voduc N, Aaron SD, Webb KA, O'Donnell DE. Physiological changes during symptom recovery from moderate exacerbations of COPD. Eur Respir J 2005;26:420–8.
71. Barnes PJ. Distribution of receptor targets in the lung. Proc Am Thorac Soc 2004;1:345–51.
72. Anthonisen NR, Connett JE, Kiley JP et al. Effects of smoking intervention and the use of an inhaled anticholinergic bronchodilator on the rate of decline of FEV1. The Lung Health Study. JAMA 1994;272:1497–505.
73. Celli BR, Thomas NE, Anderson JA, et al. Effect of pharmacotherapy on rate of decline of lung function in chronic obstructive pulmonary disease: results from the TORCH study. Am J Respir Crit Care Med 2008;178:332–338.
74. Highland KB, Strange C, Heffner JE. Long-term effects of inhaled corticosteroids on FEV1 in patients with chronic obstructive pulmonary disease. A meta-analysis. Ann Intern Med 2003;138:969–73.
75. Anthonisen NR, Connett JE, Enright PL, Manfreda J. Lung Health Study Research Group. Hospitalizations and mortality in the Lung Health Study. Am J Respir Crit Care Med 2002;166:333–9.
76. Celli BR, Cote CG, Marin JM, et al. The body-mass index, airflow obstruction, dyspnea, and exercise capacity index in chronic obstructive pulmonary disease. New Engl J Med 2004;350:1005–12.
77. Casanova C, Cote C, de Torres JP, et al. Inspiratory-to-total lung capacity ratio predicts mortality in patients with chronic obstructive pulmonary disease. Am J Respir Crit Care Med 2005;171:591–7.

78. Tantucci C, Donati P, Nicosia F, et al. Inspiratory capacity predicts mortality in patients with chronic obstructive pulmonary disease. Respir Med 2008;102:613–19.
79. Nishimura K, Izumi T, Tsukino M, Oga T. Dyspnea is a better predictor of 5-year survival than airway obstruction in patients with COPD. Chest 2002;121(5):1434–40.
80. Connors AF, Dawson NV, Thomas C, et al. Outcomes following acute exacerbation of severe chronic obstructive lung disease. The SUPPORT investigators (Study to Understand Prognoses and Preferences for Outcomes and Risks of Treatments). Am J Respir Crit Care Med 1996;154:959–67.
81. Patil SP, Krishnan JA, Lechtzin N, Diette GB. In-hospital mortality following acute exacerbations of chronic obstructive pulmonary disease. Arch Intern Med 2003;163: 1180–6.
82. Soler-Cataluña JJ, Martínez-García MA, Román Sánchez P, et al. Severe acute exacerbations and mortality in patients with chronic obstructive pulmonary disease. Thorax 2005;60: 925–31.
83. Oga T, Nishimura K, Tsukino M, Sato S, Hajiro T. Analysis of the factors related to mortality in chronic obstructive pulmonary disease: role of exercise capacity and health status. Am J Respir Crit Care Med 2003;167:544–9.
84. Decramer M, Nici L, Nardini S, Reardon J, Rochester CL, Sanguinetti CM, Troosters T. Targeting the COPD exacerbation. Respir Med 2008 Jun;102 Suppl 1:S3–15. Review.
85. Fishman A, Martinez F, Naunheim K, et al. National Emphysema Treatment Trial Research Group. A randomized trial comparing lung-volume-reduction surgery with medical therapy for severe emphysema. New Engl J Med 2003;348:2059–73.
86. Gershon AS, Wang L, To T, Luo J, Upshur RE. Survival with tiotropium compared to long-acting beta-2-agonists in chronic obstructive pulmonary disease. COPD 2008;5:229–34.
87. Suissa S. Methodologic shortcomings of the INSPIRE randomized trial. Am J Respir Crit Care Med 2008;178:1090–1.
88. Kesten S, Jara M, Wentworth C, Lanes S. Pooled clinical trial analysis of tiotropium safety. Chest 2006;130:1695–703.
89. Singh S, Loke YK, Furberg CD. Inhaled anticholinergics and risk of major adverse cardiovascular events in patients with chronic obstructive pulmonary disease: a systematic review and meta-analysis. JAMA 2008;300:1439–1450.
90. Covelli H, Bhattacharya S, Cassino C, Conoscenti C, Kesten S. Absence of electrocardiographic findings and improved function with once-daily tiotropium in patients with chronic obstructive pulmonary disease. Pharmacotherapy 2005;25:1708–18.
91. Morganroth J, Golisch W, Kesten S. Electrocardiographic monitoring in COPD patients receiving tiotropium. COPD 2004;1:181–90.
92. Boulet L-P, Becker A, Berube D, Beveridge RC, Ernst P. on behalf of the Canadian Asthma Consensus Group. Canadian asthma consensus report, 1999. Can Med Assoc J 1999;161: S1–S62.
93. Global Initiative for Asthma (GINA). Global Strategy for Asthma Management and Prevention. Global Initiative for Asthma (GINA), 2010. http://ginasthma.org/
94. National Heart, Lung, and Blood Institute, National Institutes of Health. Expert Panel Report 3 (EPR 3): Guidelines for the Diagnosis and Management of Asthma. No. 08-4051, 2007. http://www.nhlbi.nih.gov/guidelines/asthma/
95. Beveridge RC, Grunfeld AF, Hodder RV, Verbeek PR, Canadian Association of Emergency Physicians and the Canadian Thoracic Society Asthma Advisory Committee. Guidelines for the emergency management of asthma in adults. Can Med Assoc J 1996;155:25–37.

96. Westby M, Benson M, Gibson P. Anticholinergic agents for chronic asthma in adults. Cochrane Database Syst Rev 2004; Issue 3. Art. No.:CD003269. doi: 10.1002/14651858.CD003269. pub2.

97. O'Connor BJ, Towse LJ, Barnes PJ. Prolonged effect of tiotropium bromide on methacholine-induced bronchoconstriction in asthma. Am J Respir Crit Care Med 1996;154:876–80.

98. Terzano C, Petroianni A, Ricci A, D'Antoni L, Allegra L. Early protective effects of tiotropium bromide in patients with airways hyperresponsiveness. Eur Rev Med Pharmacol Sci 2004;8:259–64.

99. Israel E, Drazen JM, Liggett SB, et al. The effect of polymorphisms of the beta(2)-adrenergic receptor on the response to regular use of albuterol in asthma. Am J Respir Crit Care Med 2000;162:75–80.

100. Taylor DR, Drazen JM, Herbison GP, et al. Asthma exacerbations during long term beta agonist use: influence of beta(2) adrenoceptor polymorphism. Thorax 2000;55:762–7.

101. Palmer CN, Lipworth BJ, Lee S, et al. Arginine-16 beta2 adrenoceptor genotype predisposes to exacerbations in young asthmatics taking regular salmeterol. Thorax 2006;61:940–4.

102. Israel E, Chinchilli VM, Ford JG, et al. Use of regularly scheduled albuterol treatment in asthma: genotype-stratified, randomised, placebo-controlled cross-over trial. Lancet 2004;364; 1505–12.

103. Dow L, Carroll M. The aging lung: structural and functional aspects. In: Connolly MJ (ed.), Respiratory Disease in the Elderly Patient. Chapman and Hall, London, 1996; pp. 1–17.

104. Johnson BD, Reddan WG, Seow KC, Dempsey JA. Mechanical constraints on exercise hyperpnea in a fit aging population. Am Rev Respir Dis 1991;143:968–77.

105. Ofir D, Laveneziana P, Webb KA, Lam YM, O'Donnell DE. Sex differences in the perceived intensity of breathlessness during exercise with advancing age. J Appl Physiol 2008;104: 1583–93.

106. Connolly MJ. Ageing, late-onset asthma and the beta-adrenoceptor. Pharmacol Therapeut 1993;60:389–404.

107. van Schayck CP, Folgering H, Harbers H, Maas KL, van Weel C. Effects of allergy and age on responses to salbutamol and ipratropium bromide in moderate asthma and chronic bronchitis. Thorax 1991;46:355–9.

108. Ruffin RE, Fitzgerald JD, Rebuck AS. A comparison of the bronchodilator activity of Sch 1000 and salbutamol. J Allergy Clin Immunol 1977;59:136–41.

109. Vestal RE, Connolly MJ. Drug therapy in the elderly patient with respiratory disease. In: Connolly MJ (ed.), Respiratory Disease in the Elderly Patient. Chapman and Hall, London, 1996; pp. 231–60.

110. Magnussen, H, Bugnas B, van Noord J, et al. Improvements with tiotropium in COPD patients with concomitant asthma. Respir Med 2008;102:50–6.

111. Fardon T, Haggart K, Lee DK, Lipworth BJ. A proof of concept study to evaluate stepping down the dose of fluticasone in combination with salmeterol and tiotropium in severe persistent asthma. Respir Med 2007;101:1218–28.

112. Gosens R, Zaagsma J, Meurs H, Halayko AJ. Muscarinic receptor signaling in the pathophysiology of asthma and COPD. Respir Res 2006;7:73.

113. Gosens R, Bos IS, Zaagsma J, Meurs H. Protective effects of tiotropium bromide in the progression of airway smooth muscle remodeling. Am J Respir Crit Care Med 2005;171:1096–102.

114. Hetzel MR, Clark TJ. Comparison of normal and asthmatic circadian rhythms in peak expiratory flow rate. Thorax 1980;35:732–8.

115. Ryan G, Latimer KM, Dolovich J, Hargreave FE. Bronchial responsiveness to histamine: rela-tionship to diurnal variation of peak flow rate, improvement after bronchodilator, and airway caliber. Thorax 1982;37:423–9.

116. Morrison JF, Pearson SB, Dean HG. Parasympathetic nervous system in nocturnal asthma. Brit Med J (Clin Res edn), 1988;296:1427–9.

117. Catterall JR, Rhind GB, Whyte KF, Shapiro CM, Douglas NJ. Is nocturnal asthma caused by changes in airway cholinergic activity? Thorax 1988;43:720–4.

118. Mackay TW, Fitzpatrick MF, Douglas NJ. Non-adrenergic, non-cholinergic nervous sys-tem and overnight airway calibre in asthmatic and normal subjects. Lancet 1991;338: 1289–92.

119. American Thoracic Society. Proceedings of the ATS workshop on refractory asthma: current understanding, recommendations, and unanswered questions. American Thoracic Society. Am J Respir Crit Care Med 2000;162:2341–51.

120. Chung KF, Godard P, Adelroth E, et al. Difficult/therapy-resistant asthma: the need for an inte-grated approach to define clinical phenotypes, evaluate risk factors, understand pathophysiology and find novel therapies. ERS Task Force on Difficult/Therapy-Resistant Asthma. European Respiratory Society. Eur Respir J 1999;13:1198–208.

121. Wenzel S. Severe asthma in adults. Am J Respir Crit Care Med 2005;172:149–60.

122. Lodi U, Harding SM, Coghlan HC, Guzzo MR, Walker LH. Autonomic regulation in asthmatics with gastroesophageal reflux. Chest 1997;111:65–70.

123. Andersen LI, Schmidt A, Bundgaard A. Pulmonary function and acid application in the esoph-agus. Chest 1986;90:358–63.

124. Langdeau JB, Boulet LP. Prevalence and mechanisms of development of asthma and airway hyperresponsiveness in athletes. Sports Med 2001;31:601–16.

125. Goldsmith RL, Bigger JT, Steinman RC, Fleiss JL. Comparison of 24-hour parasympa-thetic activity in endurance-trained and untrained young men. J Am Coll Cardiol 1992;20: 552–8.

126. De Meersman RE. Respiratory sinus arrhythmia alteration following training in endurance athletes. Eur J Appl Physiol O 1992;64:434–6.

127. Lougheed MD, Fisher T, O'Donnell DE. Dynamic hyperinflation during bronchoconstriction in asthma: implications for symptom perception. Chest 2006;130:1072–81.

128. Lougheed MD, Lam M, Forkert L, Webb KA, O'Donnell DE. Breathlessness during acute bronchoconstriction in asthma: pathophysiologic mechanisms. Am Rev Respir Dis 1993;148:1452–9.

129. Lougheed MD, Webb KA, O'Donnell DE. Breathlessness during induced lung hyperinflation in asthma: the role of the inspiratory threshold load. Am J Respir Crit Care Med 1995;152: 911–20.

130. Lougheed MD, Fisher T, O'Donnell DE. Dynamic hyperinflation during bronchoconstriction in asthma: implications for symptom perception. Chest 2006;130 (4):1072–81.

131. Empey DW, Laitinen LA, Jacobs L, Gold WM, Nadel JA. Mechanisms of bronchial hy-perreactivity in normal subjects after upper respiratory tract infection. Am Rev Respir Dis 1976;113:131–9.

132. Aquilina AT, Hall WJ, Douglas RG, Utell MJ. Airway reactivity in subjects with viral upper respiratory tract infections: the effects of exercise and cold air. Am Rev Respir Dis 1980;122: 3–10.

133. Jacoby DB, Fryer AD. Interaction of viral infections with muscarinic receptors. Clin Exp Allergy 1999;29:59–64.

134. Jacoby DB. Virus-induced asthma attacks. JAMA 2002;287:755–61.
135. Jacoby DB. Virus-induced asthma attacks. J Aerosol Med 2004;17:169–73.
136. Kingham PJ, Costello RW, McLean WG. Eosinophil and airway nerve interactions. Pulm Pharmacol Ther 2003;16:9–13.
137. Jara M, Lanes SF, Wentworth III C, May C, Kesten S. Comparative safety of long-acting inhaled bronchodilators: A cohort study using the UK THIN primary care database. Drug Safety 2007;30:1151–60.

12

Phosphodiesterase inhibitors in obstructive lung disease

Jan Lötvall and Bo Lundbäck

Krefting Research Centre, University of Gothenburg, Göteborg, Sweden

12.1   Introduction

Chronic inflammatory processes play a key role in chronic obstructive pulmonary disease (COPD), which is typically characterized by an increase in neutrophils, macrophages and $CD8^+$ T-lymphocytes in both central and peripheral airways, as well as in lung parenchyma.[1] Therefore, therapeutic approaches to suppress inflammation in COPD could potentially improve symptoms, decrease the frequency of exacerbations and possibly slow progression of the disease. Indeed, inhaled glucocorticoids do have some, albeit limited, beneficial effects in COPD, as has been documented in several large multicentre studies.[2,3] Treatment of COPD is therefore often primarily treated with bronchodilating drugs, such as inhaled anticholinergics or long-acting β_2-agonists, which have weak or no anti-inflammatory effects.[4] Therefore, there is a substantial unmet need for efficient anti-inflammatory therapy in COPD, and the development of new treatments remains crucial.[5]

Currently, a substantial number of molecules with selective phosphodiesterase-4 (PDE4) inhibitory activity are being developed for the treatment of COPD; to date, one of these has been approved for clinical use.[6]

Over the last 20 years, major efforts have been made to develop phosphodiesterase (PDE) inhibitors that treat different functions of both asthma and COPD.[7] One obstacle is that several different PDE enzymes exist in different cells, thus the identification of drugs that are efficacious without having significant side effects has proven complicated.[8] A number of these drugs have been tested clinically, but several have not shown a beneficial therapeutic ratio, with side effects such as nausea and orthostatism occurring at therapeutically effective doses. However, research efforts in the last decade have resulted in increased understanding of the molecular processes in the different PDE pathways, and specifically the PDE4 pathway, which has resulted in the development of novel drugs with improved therapeutic ratios and subsequently

Advances in Combination Therapy for Asthma and COPD, First Edition. Edited by Jan Lötvall.
© 2012 John Wiley & Sons, Ltd. Published 2012 by John Wiley & Sons, Ltd.

clinically significant therapeutic effects. Roflimulast, which targets PDE4, has recently been registered in Europe for the treatment of COPD.[9, 10]

Phosphodiesterase enzymes modulate the degradation of cyclic nucleotides such as cAMP, which is a second messenger involved in many cellular responses that involve activation of adenylyl cyclase; blockers of PDE4 isoenzymes subsequently increase the intracellular cAMP concentration.[8] Theophylline, which has been utilized in the treatment of both asthma and COPD for many years, is believed to exert its main biological and clinical effects through non-specific PDE inhibition, which has prompted the development of more specific PDE4-targeting drugs. Indeed, theophylline has extensive side effects when doses are increased,[11] and drugs with similar or higher efficacy, but fewer side effects, have therefore been attractive alternatives for drug development. The PDE4 enzyme has been specifically targeted in obstructive lung diseases because it has been extensively documented that this enzyme is involved in regulation of inflammatory cell activity, and inhibition of this enzyme can reduce inflammation, as shown in preclinical models.[6, 12] The first generation of drugs targeting PDE4 had extensive clinical side effects, therefore, more recently, PDE4 inhibitors have been developed with a much wider therapeutic ratio, reducing the risk of side effects while maintaining clinical efficacy.[13]

This chapter will review the molecular anti-inflammatory mechanisms, some of the preclinical data, key clinical findings and future perspectives of current and future PDE4 inhibitors for the treatment primarily of COPD.

12.2   Phosphodiesterase enzymes

The cyclic nucleotide PDEs are a superfamily of intracellular enzymes that degrade the second messengers cAMP and cyclic guanosine monophosphate (cGMP).[8, 14] The PDE enzymes consist of 11 known subtypes, and intricately regulate the duration and degree of cyclic nucleotide signalling in cells. The classification of the PDE-enzymes is based on amino acid sequence, substrate specificity, regulatory properties and pharmacological properties as well as distribution in cells and tissue. Phosphodiesterase enzymes are possible targets for pharmacological inhibition due to their unique tissue distribution, structural properties, and functional properties in different organs and cells. From a pharmacological perspective, inhibition of PDE enzymes is relatively uncomplicated, and inhibitors prolong or enhance the effects of cAMP or cGMP in different tissues, as long as the pharmacological molecule is sufficiently isoenzyme specific.[8] For example, PDE5 inhibition enhances the vasodilatory effects of cGMP in the corpus cavernosum of the penis, and is used to treat erectile dysfunction.[15] Different PDE inhibitors have been identified as new potential therapeutics in areas such as pulmonary arterial hypertension, coronary heart disease, dementia, depression and schizophrenia. For obstructive airways diseases, the key focus has been on PDE4, in view of its role in inflammation. However, some attention is also given to PDE3 and PDE7, as blocking these isoenzymes can lead to bronchodilation.[16]

The enzyme PDE4 is especially abundant in inflammatory cells, and the suggestion is that it regulates the cellular inflammation in obstructive airways disease such as asthma and COPD. The PDE4 gene family consists of several genes that have alternative mRNA processing, which results in the expression of different PDE4 isoforms in different cells. It has been suggested that the anti-inflammatory role of PDE4 is primarily mediated via PDE4B,[17] and to some extent by PDE4A.

12.3   Different pharmacological agents blocking PDE4

A vast number of PDE inhibitors have been tested in patients with asthma or COPD over the last 25 years, but very few have had a sufficiently favourable therapeutic ratio to warrant testing in multicentre phase III clinical trials. The list of drugs in this section is therefore far from complete, but focuses on drugs that have recently been tested, are currently close to clinical testing or are clinically available, as is the case with roflimulast. Beyond asthma and COPD, PDE4 inhibitors for rheumatoid diseases and different skin diseases, including psoriasis, have also been tested. Some of these compounds are developed as oral medications, and some are developed for inhaled use in airways disease, although the first generation of PDE4 inhibitors was primarily tested by oral administration.

One of the first PDE4 inhibitors to be studied was rolipram, which has a half maximal inhibitory concentration (IC_{50}) value of approximately 300 nM. Rolipram was tested in the treatment of depression, but clinical development was abandoned due to side effects. Rolipram is, however, often used as a comparator in studies of novel PDE4 inhibitors.[18] Roflumilast (Daxas) is a selective PDE4 inhibitor with several anti-inflammatory properties that are potentially beneficial in COPD.[19,20] The drug has high oral bioavailability (approximately 80%), a long half-life (approximately 16 h) and is highly potent, with an IC_{50} of approximately 1 nM. Roflumilast has undergone extensive clinical testing, and has been approved in Europe for clinical use in severe COPD with bronchitis. The clinical results are described in more detail later in this chapter.

Cilomilast is a specific PDE4 inhibitor with an IC_{50} of approximately 260 nM that has gone through full clinical development for the treatment of COPD.[21] This drug has shown reasonable efficacy in COPD,[22] but the therapeutic ratio seems suboptimal, with some side effects appearing at clinical doses. It seems unlikely that the development of cilomilast will be pursued for clinical use in COPD.

Ronomilast (ELB353) is a potent oral PDE4 inhibitor with an IC_{50} of approximately 3.5 nM. The drug has demonstrated a good therapeutic margin in preclinical models, which has been confirmed in early clinical trials. The pharmacokinetics of ronomilast make it suitable for once-daily treatment, and it is currently being developed for treating COPD (http://www.biotie.com/en/recearch_and_development/inflammation/ronomilast).

An extensive series of PDE4 inhibitors are or have been tested in diseases other than COPD and asthma, but could enter clinical development in respiratory disease. Apremilast (CC-10004, Celgene) is a selective PDE4 inhibitor with a relatively moderate potency (IC_{50} of approximately 70 nM) that is primarily being developed for the treatment of psoriasis and other inflammatory skin diseases.[23] Revamilast (GRC 4039) is an orally active PDE4 inhibitor with high pharmacological potency (IC_{50} approximately 3 nM) and high specificity for PDE4. It is being developed primarily for rheumatoid arthritis, multiple sclerosis and other inflammatory disorders.[24] Preclinical studies have claimed a beneficial therapeutic ratio, with few events of emesis despite pharmacological effects *in vivo*. Oglemilast (GRC-3886) is a PDE4 inhibitor that has been tested in early phases of clinical development for both asthma and COPD. This drug is slightly less potent than other PDE4 inhibitors (IC_{50} value of 190 nM), but is highly specific for PDE4, and inhibits this enzyme with an IC_{50} value of 1.4 nM. Because of discouraging early clinical results, the development of Oglemilast is currently on hold.[25] OX914 is a PDE4 inhibitor that was initially tested in learning and memory disorders, but is now said to be undergoing testing in asthma and COPD.[26] It has also been tested in rhinitis, but with no clinically satisfactory results, and is therefore no longer being developed for that disease. It is claimed that OX914 causes a low frequency of nausea.

In view of the difficulty with oral PDE4 inhibitors in achieving high efficacy without some systemic side effects, such as nausea, several companies are developing PDE4 inhibitors for inhalation. By doing this, it is expected that higher concentrations are achieved in the airways, where most of the anti-inflammatory effect is expected to take place. GSK842470 was one the first PDE4 inhibitors to be tested via the inhaled route, but efficacy was shown to be low or lacking.[27] This compound is, however, being tested for local skin treatment for dermatological indications. Another PDE4 inhibitor that has been tested for inhaled administration in asthma and COPD is tofimilast. This compound has a moderate potency (IC_{50} 13 nM) but importantly has low oral bioavailability, which could be beneficial to avoid systemic side effects. However, clinical development was discontinued due to lack of efficacy on lung function parameters in early trials on asthma and COPD. Also another inhaled PDE4 inhibitor, UK-500,001, failed in a clinical study of COPD, and has shown very weak efficacy in an allergen model of asthma. Surprisingly, the frequency of nausea was relatively high with the larger doses of the inhaled drug.

GSK256066 is an exceptionally potent PDE4 inhibitor, with an IC_{50} in the 10 pM range, that is in clinical development for the treatment of allergic rhinitis, asthma and COPD. This drug does not show isoform selectivity for PDE4A and PDE4B. Early clinical data from allergen exposure in mild asthmatics show promising results.[28] RPL-554 and RPL-565 are both combined PDE3 and PDE4 inhibitors, and are therefore suggested to achieve some bronchodilating activity through PDE3 inhibition beyond the anti-inflammatory effect observed with PDE4 inhibition.[29] These drugs are therefore being developed primarily for allergic rhinitis and asthma; positive results in asthma have been claimed but have yet to be published.

12.4　Biological effects of PDE4 inhibition, preclinical information

Phosphodiesterase-4 is primarily expressed in different inflammatory cells, including macrophages and neutrophils, and it has been proposed that inhibition of this enzyme subtype could an efficient means of treating inflammatory airway diseases.[30,31] Indeed, treatment with one clinically approved PDE4 inhibitor, roflumilast, has been shown to reduce the degree of neutrophilic inflammation in the airways of patients with COPD, which implies a clinically important anti-inflammatory effect (Figure 12.1).[32] However, the exact mechanism of the reduced inflammation cannot be determined by *in vivo* human studies, thus preclinical experiments in cell culture models as well as in animal models are likely to be helpful in determining its mechanism of action, which in turn may reveal other potential indications for this drug. The anti-inflammatory effects of PDE4 inhibition have been confirmed in animal models, for example using models of allergen exposure or tobacco smoke exposure.[33,34]

Neutrophils are especially sensitive to PDE4 inhibition, and blockers of PDE4 have shown extensive direct effects in these cells, attenuating several of their inflammatory functions. One effect that may be important in COPD is suppression of the release of neutrophil elastase from human neutrophils, which when released can lead to tissue-damaging effects.[35,36] Furthermore, PDE4 inhibition can efficiently attenuate the accumulation of neutrophils into the airways. For example, in rodents, PDE4 inhibition can attenuate the often-observed influx of neutrophils to the airways induced by tobacco smoke exposure.[37,38] Most of these studies have shown the protective

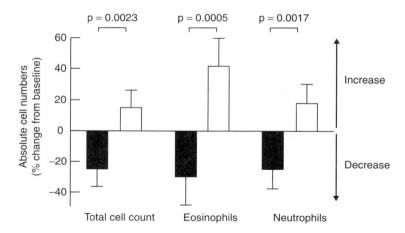

Figure 12.1　Percent change in sputum cell count in patients with COPD after treatment with roflumilast (black bars) or placebo (white bars) over 4 weeks, in a cross-over study. The results include total sputum cells, sputum eosinophils and sputum neutrophils. Reprinted with permission from Grootendorst DC, Gauw SA, Verhoosel RM, Sterk PJ, Hospers JJ, Bredenbröker D, Bethke TD, Hiemstra PS, Rabe KF. Reduction in sputum neutrophil and eosinophil numbers by the PDE4 inhibitor roflumilast in patients with COPD. Thorax. 2007 Dec;62(12):1081–7. Epub 2007 Jun 15.

effect of pretreatment with a PDE4 inhibitor on smoke-induced inflammation; however, when treatment with the PDE4 inhibitor was initiated after established smoke-induced inflammation, an attenuating effect on inflammation was observed.[38] Furthermore, influx of neutrophils induced by other stimuli, such as tobacco smoke, bleomycin and lipopolysaccharide (LPS), are also attenuated by PDE4 inhibition. PDE4 inhibition also results in reduced release of reactive oxygen species (ROS), leukotriene B_4 (LTB4) and matrix metalloproteinase-9 (MMP-9) from activated human neutrophils.[38] Of special interest could be the inhibition of LTB_4, which can function as a chemoattractant for neutrophils, and LTB_4 released from neutrophils could thus further enhance extended recruitment of neutrophils to the site of an established neutrophilic inflammation.[39]

Survival of neutrophils is prolonged by increased intracellular concentration of cAMP, and in theory PDE4 inhibition could therefore enhance neutrophilia. However, the overall *in vivo* effect is indeed inhibitory, strongly arguing that the reduction of neutrophils by PDE4 inhibition primarily is dependent on reduced recruitment rather than induction of cell death. However, PDE4 inhibition also resolves established neutrophilia through induction of cell death.[40] It is known that tobacco smoking increases the number of neutrophils in the circulation, and many of these cells accumulate in the blood vessels of the lung and are there available for prompt influx into the lungs and airways. In some animal models, it has been shown that tobacco smoke exposure will increase the expression of CD11b/CD18 on neutrophils in the lungs, which leads to greater adhesion to endothelium.[41] Importantly, cAMP, PDE3 and PDE4 have been shown to regulate inflammatory cell interaction with endothelial cells *in vitro*, as well as migration through endothelium.[42, 43] Thus, PDE4 inhibition may attenuate influx of neutrophils at least partly via interaction at the level of neutrophil adhesion and transmigration to the tissue.

Other inflammatory cells beyond the neutrophils can also be affected by PDE4 inhibition, including monocytes/macrophages and T-lymphocytes.[44] Thus, PDE4 inhibition results in reduction of LPS responses in monocyte/macrophage cultured cells, specifically related to tumor necrosis factor-α (TNF-α) release.[45] Beyond the neutrophilic inflammation induced by smoking is the role of cells of the adaptive immune response, including lymphocytes such as CD4 and CD8 cells. PDE4 inhibitors can attenuate the proliferation of both human CD4 and CD8 lymphocytes, as well as cytokine release from these cells and their influx to the airways during smoking exposure.[46, 47] In addition to the multiple inhibitory effects on inflammatory cells and impact on airway inflammation, it has also been shown that PDE4 inhibition can influence airway epithelium[48, 49] by attenuation of mucin expression, and can also regulate expression of intercellular adhesion molecule-1 (ICAM-1) on cultured human lung fibroblasts.[50] PDE4 inhibition can also increase ciliary beat frequency in epithelial cells from sinuses, trachea and bronchi, as shown in several animal models. Roflumilast has given similar results in studies of ciliated human nasal epithelial cells *in vitro*.[51, 52]

Treatment of mice with the PDE4 inhibitor roflumilast has been shown to reduce signs of lung emphysema induced by tobacco smoke exposure.[33, 53] Together, these data suggest that treatment with PDE4 inhibitors can reduce the loss of alveolar attachments and elastic recoil, important for the emphysematous component of COPD.

The cellular and molecular mechanisms by which PDE4 inhibitors can attenuate the progression of lung emphysema are not known, beyond the documented anti-inflammatory effects of these drugs. It is also possible that the imbalance between tissue injury and repair that is a key process in emphysema development may be altered by PDE4 inhibition, implied by biological effects documented in fibroblasts.[50]

Even though animal models of COPD are helpful in describing mechanisms of action of different pharmacological agents, there are limitations to how these results can be interpreted. Smoke exposure in animals does not necessarily represent all aspects and stages of COPD, and may not elicit all the pathobiological processes that are present in clinical disease. For example, few models have attempted to combine smoke exposure and bacterial overgrowth in the lung, which often can be detected in clinical disease. Furthermore, it is also difficult to assess effects and interactions of COPD mechanisms with COPD-related comorbidities in animal models of COPD.

12.5   Clinical effects of PDE4 inhibition in COPD

To date, two oral PDE4 inhibitors, cilomilast and roflumilast, have been fully tested clinically in COPD. Only roflumilast has been approved for clinical use in Europe, whereas the clinical development of cilomilast has been put on hold after it was rejected by the US Food and Drug Administration (FDA). Therefore, most of the data presented in this section relate to the evidence of clinical effects of roflumilast in COPD.

Roflumilast is used clinically as a once-daily orally administered tablet. The key clinical data that were presented for the approval of roflumilast included different primary outcomes, including exacerbation frequency, and lung function. Initially, a 6-month medium-size study with roflumilast showed a significant effect on both lung function and exacerbation frequency in COPD, with a tendency for a dose-related effect when 250 µg and 500 µg doses were compared for daily treatment.[54] Similar results were published for cilomilast in a 6-month study, showing significant effects on both lung function and exacerbation frequency.[55] The subsequent 1-year study of the effects of roflumilast treatment showed a weak effect on lung function and non-significant effects on exacerbation frequency in a broad population of COPD patients.[56] However, when retrospective analyses were performed in this longer study, a significant effect was observed in patients with more severe disease.[56] These early data therefore suggested that subgroups of COPD would be better suited for PDE4 inhibitor treatment, which helped in the design of subsequent studies. Hence, more recent publications describe the effect of roflumilast on more severe COPD, and on patients with concomitant signs of chronic bronchitis.

The key registration studies for roflumilast were thus performed in patients with more severe stages of COPD, grade III and IV.[57,58] In these patients, treatment with roflumilast had beneficial effects on several parameters. Firstly, daily treatment over a 1-year period showed significant reduction in the frequency of exacerbations. The average number of exacerbations in pooled data from two studies was 1.14 per patient per year with roflumilast treatment, and 1.37 per patient per year in the placebo group,

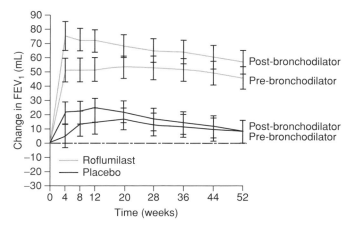

Figure 12.2   Effects on change in forced expiratory volume in 1 second (FEV₁) over 52 weeks of treatment with placebo (red) or roflumilast (blue) in patients with COPD. Reprinted from The Lancet, 374, Fabbri LM, Calverley PM, Izquierdo-Alonso JL, Bundschuh DS, Brose M, Martinez FJ, Rabe KF; M2-127 and M2-128 study groups, 695–703 (2009); with permission from Elsevier.

documenting a 17% reduction in the frequency of exacerbations with treatment.[57] In this study, COPD exacerbation was defined as an attack resulting in either oral glucocorticoid treatment, or admission to hospital, or death. In the same studies, both pre- and post-bronchodilator forced expiratory volume in 1 second (FEV₁) was significantly improved in those treated with roflumilast. Furthermore, lung function was significantly improved with roflumilast treatment (Figure 12.2).

In two additional studies of patients with moderate-to-severe COPD, again published in a single article, the effect of roflumilast treatment was explored in patients concomitantly treated with either salmeterol or tiotropium.[58] Also in these studies, additive effects could be observed during treatment with the PDE4 inhibitor, showing that lung function could be further improved by roflumilast although bronchodilators were used as baseline therapy. The effect of roflumilast on FEV₁ was, however, moderate with these treatments, with improvement in pre-bronchodilator FEV₁ generally less than 100 mL. This study was not adequately powered to determine the effect on exacerbations; the number of withdrawals was greater in the groups treated with roflumilast. The average non-significant reduction in exacerbation frequency was approximately 21% and 18% when added to salmeterol and tiotropium, respectively.[58] The greater number of withdrawals with roflumilast was related to side effects of the PDE4 inhibitor. Effects on rescue medication by roflumilast treatment seemed to be more pronounced in the study that evaluated the additive effect over tiotropium than in the study with salmeterol.

The clinical anti-inflammatory effects of roflumilast in COPD have been determined in a short-term, placebo-controlled study of patients with moderate-to-severe COPD, who received either roflumilast 500 μg/day or placebo in a 4-week cross-over study. After roflumilast, the number of neutrophils was reduced by approximately 36%

compared with placebo, whereas the number of eosinophils was reduced by approximately 50%.[32] This study also documented reduced levels of interleukin-8 (IL-8), neutrophil elastase, eosinophil cationic peptide and α_2-macroglobulin with roflumilast treatment, arguing that this PDE4 inhibitor exerts true anti-inflammatory effects *in vivo* in humans.

12.6   Effects of PDE4 inhibitors on systemic processes in COPD

COPD, and especially more severe stages of COPD, are often associated with extensive comorbidities including atheroscleorsis, diabetes, osteoporosis and muscle weakness, as well as depression and cancer. It is envisaged that the systemic inflammation observed in COPD, which can be documented as measurable differences in, for example, C-reactive protein, is associated with many of these comorbidities. Having any additional closely related disease increases the risk of a COPD patient being admitted to hospital, and increases the risk of death.[59–61]

As inflammation is common to COPD and cardiovascular disease, it makes sense to hypothesize that systemic anti-inflammatory treatment could benefit both diseases. PDE4 inhibitors have shown multiple beneficial effects on vascular injury in animal models. Overall, however, there is only circumstantial evidence to suggest a possible beneficial effect of PDE4 inhibition on systemic inflammation in COPD, and subsequent effects on cardiovascular morbidity. Large prospective studies in humans are needed to document any potential beneficial effect of PDE4 inhibition on cardiovascular comorbidities.

In experimental animal models, it has been shown that PDE4 inhibition can reduce the development of some COPD-associated comorbidity-like biological processes, for example osteoporosis, possibly by affecting osteoblast/osteoclast activity, but the anti-inflammatory effects of PDE4 inhibitors may also indirectly retain bone structure by attenuating inflammation-induced loss of bone. Furthermore, PDE4 inhibition can reduce muscle waning/muscle atrophy in animal models. PDE4 inhibitors also have the capacity to modulate insulin secretion and can affect insulin sensitivity;[62] however, the clinical relevance of these observations remains obscure. In animals, PDE4 inhibition can have an effect that mimics antidepressants, and PDE4 inhibitors have indeed initially been developed to treat such symptoms.[63] However, any antidepressive effects that could be relevant in COPD patients with such problems remain to be documented.

12.7   Side effects of PDE4 inhibitors

The dose-limiting effects of PDE4 inhibitors tested in a clinical setting are gastrointestinal side effects such as nausea and diarrhoea, as well as orthostatism. In the clinical studies that have been reported, such side effects consistently occur in at least a subgroup of patients, especially at elevated doses. Headache is also a frequently observed side effect in any clinical study. The low therapeutic ratio of PDE4 inhibitors is why doses cannot be increased. Dosing of the PDE4 inhibitor roflumilast must be seen as therapeutically optimized, and it seems unlikely that increasing the dose of this drug would increase clinical efficacy without also increasing the frequency and the degree of systemic side effects.

An alternative approach to improve the therapeutic ratio of a drug that is targeted at lung disease is to administer the drug by inhalation, which could be suitable for both COPD and asthma. When the drug is inhaled, it is envisaged that the drug concentration will become much higher in the target organ, the lung, than systemically. Indeed, several molecules inhibiting PDE4 have and are being pursued for treatment of COPD and asthma, and could in theory have such benefits. However, early studies of inhaled PDE4 inhibitors have also shown systemic side effects such as nausea; it is important that the inhaled molecule is not rapidly absorbed to the systemic circulation after inhalation, to avoid such reactions.

No important rare or dangerous side effects have been reported. In preclinical toxicology studies, vasculitis has been observed, but this has not been observed in PDE4-treated patients in published clinical studies.

12.8   PDE4 inhibitors in COPD management plans

In June 2010 roflumilast was approved in the European Union for the treatment of severe COPD associated with chronic bronchitis. Initially, it is likely that this treatment will be considered as a second-line treatment, and may primarily be given to those with frequent exacerbations despite treatment with inhaled long-acting bronchodilators and perhaps inhaled glucocorticoids.[64] PDE4 inhibition has an effect different to that of glucocorticoids, and studies determining the effects of PDE4 inhibition on top of combined inhaled glucocorticoid/long-acting beta-agonist (LABA) therapy are needed. Currently, however, the indication for PDE4 inhibition is likely to remain severe COPD with symptoms of chronic bronchitis. Roflumilast has yet to find its position in currently available guidelines for the management of COPD.

12.9   Future prospects with PDE4 inhibitors in obstructive airways disease

COPD is a complicated disease with not only extensive pathology in the lungs, but also parallel multiple systemic processes that contribute to morbidity, including systemic inflammation, osteoporosis and muscle weakness. Patients with COPD can be divided into different subgroups, depending on degree of inflammation, degree of bacterial load, degree of emphysema and several other parameters. These 'phenotypes' of disease may reflect different disease processes that may be treated with different efficiency by different treatments. The current approval of roflumilast in the treatment of COPD is limited to severe disease with concomitant bronchitis, as an add-on to other therapies.

In the future, when COPD can be better phenotyped, and subgroups of disease better identified, it is possible that patients who respond to each different treatment for COPD can be identified. It is also possible that novel approaches to managing COPD using different combinations of medications based on phenotypes of disease, may lead to greater efficacy and even better overall clinical outcomes. Lastly, it is possible that an interaction between cAMP-inducing drugs such as β_2-agonists and PDE4 inhibitors could lead to further enhanced anti-inflammatory effects; however, confirmation of such hypotheses will require further clinical investigation.

It is also possible that PDE4 inhibitors could be developed for the treatment of asthma, or at least some subgroups of asthma that may respond to such therapy. Asthma is also a disease with many different phenotypes, and the asthma syndrome consists of multiple subgroups. Some of these subgroups do not respond efficiently to inhaled glucocorticoid therapy, and could therefore be targeted with alternative anti-inflammatory therapy.[66] Therefore, studies of PDE4 inhibitors specifically in asthma patients who classically do not respond greatly to inhaled glucocorticoids, including patients with asthma but without signs of eosinophilia,[65] would be interesting to perform.

12.10   Summary

PDE4 inhibitors have anti-inflammatory effects that primarily relate to cells that are less responsive to glucocorticoids, such as neutrophils. Also, PDE4-related effects have been documented on other inflammatory cells such as monocytes and macrophages, as well as CD8 T-cells. The clinical effects on lung function in COPD are modest with most available treatments, and this is also the case for all tested PDE4 inhibitors. However, beneficial effects are observed on exacerbation frequency in subgroups of COPD, which is the key reason for this class of treatment having achieved marketing approval. These findings may also argue that some but not all patients with COPD will benefit from drugs that target PDE4 enzymes. It should also be noted that systemic side effects, such as nausea, are quite frequent and dose limiting for PDE4 inhibitors.

To date, one PDE4 inhibitor, roflumilast, is available for the treatment of COPD, but several additional drugs will most likely be introduced to the marketplace in the years to come. Some of these novel drugs may be given by inhalation, which might reduce systemic side effects. It is also possible that the anti-inflammatory effects of PDE4 inhibitors could affect disease mechanisms that current therapies are unable to treat. It will become clearer in the future whether treatments with PDE4 inhibitors have beneficial effects on COPD-related mortality, systemic processes and comorbid diseases.

References

1. Barnes PJ. Immunology of asthma and chronic obstructive pulmonary disease. Nat Rev Immunol 2008;8:183–92.
2. Calverley PM, Anderson JA, Celli B, et al. Salmeterol and fluticasone propionate and survival in chronic obstructive pulmonary disease. New Engl J Med 2007;356:775–89.

3. Pauwels RA, Löfdahl CG, Laitinen LA, et al. Long-term treatment with inhaled budesonide in persons with mild chronic obstructive pulmonary disease who continue smoking. European Respiratory Society Study on Chronic Obstructive Pulmonary Disease. New Engl J Med 1999;340:1948–53.

4. Pauwels RA, Buist AS, Calverley PM, Jenkins CR, Hurd SS; GOLD Scientific Committee. Global strategy for the diagnosis, management, and prevention of chronic obstructive pulmonary disease. NHLBI/WHO Global Initiative for Chronic Obstructive Lung Disease (GOLD) Workshop summary. Am J Respir Crit Care Med 2001;163:1256–76.

5. Calverley PM. COPD: what is the unmet need? Br J Pharmacol 2008;155:487–93.

6. Pagès L, Gavaldà A, Lehner MD. PDE4 inhibitors: a review of current developments (2005–2009). Expert Opin Ther Pat 2009;19:1501–19.

7. Teixeira MM, Gristwood RW, Cooper N, Hellewell PG. Phosphodiesterase (PDE)4 inhibitors: anti-inflammatory drugs of the future? Trends Pharmacol Sci 1997;18:164–71.

8. Conti M, Beavo J. Biochemistry and physiology of cyclic nucleotide phosphodiesterases: essential components in cyclic nucleotide signaling. Annu Rev Biochem 2007;76:481–511 [review].

9. Cazzola M. The divergent opinions of regulatory authorities on roflumilast are puzzling but we need new drugs for treating chronic obstructive pulmonary disease. Ther Adv Respir Dis 2010;4:195–8.

10. Sanford M. Roflumilast: in chronic obstructive pulmonary disease. Drugs 2010;70:1615–27.

11. Truitt EB Jr. Therapeutic risks of aminophylline. GP 1959;20:101.

12. Churg A, Wright JL. Testing drugs in animal models of cigarette smoke-induced chronic obstructive pulmonary disease. Proc Am Thorac Soc 2009;6:550–2.

13. Kroegel C, Foerster M. Phosphodiesterase-4 inhibitors as a novel approach for the treatment of respiratory disease: cilomilast. Expert Opin Investig Drugs 2007;16:109–24.

14. Boswell-Smith V, Spina D, Page CP. Phosphodiesterase inhibitors. Br J Pharmacol 2006; 147:S252–S257.

15. Seftel AD. Phosphodiesterase type 5 inhibitor differentiation based on selectivity, pharmacokinetic, and efficacy profiles. Clin Cardiol 2004;27(4 Suppl 1):I14–19 [review].

16. Fan Chung K. Phosphodiesterase inhibitors in airways disease. Eur J Pharmacol 2006;533:110–7.

17. Jin SL, Goya S, Nakae S, et al. Phosphodiesterase 4B is essential for T(H)2-cell function and development of airway hyperresponsiveness in allergic asthma. J Allergy Clin Immunol 2010;126:1252.

18. Toward TJ, Broadley KJ. Airway function, oedema, cell infiltration and nitric oxide generation in conscious ozone-exposed guinea-pigs: effects of dexamethasone and rolipram. Br J Pharmacol 2002;136:735–45.

19. Boswell-Smith V, Page CP. Roflumilast: a phosphodiesterase-4 inhibitor for the treatment of respiratory disease. Expert Opin Investig Drugs 2006;15:1105–13.

20. Karish SB, Gagnon JM. The potential role of roflumilast: the new phosphodiesterase-4 inhibitor. Ann Pharmacother 2006;40:1096–104.

21. Martina SD, Ismail MS, Vesta KS. Cilomilast: orally active selective phosphodiesterase-4 inhibitor for treatment of chronic obstructive pulmonary disease. Ann Pharmacother 2006; 40:1822–8.

22. Rennard SI, Schachter N, Strek M, Rickard K, Amit O. Cilomilast for COPD: results of a 6-month, placebo-controlled study of a potent, selective inhibitor of phosphodiesterase 4. Chest 2006;129:56–66.

23. Man HW, Schafer P, Wong LM, et al. Discovery of (S)-N-[2-[1-(3-ethoxy-4-methoxyphenyl)-2-methanesulfonylethyl]-1,3-dioxo-2,3-dihydro-1H-isoindol-4-yl] acetamide (apremilast), a potent

and orally active phosphodiesterase 4 and tumor necrosis factor-alpha inhibitor. J Med Chem 2009;52:1522–4.

24. BioCentury Online Intelligence. Revamilist GRC 4039, http://www.biocentury.com/products/grc_4039 (accessed 12 May 2011).

25. Dance with Shadows. Glenmark stops oglemilast (GRC3886) development programme for COPD & asthma with Forest, http://www.dancewithshadows.com/pillscribe/glenmark-stops-oglemilast-grc3886-development-programme-for-copd-asthma-with-forest/ (accessed 12 May 2011).

26. Orexo. OX914 – against COPD and asthma, http://www.orexo.com/en/Portfolio/OX-914/ (accessed 12 May 2011).

27. GlaxoSmithKline. Clinical Study Register, http://www.gsk-clinicalstudyregister.com/ (accessed 12 May 2011).

28. Singh D, Petavy F, Macdonald AJ, Lazaar AL, O'Connor BJ. The inhaled phosphodiesterase 4 inhibitor GSK256066 reduces allergen challenge responses in asthma. Respir Res 2010;11:26.

29. Boswell-Smith V, Spina D, Oxford AW, Comer MB, Seeds EA, Page CP. The pharmacology of two novel long-acting phosphodiesterase 3/4 inhibitors, RPL554 [9,10-dimethoxy-2(2,4,6-trimethylphenylimino)-3-(n-carbamoyl-2-aminoethyl)-3,4,6,7-tetrahydro-2H-pyrimido[6,1-a]isoquinolin-4-one] and RPL565 [6,7-dihydro-2-(2,6-diisopropylphenoxy)-9,10-dimethoxy-4H-pyrimido[6,1-a]isoquinolin-4-one]. J Pharmacol Exp Ther 2006;318:840–8.

30. Souness JE, Griffin M, Maslen C, et al. Evidence that cyclic AMP phosphodiesterase inhibitors suppress TNF alpha generation from human monocytes by interacting with a 'low-affinity' phosphodiesterase 4 conformer. Br J Pharmacol 1996;118:649–58.

31. Verghese MW, McConnell RT, Lenhard JM, Hamacher L, Jin SL. Regulation of distinct cyclic AMP-specific phosphodiesterase (phosphodiesterase type 4) isozymes in human monocytic cells. Mol Pharmacol 1995;47:1164–71.

32. Grootendorst DC, Gauw SA, Verhoosel RM, et al. Reduction in sputum neutrophil and eosinophil numbers by the PDE4 inhibitor roflumilast in patients with COPD. Thorax 2007;62:1081–7.

33. Martorana PA, Beume R, Lucattelli M, Wollin L, Lungarella G. Roflumilast fully prevents emphysema in mice chronically exposed to cigarette smoke. Am J Respir Crit Care Med 2005;172:848–53.

34. Kuss H, Hoefgen N, Johanssen S, Kronbach T, Rundfeldt C. In vivo efficacy in airway disease models of N-(3,5-dichloropyrid-4-yl)-[1-(4-fluorobenzyl)-5-hydroxy-indole-3-yl]-glyoxylic acid amide (AWD 12-281), a selective phosphodiesterase 4 inhibitor for inhaled administration. J Pharmacol Exp Ther 2003;307:373–85.

35. Jones NA, Boswell-Smith V, Lever R, Page CP. The effect of selective phosphodiesterase isoenzyme inhibition on neutrophil function in vitro. Pulm Pharmacol Ther 2005;18:93–101.

36. Johnson FJ, Reynolds LJ, Toward TJ. Elastolytic activity and alveolar epithelial type-1 cell damage after chronic LPS inhalation: effects of dexamethasone and rolipram. Toxicol Appl Pharmacol 2005;207:257–65.

37. Leclerc O, Lagente V, Planquois JM, et al. Involvement of MMP-12 and phosphodiesterase type 4 in cigarette smoke-induced inflammation in mice. Eur Respir J 2006;27:1102–9.

38. Hatzelmann A, Morcillo EJ, Lungarella G, et al. The preclinical pharmacology of roflumilast – a selective, oral phosphodiesterase 4 inhibitor in development for chronic obstructive pulmonary disease. Pulm Pharmacol Ther 2010;23:235–56.

39. Wollin L, Marx D, Wohlsen A, Beume R. Roflumilast inhibition of pulmonary leukotriene production and bronchoconstriction in ovalbumin-sensitized and -challenged Guinea pigs. J Asthma 2005;42:873–8.

40. Sousa LP, Lopes F, Silva DM, et al. PDE4 inhibition drives resolution of neutrophilic inflammation by inducing apoptosis in a PKA-PI3K/Akt-dependent and NF-kappaB-independent manner. J Leukoc Biol 2010;87:895–904.

41. Klut ME, Doerschuk CM, Van Eeden SF, Burns AR, Hogg JC. Activation of neutrophils within pulmonary microvessels of rabbits exposed to cigarette smoke. Am J Respir Cell Mol Biol 1993;9:82–9.

42. Blease K, Burke-Gaffney A, Hellewell PG. Modulation of cell adhesion molecule expression and function on human lung microvascular endothelial cells by inhibition of phosphodiesterases 3 and 4. Br J Pharmacol 1998;124:229–37.

43. Netherton SJ, Sutton JA, Wilson LS, Carter RL, Maurice DH. Both protein kinase A and exchange protein activated by cAMP coordinate adhesion of human vascular endothelial cells. Circ Res 2007;101:768–7.

44. Barber R, Baillie GS, Bergmann R, et al. Differential expression of PDE4 cAMP phosphodiesterase isoforms in inflammatory cells of smokers with COPD, smokers without COPD, and nonsmokers. Am J Physiol Lung Cell Mol Physiol 2004;287:L332–43.

45. Seldon PM, Meja KK, Giembycz MA. Rolipram, salbutamol and prostaglandin E2 suppress TNFalpha release from human monocytes by activating Type II cAMP-dependent protein kinase. Pulm Pharmacol Ther 2005;18:277–84.

46. Hidi R, Timmermans S, Liu E, et al. Phosphodiesterase and cyclic adenosine monophosphate-dependent inhibition of T-lymphocyte chemotaxis. Eur Respir J 2000;15:342–9.

47. Giembycz MA, Corrigan CJ, Seybold J, Newton R, Barnes PJ. Identification of cyclic AMP phosphodiesterases 3, 4 and 7 in human CD4+ and CD8+ T-lymphocytes: role in regulating proliferation and the biosynthesis of interleukin-2. Br J Pharmacol 1996;118:1945–58.

48. Tang HF, Chen JQ, Xie QM, et al. The role of PDE4 in pulmonary inflammation and goblet cell hyperplasia in allergic rats. Biochim Biophys Acta 2006;1762:525–32. Erratum in Biochim Biophys Acta 2006;1762:781.

49. Barnes AP, Livera G, Huang P, et al. Phosphodiesterase 4D forms a cAMP diffusion barrier at the apical membrane of the airway epithelium. J Biol Chem 2005;280:7997–8003.

50. Sabatini F, Petecchia L, Boero S, et al. A phosphodiesterase 4 inhibitor, roflumilast N-oxide, inhibits human lung fibroblast functions in vitro. Pulm Pharmacol Ther 2010;23:283–91.

51. Wohlsen A, Hirrle A, Tenor H, Marx D, Beume R. Effect of cyclic AMP-elevating agents on airway ciliary beat frequency in central and lateral airways in rat precision-cut lung slices. Eur J Pharmacol 2010;635:177–8.

52. Cervin A, Lindgren S. The effect of selective phosphodiesterase inhibitors on mucociliary activity in the upper and lower airways in vitro. Auris Nasus Larynx 1998;25:269–76.

53. Mori H, Nose T, Ishitani K, et al. Phosphodiesterase 4 inhibitor GPD-1116 markedly attenuates the development of cigarette smoke-induced emphysema in senescence-accelerated mice P1 strain. Am J Physiol Lung Cell Mol Physiol 2008;294:L196–204.

54. Rabe KF, Bateman ED, O'Donnell D, Witte S, Bredenbröker D, Bethke TD. Roflumilast – an oral anti-inflammatory treatment for chronic obstructive pulmonary disease: a randomised controlled trial. Lancet 2005;366:563–71.

55. Rennard SI, Schachter N, Strek M, Rickard K, Amit O. Cilomilast for COPD: results of a 6-month, placebo-controlled study of a potent, selective inhibitor of phosphodiesterase 4. Chest 2006;129:56–66.

56. Calverley PM, Sanchez-Toril F, McIvor A, Teichmann P, Bredenbroeker D, Fabbri LM. Effect of 1-year treatment with roflumilast in severe chronic obstructive pulmonary disease. Am J Respir Crit Care Med 2007;176:154–61.

57. Calverley PM, Rabe KF, Goehring UM, Kristiansen S, Fabbri LM, Martinez FJ; M2-124 and M2-125 study groups. Roflumilast in symptomatic chronic obstructive pulmonary disease: two randomised clinical trials. Lancet 2009;374:685–94.

58. Fabbri LM, Calverley PM, Izquierdo-Alonso JL, et al.; M2-127 and M2-128 study groups. Roflumilast in moderate-to-severe chronic obstructive pulmonary disease treated with longacting bronchodilators: two randomised clinical trials. Lancet 2009;374:695–703.

59. Bustamante-Fermosel A, De Miguel-Yanes JM, Duffort-Falcó M, Muñoz J. Mortality-related factors after hospitalization for acute exacerbation of chronic obstructive pulmonary disease: the burden of clinical features. Am J Emerg Med 2007;25:515–22.

60. Mohan A, Premanand R, Reddy LN, et al. Clinical presentation and predictors of outcome in patients with severe acute exacerbation of chronic obstructive pulmonary disease requiring admission to intensive care unit. BMC Pulm Med 2006;6:27.

61. Roca B, Almagro P, López F, et al.; For the ECCO Working Group on COPD, Spanish Society of Internal Medicine. Factors associated with mortality in patients with exacerbation of chronic obstructive pulmonary disease hospitalized in General Medicine departments. Intern Emerg Med 2011;6:47–54.

62. Waddleton D, Wu W, Feng Y, et al. Phosphodiesterase 3 and 4 comprise the major cAMP metabolizing enzymes responsible for insulin secretion in INS-1 (832/13) cells and rat islets. Biochem Pharmacol 2008;76:884–93.

63. Zhang HT. Cyclic AMP-specific phosphodiesterase-4 as a target for the development of antidepressant drugs. Curr Pharm Des 2009;15:1688–98.

64. O'Byrne PM, Gauvreau G. Phosphodiesterase-4 inhibition in COPD. Lancet 2009;374:665–7.

65. Berry M, Morgan A, Shaw DE, et al. Pathological features and inhaled corticosteroid response of eosinophilic and non-eosinophilic asthma. Thorax 2007;62:1043–9.

13

Biological therapies in development for COPD

J. Morjaria* and R. Polosa†

*Department of Infection, Inflammation and Repair, University of Southampton, Southampton, UK
†Dipartimento di Medicina Interna e Specialistica, Centro Antifumo Universitario, Università di Catania, Catania, Italy

13.1   Introduction

Chronic obstructive pulmonary disease (COPD) is a progressive and debilitating disease that affects millions of people and is projected to become the third most common cause of death worldwide by 2020.[1] COPD is characterized by a persistent inflammatory response that cannot be reversed and generally leads to progressive decline in lung function, respiratory failure, cor pulmonale and death.[2] The persistent inflammatory response of the airways in COPD is typically associated with smoking,[3,4] but environmental pollutants are also important causes in developing countries.[5]

Studies have reported that smokers have a more rapid rate of decline in forced expiratory volume in 1 second (FEV_1).[6] Although smoking has been closely associated with development of COPD, only 10–20% of smokers develop the condition,[7,8] suggesting that genetic predispositions and other environmental factors play a role in the disease pathogenesis.

The tragedy of COPD is that in most cases the cause of the disease and best way to prevent its incidence and development are already known – smoking cessation, at least in the early stages. However, the addictive properties of tobacco make smoking cessation difficult despite intensive interventions. Furthermore, it is known that once inflammation is established in COPD, it persists even when smoking has stopped. This inflammation responds marginally or not at all to current anti-inflammatory drugs including high-dose inhaled corticosteroids.[9]

The inflammatory infiltrate in the airways or alveoli of patients with COPD is distinctive compared to asthma. It is characterized by elevated numbers of neutrophils, monocytes/macrophages, $CD8^+$ and $CD4^+$ T-cells, B-cells, dendritic cells (DCs),

Advances in Combination Therapy for Asthma and COPD, First Edition. Edited by Jan Lötvall.
© 2012 John Wiley & Sons, Ltd. Published 2012 by John Wiley & Sons, Ltd.

natural killer (NK) cells and/or mast cells in the airway walls, alveolar compartments and vascular smooth muscle.[10–12] This chronic inflammation of the lung typically results in disease progression leading to mucus hypersecretion and structurally irreversible lung lesions.

As our understanding of the pathology of COPD has increased it has been established that the progressive pulmonary inflammation that is associated with COPD is likely to be a key target for novel therapeutics. Thus, it is anticipated that drugs that reduce pulmonary inflammation may provide effective, disease-modifying therapies. Unfortunately, airways inflammation in COPD responds poorly to corticosteroids.[13,14] Indeed, corticosteroids are known to prolong neutrophil survival by inhibiting their apoptosis.[15,16] Here, we specifically consider the potential of biological therapies that are currently in clinical development for COPD and discuss how these drugs might modulate pulmonary inflammation and remodelling in this disease. Figure 13.1 summarizes the inflammatory cells and mediators thought to be involved in the pathogenesis of COPD.

13.2   Inflammatory cells involved in the pathogenesis of COPD

The innate defence system of the lung includes the mucociliary clearance apparatus and the epithelial barrier, in addition to the coagulation and inflammatory cascades.[11,17,18] Although the innate immunity is swift in onset, it is uniform, non-specific and has no memory. Smoking impedes the innate immune system by increasing mucus production and reducing mucociliary clearance, by damaging the epithelial barrier and stimulating the migration of various cells into the injured tissues. Furthermore, smoking stimulates the humoral and cellular components of the adaptive immune response to provide a much more specific and very diverse reaction that has exquisite memory for prior interaction to foreign material to the lung.[10,19] There is compelling evidence implicating macrophages and neutrophils in the pathogenesis of COPD.

Macrophages

Macrophages are the most abundant cell type in bronchoalveolar lavage fluid (BALF) of COPD patients.[20,21] Also there is a 5–10-fold increase in macrophage numbers in sputum, airways and lung parenchyma,[22,23] and their numbers correlate with severity of the disease.[20,21] Smoking and other noxious particles activate macrophages to produce tumor necrosis factor-α (TNF-α), monocyte chemotactic peptide-1 (MCP-1), reactive oxygen species and neutrophil chemotactic factors such as interleukin-8 (IL-8) and leukotriene B_4 (LTB$_4$), which are elevated in sputum from COPD patients.[22] In addition to this, macrophages also secrete elastolytic enzymes including matrix metalloproteinases (MMP)-1, MMP-2, MMP-9, MMP-12 and cathepsins K, L and S, which together mediate the lung parenchymal damage.[6] Healthy smokers express more MMP-9 than normal subjects.[24] Moreover, in COPD patients there is a marked

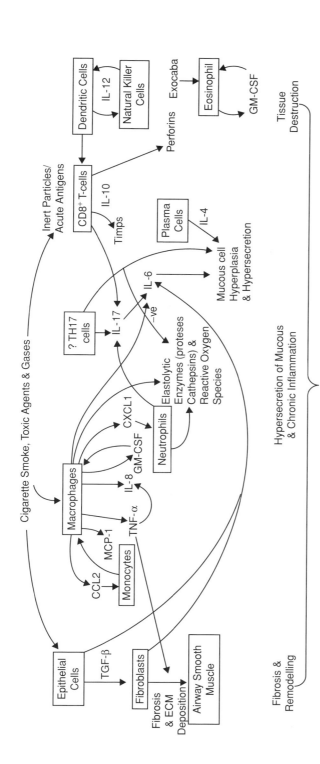

Figure 13.1 Effects of cigarette smoking and noxious gases on the lungs. Cigarette smoke (and other irritants) activate epithelial cells to generate transforming growth factor-β (TGF-β), which in turn stimulates fibroblasts to cause fibrosis and extracellular matrix (ECM) deposition, besides producing inflammatory cytokines involved in the inflammatory process. Macrophages when activated by cigarette smoke initiate a myriad of cytokines and chemokines involved in inflammation, mucus secretion, tissue destruction and fibrosis. This is accomplished directly, or indirectly by attracting other inflammatory cells that in turn release proteolytic enzymes, such as neutrophil elastase and matrix metalloproteinases. The noxious gases also stimulate CD8⁺ T-cells, which are involved in the alveolar wall destruction leading to emphysema. More recently, T-helper-17 (Th17) cells have been implicated in the inflammatory and mucus hypersecretory pathogenesis of COPD. MCP-1, monocyte chemotactic protein-1; TNF-α, tumor necrosis factor-α; IL, interleukin; GM-CSF, granulocyte-monocyte colony-stimulating factor; TIMPs, tissue inhibitors of metalloproteinases.

increase in macrophages with their augmented elastolytic activity.[25,26] Normal alveolar macrophages (AM) demonstrated a distinct reduction in the ability to consume apoptotic cells in relation to consumption of inert articles and pathogens.[27-29] This ability has been reported to be further diminished in COPD, where there is an attendant increase in the apoptotic cell build-up.[30,31] It is postulated that the apoptotic cells induce an inflammatory state in macrophages on recognition,[32,33] hence resulting in an abnormal clearance of these cells. This autoimmunity induced by the apoptotic cells may result in the promotion of inflammation.

Activation of AM is inhibited by transforming growth factor-β1 (TGF-β1) bound to $\alpha_v\beta_6$-intergrin on alveolar epithelial cells. Lack of this inhibition stimulates MMP-12 production and emphysema in mice.[34,35] Furthermore, restraint in the propagation of inflammation is achieved by the controlled synthesis of proinflammatory mediators through regulated DNA binding with transcription factors – Ref-1 and activator protein-1 (AP-1)[36] – and the lack of ability to stimulate naive T-cells despite their ability to migrate to local lymph nodes.[37] Of note, AM lack the autocrine amplification of inflammation unlike other phagocytic cells via the production of interferon (IFN)-β and AP-1 activation. They require exogenous IFN-β to mount a second phase of defence,[38,39] hence AM response is swift but confined to synthesizing destructive mediators without added signals.

Neutrophils

Sputum, BALF and bronchial biopsies from COPD patients have elevated neutrophil numbers. Moreover, smoking has been demonstrated to induce neutrophilia systemically with sequestration into the pulmonary capillaries.[22,23,40,41] Chemoattractants such as IL-8, LTB$_4$ and granulocyte-macrophage colony-stimulating factor (GM-CSF) are involved in the mobilization of neutrophils into the lung interstitium, and hence also their levels are increased in the airways of COPD patients.[42-44] Furthermore, neutrophil survival in the airways may be prolonged by GM-CSF and granulocyte colony-stimulating factor (G-CSF).[6] Neutrophils are a rich source of inflammatory mediators including reactive oxidant species (ROS), lipid mediators and tissue proteases; these include neutrophil elastase (NE), cathepsin G, protease-3, MMP-8 and MMP-9.[6,45,46] Of note, neutrophil numbers in airways not only correlate with disease severity,[20,22] but also with rate of decline in lung function.[47]

CD8$^+$ T-cells

It has been reported that CD8$^+$ T-cell numbers in the lungs of COPD patients are an excellent predictor of decline in lung function and morbidity.[10,48,49] It is thought their presence in COPD lungs contributes to the activation of macrophages to release neutrophilic chemotactic factors and proteases.[10,48] Furthermore, granzymes, which are effector protease molecules of CD8$^+$ T-cells, have an increased expression in type II pneumocytes in patients with severe COPD.[50]

Eosinophils

Eosinophils have been demonstrated to be elevated markedly during COPD exacerbations.[51] Furthermore, inflammatory mediators implicated in the pathogenesis of COPD induce synthesis of GM-CSF by eosinophils in an autocrine mechanism.[52]

Dendritic cells (DCs) and natural killer (NK) cells

Normal lung tissue contains potent antigen-presenting cells in the form of DCs,[53] which, using the CC chemokine receptor 7 (CCR7), migrate to the regional lymph nodes, where they activate the proliferation of naive T-cells. All four types of DCs found in the systemic circulation have been detected in the lungs.[54,55] DCs and NK cells are suggested to regulate each other's maturation reciprocally.[56] Thus, NK cells exposed to DC-produced IL-12 stimulate DC maturation and their capacity to secrete IL-12.[57]

Plasma cells

There are elevated numbers of inflammatory cells in the airway submucosal glands as well as increased mucus in the larger airways of smokers with chronic bronchitis. Plasma cells associated with these glands express IL-4, which is thought to perpetuate this increased mucus production.[58]

Epithelial cells and fibroblasts

The role in COPD of epithelial cells and interactions in the underlying cell layers is poorly understood.[59-61] Cigarette smoke may not only stimulate release of proinflammatory mediators, but also disrupt the interface with fibroblast and smooth muscle cells.[62] Smoking may injure epithelial cells, possibly leading to a lack of fibroblast proliferation-limiting factors, and hence subsequent progression to fibrosis and extracellular matrix (ECM) disposition. Also, it has been reported that senescence of lung fibroblasts is induced by smoking.[63] Thus, there is linkage between deregulated cell function and deregulated expression and activity of the transcription factor family of the CCAAT/enhancer binding proteins (C/EBP). This family of proteins, which are pivotal controllers of cell differentiation and apoptosis, have been demonstrated to be deregulated in asthma and COPD.[64-67]

13.3   Cytokines and chemokines in COPD

Smoking and noxious airway irritants have been proposed to induce AM, alveolar epithelial cells, T-cells and DCs to produce chemotactic factors for inflammatory cells. Transnasal administration of lipopolysaccahride (LPS) causes marked lung inflammation consisting of neutrophilia, accumulation of AM, and increased expression of cytokines (TNF-α, GM-CSF, G-CSF), chemokines (macrophage inhibitor protein-2, or MIP-2), proteases (MMP-9) and Toll-like receptor (TLR)-4.[68,69] Other cytokines and chemokines have also been implicated in the pathogenesis of COPD.[70] Although the mechanisms of action of the cytokines and chemokines are intertwined, involving various types of cells in the airways, we discuss them individually below.

Cytokines

Tumor necrosis factor-α (TNF-α)

Tumor necrosis factor-α is an extremely potent proinflammatory mediator. There have been reports that TNF-α expression in patients with COPD is elevated, due to either induction by cigarette smoke or genetic aberrations.[71–73] TNF-α has the capacity to induce inflammation not only by direct mechanisms, but also by indirect ones. The activation of TNF-alpha receptor (TNFR) induces the production and release of a number of inflammatory mediators, which in turn induce further inflammatory effects. These include a broad spectrum of proinflammatory cytokines (GM-CSF, IL-1, TNF-α, IL-6),[74,75] chemokines (CXCL8, MCP-1), proteases (MMP-9, MMP-12)[74–76] and adhesion molecules (intercellular adhesion molecule-1 (ICAM-1), p-selectin).[77,78] Furthermore, TNF-α has been implicated in various *in vitro* and *in vivo* studies in the induction of airway mucous cell metaplasia and hypersecretion,[79,80] decreased interepithelial binding and cell death,[81,82] emphysematous lesions and alveolar collagen deposition in murine alveolar walls,[83] and induction of IFN-γ receptors on epithelial cells.[84] IFN-γ in turn inhibits the proliferation of and decreases desmosome formation between epithelial cells.[82]

In healthy smokers sputum TNF-α levels were comparable with those in smoking-related COPD patients, but elevated neutrophil numbers and levels of soluble (s) TNFR-55 were noted in the diseased patients.[85] Furthermore, the sputum sTNFR correlated with the degree of airflow limitation. TNF-α may also be involved in the progression of COPD and disability as circulating TNF-α levels have been found to be associated with increased dyspnoea severity and inversely correlated with Po_2.[86,87] Not only does TNF-α have a pivotal role in lung inflammation perpetuated by neutrophilia in bronchial airways and parenchyma, but also it is involved systematically in 'inflammatory weight loss'.[88] Systemic TNF-α levels in patients with COPD and weight loss were reported to be significantly elevated when compared to COPD patients with stable weight or with age- and gender-matched healthy volunteers.[89]

Hence antagonizing the effects of TNF-α, the multifunctional cytokine, may have a role in the treatment of COPD. Trials of TNF-α antagonism are discussed later in this chapter.

Interleukin-6 (IL-6)

Interleukin-6 is a potent proinflammatory mediator, produced by a variety of cells, and manifests its action by stimulating epithelial and other structural cells as well as leucocytes.[70,90] Also, IL-6 is pivotal inducer of acute-phase protein synthesis from the liver including C-reactive protein (CRP), fibrinogen, haptoglobin and serum amyloid

A.[90–92] Furthermore, IL-6 is not only involved in the activation, growth, differentiation and survival of T-cells,[93–95] but also in antibody synthesis by B-cells.[96]

Levels of IL-6 are elevated in exhaled breath condensate, induced sputum, BALF and blood in COPD patients[91,97,98] during stable disease, and increase further during exacerbations.[92,99] *In vivo* studies confirm a role for IL-6 in augmentation of leucocyte recruitment to inflammatory sites.[100] Furthermore, it is suggested that levels of IL-6 in BALF correlate with the severity of COPD.[98] Based on these reports, IL-6 inhibition may have a role in the treatment of COPD patients. In rheumatoid arthritis (RA), IL-6 blockade has been shown to be helpful.[101] Unfortunately, there are as yet no published clinical trials in the literature on the antagonism of IL-6 in COPD patients.

Interleukin-10 (IL-10)

Interleukin-10 is considered to be a mainly anti-inflammatory cytokine because it inhibits the synthesis of many inflammatory mediators and the activity of CD4$^+$ T-cells.[70] Also, IL-10 inhibits certain proteases (MMP-9) and increases the release of tissue inhibitors of MMPs (TIMPs), the endogenous inhibitors of MMPs.[102] Bronchial biopsies of COPD patients show increased expression of IL-10.[103] Furthermore, CD8$^+$ T-cells, which are known to synthesize IL-10, have been reported to be elevated in BALF of patients with COPD compared to healthy smokers and non-smokers.[104] In addition, it has been reported that increased systemic IL-10 levels, in patients with a minimal threshold level of systemic TNF-α, correlate with the severity of COPD.[105]

Although there are no studies in the literature of increasing IL-10 levels locally or systemically in COPD using recombinant (rh) IL-10, reports suggest it to be efficacious in other inflammatory conditions. Thus, rhIL-10 drugs that activate the unique signal transduction pathways activated by IL-10 receptor or drugs that increase endogenous IL-10 synthesis may prove to be of therapeutic relevance.

Granulocyte-macrophage colony-stimulating factor (GM-CSF)

Granulocyte-macrophage colony-stimulating factor is a multifunctional proinflammatory cytokine produced by mesenchymal cells, endothelium, epithelial cells and monocytes/macrophages as well as an autocrine mechanism.[106] Its functions include accelerated myelopoeisis; priming of leucocytes for activation and survival at inflammatory sites;[107,108] development of small airway fibrosis;[109,110] priming for sensitization to aeroallergens; direct inflammatory responses to the PP10 fraction (particles $<$10 μm), which has been implicated in COPD exacerbations;[111] and driving the terminal differentiation of AM by activating the transcription factor PU-1.[112] Concentrations of GM-CSF in BALF are elevated in stable disease[113] and during exacerbations.[114] Smoking has been reported to upregulate GM-CSF mRNA.[115] Of note, although *in vitro* GM-CSF levels from COPD lung tissue are in plentiful, its release is not antagonized by steroids.[106] As glucocorticosteroids require intact histone deacetylase (HDAC), the reduced HDAC 2, 5 and 8 in COPD[116] may explain the glucocorticosteroid refractoriness observed in COPD.

Murine model studies of subchronic exposure to cigarette smoke (4 days) have shown an increase in inflammatory cells, cytokines, chemokines, proteases and TLRs in BALF.[117] Furthermore, intrinsically administered GM-CSF antagonism to these mice significantly attenuated BALF macrophages and neutrophils, as well as whole lung proteases' mRNA, cytokines and chemokines.[115] Moreover, there was dampening of cigarette smoke-induced macrophage proliferation. Hence, anti-GM-CSF antibody is efficacious in animal models of COPD where corticosteroids have little or no effect. Antagonism of GM-CSF is also effective in experimental exacerbations of COPD triggered by bacterial surrogates and live viruses.[118] Of note, GM-CSF blockade results in the development of alveolar proteinosis because surfactant clearance is dependent on a mature PU-1-dependent macrophage pool in the lung,[112,119,120] which is reversible on stopping the blockade. Thus attenuating, but not entirely inhibiting, inflammation by targeting GM-CSF with clinically titrated doses could provide a novel and useful therapeutic strategy to combat COPD, its acute exacerbations and their sequelae. However, as yet, there have been no clinical trials of GM-CSF antagonism.

Interleukin-17 (IL-17), interleukin-18 (IL-18) and interleukin-23 (IL-23)

The inflammation in COPD has primarily been considered to be T-helper-1 cell (Th1) mediated; however, recent developments in the understanding of cytokine biology have brought to light the presence of another discrete subpopulation of CD4$^+$ T-cells, the Th17 phenotype.[121] By their designated name of Th17 cells, the cells synthesize the cytokines IL-17A and IL-17F. IL-17 is also produced by the other cells including CD8$^+$ T-cells, $\gamma\delta$ T-cells, NK cells and neutrophils, but not by Th1 or Th2 CD4$^+$ T-cells.[122] Besides the production of IL-17A and IL-17F, Th17 cells also produce IL-6, TNF-α and GM-CSF and express receptors for IL-18 and IL-23, which are mainly produced by monocytes, AM and DCs.

Interleukin-17 stimulates mesenchymal and bronchial epithelial cells to produce IL-6;[123] both of these cytokines have been implicated in increased production of mucus via induction of *MUC5AC* and *MUC5B* genes in bronchial epithelial goblet cells and submucosal glands.[124] Moreover, IL-17 potently stimulates bronchial epithelial cells to generate CXCL8 (IL-8), a chemoattractant for neutrophils,[125,126] and the overexpression of IL-17 in mice displays lung inflammation.[127] Of note, IL-17A is itself generated by IL-23, a cytokine of the innate immune system, suggesting the existence of a positive feedback loop.[128–130] This feedback loop involving IL-17 and IL23 may explain the persistent and refractory inflammation in COPD despite smoking cessation.

Th17 cells have potent inflammatory properties and have been demonstrated to play a pivotal part in other inflammatory and autoimmune conditions such as RA and psoriasis.[121,127,131] From murine model studies it has been reported that the lack of IL-23 receptors and IL-17 knockout mice are resistant to several autoimmune conditions of collagen-induced arthritis.[132–134] It has been suggested that COPD is an autoimmune condition.[135] Given the importance of Th17 cells in COPD and other autoimmune diseases it may be inferred that Th17 cells could be pivotal in the development of COPD;

more work needs to be done to establish the function of these cells in inflammatory pathways, and the potential of therapeutic options involving inhibition of the IL-17/IL-23 feedback loops. Currently, no clinical studies of antagonism of either of these cytokines have been reported.

Chemokines and chemokine receptors

CXC chemokines and receptors

The chemokines CXCL8 (IL-8) and CXCL1 (growth-related oncogene-1 (GRO-1)) are expressed by mesenchymal, structural and inflammatory cells, and their expression can be stimulated by TNF-α, cigarette smoke and endotoxins.[70,136] They act via the receptors CXCR1 and CXCR2. They are key mediators of neutrophil and monocyte chemotaxis, and degranulation – via CXCR1 and CXCR2[70,136] – and of wound re-pair, angiogenesis, epithelial proliferation and migration, endothelial migration and neovascularization – via CXCR2.[137–139] Levels of CXCL8 and CXCL1 are elevated in induced sputum and BALF in COPD patients compared to healthy smokers and non-smokers.[22,42,98] In murine models of cigarette smoke exposure, CXCR2 antagonism resulted in attenuated polymorphonuclear (PMN) leucocyte accumulation,[140,141] and likewise in other experimental murine models with IL-8 antagonism.[142,143]

Since CXCL8 and CXCL1 are capable of inducing epithelial repair via CXCR2, the use of antagonists to CXCR2 may impair repair and hence not be of much benefit. The use of CXCR1 inhibitors may have a role in COPD as they inhibit the proinflammatory and destructive mediators from inflammatory cells. Moreover, CXCL8 blockage may also be a potential therapeutic target in COPD, and clinical trials of the antagonism of IL-8 are discussed later in this chapter.

CC chemokines and receptors

Macrophages and monocytes express multiple chemokine receptors (CCR1, CCR2 and CCR5), which when bound by ligands (MIP-α/CCL3, MIP-β/CCL4, MCP-1/CCL2, MCP-2/CCL8, MCP-3/CCL7, MCP-4/CCL13) stimulate these cells to migrate *in vitro*.[144–147] However, *in vivo* MCP-1 and CCR2 are important chemoattractants for the above mentioned two cell types (macrophages and monocytes), and the for-mer can also activate and attract mast cells and T-cells.[148,149] CCR2 is the only known receptor for MCP-1.[150] MCP-1 is synthesized by various cells including AM, and mesenchymal and structural cells of the airways;[151,152] and its expression is in-duced by other chemokines (TNF-α and IFN-γ).[76,153] However, IFN-γ inhibits CCR2 expression,[154] suggesting a probable natural inhibitory mechanism for the accumu-lation of macrophages. Multiple studies *in vivo* support distinct roles of MCP-1 and CCR2 in macrophage migration and the specificity of the MCP-1/CCR2 system rather than MIP-1α.[144–147,155–157] MCP-1 is also involved in the stimulation of endothelial wound healing by inducing endothelial migration,[158] angiogenesis,[159] induction of vas-cular smooth muscle hyperplasia,[160] collagen and TGF-β expression by fibroblasts,[161] and expression of adhesion molecules CD11c and CD11b as well as IL-1 and IL-6 by blood monocytes.[162] Also, CCR2 is expressed on human bronchial epithelial cells and MCP-1 may have an autocrine effect on epithelial cells.[151]

Hence, these data confirm a pivotal role for MCP-1 and CCR2 in airway remodelling and inflammation directly or via macrophages/monocytes. Taking this into consideration, various antagonists of both MCP-1 and CCR2 have been developed and tested in murine models,[147,163–165] with clinical and histological improvements in airway inflammation and hyperresponsiveness and bacterial clearance.[145, 156] However, there have been no clinical trials to assess the efficacy of the antagonism of this ligand or its receptor. Caution is needed in their use because in murine models of *Mycobacterium tuberculosis* infection they are ineffective;[146] also it is known that MCP-1 is involved in wound repair and can retard healing.[136]

13.4   Development of biological agents in COPD

Current management of COPD focuses mainly on reducing symptoms using short-acting and long-acting bronchodilators, either as monotherapies or combinations of long-acting β_2-adrenoceptor agonist bronchodilators with inhaled corticosteroids (ICS). The disappointing anti-inflammatory data for ICS either alone or in combination with β_2-adrenoceptor agonists have intensified the search for an effective anti-inflammatory drug for COPD and this remains a key objective for the pharmaceutical industry. In particular drugs that reduce pulmonary inflammation may provide effective, disease-modifying therapies.

Emerging anti-inflammatory therapies currently under clinical investigation may attenuate the chronic pulmonary inflammation targeting a plethora of different molecules. In the next section, we specifically review the status of biological therapies that are currently in clinical development for COPD. Other anti-inflammatory mechanisms in development for COPD such as 5-lipoxygenase inhibition, LTB_4 antagonism, adhesion molecule block, phosphodiesterase-4 inhibition, anaphylatoxin antagonism, inhibition of signal transduction proteins, adenosine signalling modulation, inducible nitric oxide synthase (iNOS) inhibition and antioxidants will not be discussed here.

Anti-TNF-α drugs

As mentioned earlier TNF-α has been implicated in the pathogenesis of COPD both locally and systemically. There have been three studies to assess the efficacy of TNF-α antagonism in COPD;[166–168] these are discussed below, and include both short- and long-term trials. All the trials discussed used infliximab, a monoclonal antibody with a human component (constant region of human IgG1) and a murine component (Fv region of murine anti-human TNF-α antibody). Infliximab works by inhibiting the binding of soluble TNF-α to TNFRs; it neutralizes soluble and membrane-bound TNF-α, and has the potential to dissociate soluble TNFR (sTNFR) complexes.

In the first study, van der Vaart and colleagues[166] performed an exploratory double-blind, placebo-controlled, randomized trial in 22 (14 infliximab; 8 placebo) current smokers with mild-to-moderate COPD. Subjects received three infusions of 5 mg/kg of infliximab or placebo at weeks 0, 2 and 6; the primary outcome measure was percent sputum neutrophil reduction, besides various secondary endpoints of lung function, quality of life (QoL), bronchial hyperresponsiveness (BHR) and exhaled nitric oxide. It was reported that infliximab had no overall positive effect on the percent of sputum neutrophils, lung function, resting energy expenditure or QoL. There were eight subjects in the infliximab group who developed an increasing cough, but no serious adverse events or increase in respiratory infections were reported during 9 weeks of follow-up.

In another small study, TNF-α antagonism using infliximab was assessed in COPD subjects with cachexia, which is characterized by inflammation reflected by elevated TNF-α levels.[167] Not only was systemic inflammation evaluated, but also localized inflammation was monitored using exhaled breath condensate (EBC). In this double-blind, placebo-controlled, randomized study, 41 (16 infliximab; 25 placebo) cachectic moderate-to-severe COPD patients were randomized to receive infliximab at 5 mg/kg or placebo at weeks 0, 2 and 6. Subjects were reviewed at weeks 8, 12 and 26 as well. Although it was noted that in the EBC there were elevated levels of MIP, IL-12, RANTES and sICAM-1 in cachectic COPD patients compared to placebo, treatment with infliximab had no effect on these markers. Furthermore, there were no changes in systemic acute-phase proteins (CRP, fibrinogen and lipopolysaccharide-binding protein), cytokine (IL-6) or sTNFR55. Hence, TNF-α blockade demonstrated no observable reduction in local or systemic markers of inflammation.

Lastly, the longest and largest clinical trial of TNF-α blockade in COPD was conducted to determine the clinical benefit and safety in GOLD-staged moderate-to-severe subjects.[168] This was a multicentre, double-blind, placebo-controlled, randomized trial in which subjects were given infliximab at 3 mg/kg ($n = 78$) or 5 mg/kg ($n = 79$), or placebo ($n = 77$) at weeks 0, 2, 6, 12, 18 and 24. The primary endpoint was a change in the QoL from baseline as measured using the Chronic Respiratory Questionnaire along with other secondary endpoints of lung function, 6-minute walk distance (6MWD) test, transition dyspnoea index (TDI), COPD exacerbations and short form (SF)-36 physical scores. Subjects were followed up till Week 44. Unfortunately, as in to the other clinical trials of TNF-α antagonism in COPD, there were no significant improvements in the primary or secondary endpoints assessed. However, unlike the study of Dentener et al.,[167] a post-hoc analysis reported that younger or cachectic COPD subjects at baseline had significant increases in 6MWD as a result of treatment with infliximab. However, it was also reported that 9 out of 157 in the infliximab-treated arm were diagnosed to have a malignancy during the course of the trial, compared with 1 of 77 of the placebo-treated subjects. Also, there was an increased incidence of pneumonias in the infliximab group compared to placebo, but no infection-related mortality was noted. There was a higher rate of study dropouts in the infliximab group (20–27%) compared to placebo (9%).

Overall, although there is considerable evidence suggesting that TNF-α may play a role in COPD, administration of TNF-α blockade using infliximab for up to 6 months in clinical trials has not shown any subjective or objective improvements. This raises the question as to whether TNF-α is a pivotal cytokine in the pathogenesis of COPD. TNF-α may be useful in small subgroups of COPD patients and hence appropriate selection criteria of these subjects and outcome measures to assess efficacy should be carefully chosen in future trials. Clearly the use of infliximab routinely in moderate-to-severe COPD is not indicated. Besides, TNF-α antagonists in COPD and other inflammatory diseases, such as RA,[169] have shown increased incidences of malignancies and severe infections, and hence the use of these agents needs careful evaluation not only for efficacy but also for safety issues.

IL-8 antagonism

Interleukin-8 is responsible for developing the chemotactic activity of neutrophils and CD8[+] cells; it activates neutrophils by promoting degranulation and elastase release. Mahler and colleagues examined the efficacy and safety of ABX-IL8, a fully human monoclonal IgG2 antibody directed against human IL-8 (CXCL8), in moderate-to-severe COPD subjects, all of whom had a component of chronic bronchitis.[170] They conducted a double-blind, placebo-controlled, multicentre trial in which 109 (59 ABX-IL8, 60 placebo) were enrolled to receive three intravenous infusions of either ABX-IL8 (800 mg loading dose and 400 mg subsequent doses) or placebo over a 3-month period. The primary outcome measure was a reduction in dyspnoea as measured by the TDI, and secondary measures of health status, lung function, 6MWD and rescue inhaler use were also made. It was observed that ABX-IL8 reduced the severity of the dyspnoea, using TDI, at 2 weeks after the initial infusion and this persisted for a 2-month period compared to placebo. However, there were no significant differences in lung function, health status or rescue inhaler use between the two groups. The pilot study did show that treatment with ABX-IL8 is safe and well tolerated as the numbers of adverse events were similar between the two groups. Although the trial showed an improvement in the dyspnoea, the exact mechanism(s) are unclear. Furthermore, it seems that the effect is short-lived as the significant improvement was seen only at week 2 in the follow-up period. Further trials of IL-8 antagonism should probably be better employing an inhalational agent with optimal doses and appropriate endpoints.

Other drug candidates in development

Elevated levels of IL-1β have been measured in the sputum of stable COPD patients, and these correlate with neutrophil number, IL-8 and TNF-α.[171] Most of the evidence for an important role of IL-1β in COPD has originated from work in rodents. Firstly, mice that overexpress IL-1β in lung epithelium during adulthood develop pulmonary inflammation, emphysema and airway remodelling.[172] Secondly, pulmonary inflammation induced by multiple exposure to tobacco smoke in mice is inhibited by treatment with an anti-IL-1β monoclonal antibody.[173] Lastly, IL-1 receptor-knockout mice have significantly reduced emphysema following chronic exposure to tobacco smoke.[174] A monoclonal antibody against IL-1 is currently under clinical development by Novartis.

Also MCP-1 levels are elevated in the sputum from COPD patients and correlate with neutrophil number and lung function (FEV_1).[42] Furthermore, MCP-1 and its receptor, CCR2, appear to be increased on macrophages and epithelial cells obtained from COPD patients.[151] In view of this, Novartis is seeking neutralization of MCP-1 in COPD by means of an anti-MCP-1 monoclonal antibody – ABN912.

13.5 Conclusions

There are several mediators involved in the pathogenesis of COPD, some of which are potential target cytokines (TNF-α, IFN-γ, IL-6, GM-CSF, IL-17/IL-23), chemokines (CXCL8/IL-8, CXCL1, CCL2, CCL3, CCL13) and their receptors, and proteinases (MMPs, neutrophil elastase) and all are potentially rational targets for the development of new treatments for COPD. However, blockade of individual mediators may not be an ideal strategy and may require multiple biological agent combinations to be effective. Future trials should not only look into the best method of administration, optimal dosage and the duration of treatment, but also use appropriate outcome measures and subject selection, and include biomarkers to determine the efficacy as well as mechanism of action of biological agents in COPD. Besides the therapeutic efficacy of future biological agents, it is vital that the benefits of individual or combined mediator-based biological therapy are balanced with the risks of treatments in view of the possibility of increased infections and malignancies. Similarly, vigilance of long-term treatment of biological agents would be of paramount importance whether single or multiple agents are used.

References

1. Lopez AD, Murray CC. The global burden of disease, 1990–2020. Nat Med 1998;4:1241–3.
2. Pauwels RA, Buist AS, Calverley PM, Jenkins CR, Hurd SS. Global strategy for the diagnosis, management, and prevention of chronic obstructive pulmonary disease. NHLBI/WHO Global Initiative for Chronic Obstructive Lung Disease (GOLD) Workshop summary. Am J Respir Crit Care Med 2001;163:1256–76.
3. MacNee W. Oxidants and COPD. Curr Drug Targets Inflamm Allergy 2005;4:627–41.
4. Spurzem JR, Rennard SI. Pathogenesis of COPD. Semin Respir Crit Care Med 2005;26:142–53.
5. Xu X, Weiss ST, Rijcken B, Schouten JP. Smoking, changes in smoking habits, and rate of decline in FEV1: new insight into gender differences. Eur Respir J 1994;7:1056–61.
6. Barnes PJ, Shapiro SD, Pauwels RA. Chronic obstructive pulmonary disease: molecular and cellular mechanisms. Eur Respir J 2003;22:672–88.
7. Cigarette smoking and health. Am J Respir Crit Care Med 1996;153:861–5.
8. Lokke A, Lange P, Scharling H, Fabricius P, Vestbo J. Developing COPD: a 25 year follow up study of the general population. Thorax 2006;61:935–9.
9. Pauwels RA, Lofdahl CG, Laitinen LA, et al. Long-term treatment with inhaled budesonide in persons with mild chronic obstructive pulmonary disease who continue smoking. European Respiratory Society Study on Chronic Obstructive Pulmonary Disease. New Engl J Med 1999;340:1948–53.
10. Hogg JC, Chu F, Utokaparch S, et al. The nature of small-airway obstruction in chronic obstructive pulmonary disease. New Engl J Med 2004;350:2645–53.
11. Kumar V, Abbas AK, Fausto N. Acute and Chronic Inflammation. In: Robbins and Cortran pathological basis of disease. Elsevier Saunders, Philadelphia, 2005;47–86.

12. Grashoff WF, Sont JK, Sterk PJ, et al. Chronic obstructive pulmonary disease: role of bronchiolar mast cells and macrophages. Am J Pathol 1997;151:1785–90.
13. Culpitt SV, Maziak W, Loukidis S, Nightingale JA, Matthews JL, Barnes PJ. Effect of high dose inhaled steroid on cells, cytokines, and proteases in induced sputum in chronic obstructive pulmonary disease. Am J Respir Crit Care Med 1999;160:1635–9.
14. Loppow D, Schleiss MB, Kanniess F, Taube C, Jorres RA, Magnussen H. In patients with chronic bronchitis a four week trial with inhaled steroids does not attenuate airway inflammation. Respir Med 2001;95:115–21.
15. Cox G. Glucocorticoid treatment inhibits apoptosis in human neutrophils. Separation of survival and activation outcomes. J Immunol 1995;154:4719–25.
16. Meagher LC, Cousin JM, Seckl JR, Haslett C. Opposing effects of glucocorticoids on the rate of apoptosis in neutrophilic and eosinophilic granulocytes. J Immunol 1996;156:4422–8.
17. Knowles MR, Boucher RC. Mucus clearance as a primary innate defense mechanism for mammalian airways. J Clin Invest 2002;109:571–7.
18. Simani AS, Inoue S, Hogg JC. Penetration of the respiratory epithelium of guinea pigs following exposure to cigarette smoke. Lab Invest 1974;31:75–81.
19. Buzatu L, Chu FSF, Javadifard A, et al. The accumulation of dendritic and natural killer cells in the small airways at different levels of COPD severity. Proc Am Thorac Soc 2005;2:A135 [abstract].
20. Di Stefano A, Capelli A, Lusuardi M, et al. Severity of airflow limitation is associated with severity of airway inflammation in smokers. Am J Respir Crit Care Med 1998;158:1277–85.
21. MacNee W. Pathogenesis of chronic obstructive pulmonary disease. Proc Am Thorac Soc 2005;2:258–66; discussion 90–1.
22. Keatings VM, Collins PD, Scott DM, Barnes PJ. Differences in interleukin-8 and tumor necrosis factor-alpha in induced sputum from patients with chronic obstructive pulmonary disease or asthma. Am J Respir Crit Care Med 1996;153:530–4.
23. Pesci A, Balbi B, Majori M, et al. Inflammatory cells and mediators in bronchial lavage of patients with chronic obstructive pulmonary disease. Eur Respir J 1998;12:380–6.
24. Lim S, Roche N, Oliver BG, Mattos W, Barnes PJ, Chung KF. Balance of matrix metalloprotease-9 and tissue inhibitor of metalloprotease-1 from alveolar macrophages in cigarette smokers. Regulation by interleukin-10. Am J Respir Crit Care Med 2000;162:1355–60.
25. Russell RE, Culpitt SV, DeMatos C, et al. Release and activity of matrix metalloproteinase-9 and tissue inhibitor of metalloproteinase-1 by alveolar macrophages from patients with chronic obstructive pulmonary disease. Am J Respir Cell Mol Biol 2002;26:602–9.
26. Russell RE, Thorley A, Culpitt SV, et al. Alveolar macrophage-mediated elastolysis: roles of matrix metalloproteinases, cysteine, and serine proteases. Am J Physiol Lung Cell Mol Physiol 2002;283:L867–73.
27. Newman SL, Henson JE, Henson PM. Phagocytosis of senescent neutrophils by human monocyte-derived macrophages and rabbit inflammatory macrophages. J Exp Med 1982;156:430–42.
28. Hu B, Sonstein J, Christensen PJ, Punturieri A, Curtis JL. Deficient in vitro and in vivo phagocytosis of apoptotic T cells by resident murine alveolar macrophages. J Immunol 2000;165:2124–33.
29. Hodge S, Hodge G, Scicchitano R, Reynolds PN, Holmes M. Alveolar macrophages from subjects with chronic obstructive pulmonary disease are deficient in their ability to phagocytose apoptotic airway epithelial cells. Immunol Cell Biol 2003;81:289–96.

30. Vandivier RW, Henson PM, Douglas IS. Burying the dead: the impact of failed apoptotic cell removal (efferocytosis) on chronic inflammatory lung disease. Chest 2006;129:1673–82.

31. Fadok VA, Bratton DL, Konowal A, Freed PW, Westcott JY, Henson PM. Macrophages that have ingested apoptotic cells in vitro inhibit proinflammatory cytokine production through autocrine/paracrine mechanisms involving TGF-beta, PGE2, and PAF. J Clin Invest 1998;101:890–8.

32. Johann AM, von Knethen A, Lindemann D, Brune B. Recognition of apoptotic cells by macrophages activates the peroxisome proliferator-activated receptor-gamma and attenuates the oxidative burst. Cell Death Differ 2006;13:1533–40.

33. Patel VA, Longacre A, Hsiao K, et al. Apoptotic cells, at all stages of the death process, trigger characteristic signaling events that are divergent from and dominant over those triggered by necrotic cells: Implications for the delayed clearance model of autoimmunity. J Biol Chem 2006;281:4663–70.

34. Mu D, Cambier S, Fjellbirkeland L, et al. The integrin alpha(v)beta8 mediates epithelial home-ostasis through MT1-MMP-dependent activation of TGF-beta1. J Cell Biol 2002;157:493–507.

35. Morris DG, Huang X, Kaminski N, et al. Loss of integrin alpha(v)beta6-mediated TGF-beta activation causes Mmp12-dependent emphysema. Nature 2003;422:169–73.

36. Monick MM, Carter AB, Hunninghake GW. Human alveolar macrophages are markedly deficient in REF-1 and AP-1 DNA binding activity. J Biol Chem 1999;274:18075–80.

37. Harmsen AG, Muggenburg BA, Snipes MB, Bice DE. The role of macrophages in particle translocation from lungs to lymph nodes. Science 1985;230:1277–80.

38. Condos R, Raju B, Canova A, et al. Recombinant gamma interferon stimulates signal transduction and gene expression in alveolar macrophages in vitro and in tuberculosis patients. Infect Immun 2003;71:2058–64.

39. Punturieri A, Alviani RS, Polak T, Copper P, Sonstein J, Curtis JL. Specific engagement of TLR4 or TLR3 does not lead to IFN-beta-mediated innate signal amplification and STAT1 phosphorylation in resident murine alveolar macrophages. J Immunol 2004;173:1033–42.

40. Peleman RA, Rytila PH, Kips JC, Joos GF, Pauwels RA. The cellular composition of induced sputum in chronic obstructive pulmonary disease. Eur Respir J 1999;13:839–43.

41. Rutgers SR, Postma DS, ten Hacken NH, et al. Ongoing airway inflammation in patients with COPD who do not currently smoke. Chest 2000;117(5 Suppl 1): 262S.

42. Traves SL, Culpitt SV, Russell RE, Barnes PJ, Donnelly LE. Increased levels of the chemokines GROalpha and MCP-1 in sputum samples from patients with COPD. Thorax 2002;57:590–5.

43. Gomez-Cambronero J, Horn J, Paul CC, Baumann MA. Granulocyte-macrophage colony-stimulating factor is a chemoattractant cytokine for human neutrophils: involvement of the ribosomal p70 S6 kinase signaling pathway. J Immunol 2003;171:6846–55.

44. Tanino M, Betsuyaku T, Takeyabu K, et al. Increased levels of interleukin-8 in BAL fluid from smokers susceptible to pulmonary emphysema. Thorax 2002;57:405–11.

45. Hiemstra PS, van Wetering S, Stolk J. Neutrophil serine proteinases and defensins in chronic obstructive pulmonary disease: effects on pulmonary epithelium. Eur Respir J 1998;12:1200–8.

46. Stockley RA. Neutrophils and protease/antiprotease imbalance. Am J Respir Crit Care Med 1999;160:S49–52.

47. Stanescu D, Sanna A, Veriter C, et al. Airways obstruction, chronic expectoration, and rapid decline of FEV1 in smokers are associated with increased levels of sputum neutrophils. Thorax 1996;51:267–71.

48. Saetta M, Di Stefano A, Turato G, et al. CD8+ T-lymphocytes in peripheral airways of smokers with chronic obstructive pulmonary disease. Am J Respir Crit Care Med 1998;157:822–6.

49. Turato G, Zuin R, Miniati M, et al. Airway inflammation in severe chronic obstructive pulmonary disease: relationship with lung function and radiologic emphysema. Am J Respir Crit Care Med 2002;166:105–10.

50. Vernooy JH, Moller GM, van Suylen RJ, et al. Increased granzyme A expression in type II pneumocytes of patients with severe chronic obstructive pulmonary disease. Am J Respir Crit Care Med 2007;175:464–72.

51. Fujimoto K, Yasuo M, Urushibata K, Hanaoka M, Koizumi T, Kubo K. Airway inflammation during stable and acutely exacerbated chronic obstructive pulmonary disease. Eur Respir J 2005;25:640–6.

52. Shinagawa K, Trifilieff A, Anderson GP. Involvement of CCR3-reactive chemokines in eosinophil survival. Int Arch Allergy Immunol 2003;130:150–7.

53. Vermaelen K, Pauwels R. Pulmonary dendritic cells. Am J Respir Crit Care Med 2005;172:530–51.

54. Demedts IK, Brusselle GG, Vermaelen KY, Pauwels RA. Identification and characterization of human pulmonary dendritic cells. Am J Respir Cell Mol Biol 2005;32:177–84.

55. Demedts IK, Bracke KR, Maes T, Joos GF, Brusselle GG. Different roles for human lung dendritic cell subsets in pulmonary immune defense mechanisms. Am J Respir Cell Mol Biol 2006;35:387–93.

56. Gerosa F, Gobbi A, Zorzi P, et al. The reciprocal interaction of NK cells with plasma-cytoid or myeloid dendritic cells profoundly affects innate resistance functions. J Immunol 2005;174:727–34.

57. Marcenaro E, Della Chiesa M, Bellora F, et al. IL-12 or IL-4 prime human NK cells to mediate functionally divergent interactions with dendritic cells or tumors. J Immunol 2005;174:3992–8.

58. Zhu J, Qiu Y, Valobra M, et al. Plasma cells and IL-4 in chronic bronchitis and chronic obstructive pulmonary disease. Am J Respir Crit Care Med 2007;175:1125–33.

59. Lapperre TS, Sont JK, van Schadewijk A, et al. Smoking cessation and bronchial epithelial remodelling in COPD: a cross-sectional study. Respir Res 2007;8:85.

60. Waters CM, Sporn PH, Liu M, Fredberg JJ. Cellular biomechanics in the lung. Am J Physiol Lung Cell Mol Physiol 2002;283:L503–9.

61. Horowitz JC, Thannickal VJ. Epithelial-mesenchymal interactions in pulmonary fibrosis. Semin Respir Crit Care Med 2006;27:600–12.

62. Wang H, Liu X, Umino T, et al. Cigarette smoke inhibits human bronchial epithelial cell repair processes. Am J Respir Cell Mol Biol 2001;25:772–9.

63. Nyunoya T, Monick MM, Klingelhutz A, Yarovinsky TO, Cagley JR, Hunninghake GW. Cigarette smoke induces cellular senescence. Am J Respir Cell Mol Biol 2006;35:681–8.

64. Roth M, Johnson PR, Borger P, et al. Dysfunctional interaction of C/EBPalpha and the glucocorticoid receptor in asthmatic bronchial smooth-muscle cells. New Engl J Med 2004;351:560–74.

65. Hersh CP, Demeo DL, Lazarus R, et al. Genetic association analysis of functional impairment in chronic obstructive pulmonary disease. Am J Respir Crit Care Med 2006;173:977–84.

66. Didon L, Qvarfordt I, Andersson O, Nord M, Riise GC. Decreased CCAAT/enhancer binding protein transcription factor activity in chronic bronchitis and COPD. Chest 2005;127:1341–6.

67. Myerburg MM, Latoche JD, McKenna EE, et al. Hepatocyte growth factor and other fibroblast secretions modulate the phenotype of human bronchial epithelial cells. Am J Physiol Lung Cell Mol Physiol 2007;292:L1352–60.

68. Bozinovski S, Jones JE, Vlahos R, Hamilton JA, Anderson GP. Granulocyte/macrophage-colony-stimulating factor (GM-CSF) regulates lung innate immunity to lipopolysaccharide through Akt/Erk activation of NFkappa B and AP-1 in vivo. J Biol Chem 2002;277:42808–14.

69. Bozinovski S, Jones J, Beavitt SJ, Cook AD, Hamilton JA, Anderson GP. Innate immune responses to LPS in mouse lung are suppressed and reversed by neutralization of GM-CSF via repression of TLR-4. Am J Physiol Lung Cell Mol Physiol 2004;286:L877–85.
70. Kim V, Rogers TJ, Criner GJ. New concepts in the pathobiology of chronic obstructive pulmonary disease. Proc Am Thorac Soc 2008;5:478–85.
71. Mio T, Romberger DJ, Thompson AB, Robbins RA, Heires A, Rennard SI. Cigarette smoke induces interleukin-8 release from human bronchial epithelial cells. Am J Respir Crit Care Med 1997;155:1770–6.
72. Keatings VM, Cave SJ, Henry MJ, et al. A polymorphism in the tumor necrosis factor-alpha gene promoter region may predispose to a poor prognosis in COPD. Chest 2000;118:971–5.
73. Sakao S, Tatsumi K, Igari H, Shino Y, Shirasawa H, Kuriyama T. Association of tumor necrosis factor alpha gene promoter polymorphism with the presence of chronic obstructive pulmonary disease. Am J Respir Crit Care Med 2001;163:420–2.
74. Cromwell O, Hamid Q, Corrigan CJ, et al. Expression and generation of interleukin-8, IL-6 and granulocyte-macrophage colony-stimulating factor by bronchial epithelial cells and enhancement by IL-1 beta and tumour necrosis factor-alpha. Immunology 1992;77:330–7.
75. von Asmuth EJ, Dentener MA, Ceska M, Buurman WA. IL-6, IL-8 and TNF production by cytokine and lipopolysaccharide-stimulated human renal cortical epithelial cells in vitro. Eur Cytokine Netw 1994;5:301–10.
76. Standiford TJ, Kunkel SL, Phan SH, Rollins BJ, Strieter RM. Alveolar macrophage-derived cytokines induce monocyte chemoattractant protein-1 expression from human pulmonary type II-like epithelial cells. J Biol Chem 1991;266:9912–8.
77. Di Stefano A, Maestrelli P, Roggeri A, et al. Upregulation of adhesion molecules in the bronchial mucosa of subjects with chronic obstructive bronchitis. Am J Respir Crit Care Med 1994;149:803–10.
78. Mulligan MS, Polley MJ, Bayer RJ, Nunn MF, Paulson JC, Ward PA. Neutrophil-dependent acute lung injury. Requirement for P-selectin (GMP-140). J Clin Invest 1992;90:1600–7.
79. Takeyama K, Dabbagh K, Lee HM, et al. Epidermal growth factor system regulates mucin production in airways. Proc Natl Acad Sci U S A 1999;96:3081–6.
80. Takeyama K, Jung B, Shim JJ, et al. Activation of epidermal growth factor receptors is responsible for mucin synthesis induced by cigarette smoke. Am J Physiol Lung Cell Mol Physiol 2001;280:L165–72.
81. Schmitz H, Fromm M, Bentzel CJ, et al. Tumor necrosis factor-alpha (TNFalpha) regulates the epithelial barrier in the human intestinal cell line HT-29/B6. J Cell Sci 1999;112:137–46.
82. Kampf C, Relova AJ, Sandler S, Roomans GM. Effects of TNF-alpha, IFN-gamma and IL-beta on normal human bronchial epithelial cells. Eur Respir J 1999;14:84–91.
83. Miyazaki Y, Araki K, Vesin C, et al. Expression of a tumor necrosis factor-alpha transgene in murine lung causes lymphocytic and fibrosing alveolitis. A mouse model of progressive pulmonary fibrosis. J Clin Invest 1995;96:250–9.
84. Wu AJ, Chen ZJ, Tsokos M, O'Connell BC, Ambudkar IS, Baum BJ. Interferon-gamma induced cell death in a cultured human salivary gland cell line. J Cell Physiol 1996;167:297–304.
85. Vernooy JH, Kucukaycan M, Jacobs JA, et al. Local and systemic inflammation in patients with chronic obstructive pulmonary disease: soluble tumor necrosis factor receptors are increased in sputum. Am J Respir Crit Care Med 2002;166:1218–24.
86. Takabatake N, Nakamura H, Abe S, et al. The relationship between chronic hypoxemia and activation of the tumor necrosis factor-alpha system in patients with chronic obstructive pulmonary disease. Am J Respir Crit Care Med 2000;161:1179–84.

87. Garrod R, Marshall J, Barley E, Fredericks S, Hagan G. The relationship between inflammatory markers and disability in chronic obstructive pulmonary disease (COPD). Prim Care Respir J 2007;16:236–40.

88. Di Francia M, Barbier D, Mege JL, Orehek J. Tumor necrosis factor-alpha levels and weight loss in chronic obstructive pulmonary disease. Am J Respir Crit Care Med 1994;150:1453–5.

89. de Godoy I, Donahoe M, Calhoun WJ, Mancino J, Rogers RM. Elevated TNF-alpha production by peripheral blood monocytes of weight-losing COPD patients. Am J Respir Crit Care Med 1996;153:633–7.

90. Park JY, Pillinger MH. Interleukin-6 in the pathogenesis of rheumatoid arthritis. Bull NYU Hosp Jt Dis 2007;65(Suppl. 1): S4–10.

91. Man SF, Connett JE, Anthonisen NR, Wise RA, Tashkin DP, Sin DD. C-reactive protein and mortality in mild to moderate chronic obstructive pulmonary disease. Thorax 2006;61:849–53.

92. Wedzicha JA, Seemungal TA, MacCallum PK, et al. Acute exacerbations of chronic obstructive pulmonary disease are accompanied by elevations of plasma fibrinogen and serum IL-6 levels. Thromb Haemost 2000;84:210–5.

93. Garman RD, Jacobs KA, Clark SC, Raulet DH. B-cell-stimulatory factor 2 (beta 2 interferon) functions as a second signal for interleukin 2 production by mature murine T cells. Proc Natl Acad Sci U S A 1987;84:7629–33.

94. Noma T, Mizuta T, Rosen A, Hirano T, Kishimoto T, Honjo T. Enhancement of the interleukin 2 receptor expression on T cells by multiple B-lymphotropic lymphokines. Immunol Lett 1987;15:249–53.

95. Takai Y, Wong GG, Clark SC, Burakoff SJ, Herrmann SH. B cell stimulatory factor-2 is involved in the differentiation of cytotoxic T lymphocytes. J Immunol 1988;140:508–12.

96. Muraguchi A, Hirano T, Tang B, et al. The essential role of B cell stimulatory factor 2 (BSF-2/IL-6) for the terminal differentiation of B cells. J Exp Med 1988;167:332–44.

97. Bhowmik A, Seemungal TA, Sapsford RJ, Wedzicha JA. Relation of sputum inflammatory markers to symptoms and lung function changes in COPD exacerbations. Thorax 2000;55:114–20.

98. Soler N, Ewig S, Torres A, Filella X, Gonzalez J, Zaubet A. Airway inflammation and bronchial microbial patterns in patients with stable chronic obstructive pulmonary disease. Eur Respir J 1999;14:1015–22.

99. Bucchioni E, Kharitonov SA, Allegra L, Barnes PJ. High levels of interleukin-6 in the exhaled breath condensate of patients with COPD. Respir Med 2003;97:1299–302.

100. Romano M, Sironi M, Toniatti C, et al. Role of IL-6 and its soluble receptor in induction of chemokines and leukocyte recruitment. Immunity 1997;6:315–25.

101. Ohsugi Y, Kishimoto T. The recombinant humanized anti-IL-6 receptor antibody tocilizumab, an innovative drug for the treatment of rheumatoid arthritis. Expert Opin Biol Ther 2008;8:669–81.

102. Lacraz S, Nicod LP, Chicheportiche R, Welgus HG, Dayer JM. IL-10 inhibits metalloproteinase and stimulates TIMP-1 production in human mononuclear phagocytes. J Clin Invest 1995;96:2304–10.

103. Panzner P, Lafitte JJ, Tsicopoulos A, Hamid Q, Tulic MK. Marked up-regulation of T lymphocytes and expression of interleukin-9 in bronchial biopsies from patients with chronic bronchitis with obstruction. Chest 2003;124:1909–15.

104. Barcelo B, Pons J, Fuster A, et al. Intracellular cytokine profile of T lymphocytes in patients with chronic obstructive pulmonary disease. Clin Exp Immunol 2006;145:474–9.

105. Ciccolella DE, Rogers TJ, Crinor GJ. Systemic levels of IL-8 are elevated in patients with COPD exacerbation. Proc Am Thorac Soc 2006;3:A626 [abstract].

106. Vlahos R, Bozinovski S, Hamilton JA, Anderson GP. Therapeutic potential of treating chronic obstructive pulmonary disease (COPD) by neutralising granulocyte macrophage-colony stimulating factor (GM-CSF). Pharmacol Ther 2006;112:106–15.

107. Hamilton JA. GM-CSF in inflammation and autoimmunity. Trends Immunol 2002;23:403–8.

108. Hamilton JA, Anderson GP. GM-CSF biology. Growth Factors 2004;22:225–31.

109. Piguet PF, Grau GE, de Kossodo S. Role of granulocyte-macrophage colony-stimulating factor in pulmonary fibrosis induced in mice by bleomycin. Exp Lung Res 1993;19:579–87.

110. Xing Z, Ohkawara Y, Jordana M, Graham F, Gauldie J. Transfer of granulocyte-macrophage colony-stimulating factor gene to rat lung induces eosinophilia, monocytosis, and fibrotic reactions. J Clin Invest 1996;97:1102–10.

111. Stampfli MR, Wiley RE, Neigh GS, et al. GM-CSF transgene expression in the airway allows aerosolized ovalbumin to induce allergic sensitization in mice. J Clin Invest 1998;102: 1704–14.

112. Shibata Y, Berclaz PY, Chroneos ZC, Yoshida M, Whitsett JA, Trapnell BC. GM-CSF regulates alveolar macrophage differentiation and innate immunity in the lung through PU.1. Immunity 2001;15:557–67.

113. Balbi B, Bason C, Balleari E, et al. Increased bronchoalveolar granulocytes and granulocyte/macrophage colony-stimulating factor during exacerbations of chronic bronchitis. Eur Respir J 1997;10:846–50.

114. Tsoumakidou M, Tzanakis N, Chrysofakis G, Siafakas NM. Nitrosative stress, heme oxygenase-1 expression and airway inflammation during severe exacerbations of COPD. Chest 2005;127:1911–8.

115. Vlahos R, Bozinovski S, Irving L, Smallwood DM, Hamilton JA, Anderson GP. GM-CSF is a pathogenic mediator in experimental COPD. Am J Respir Crit Care Med 2005: A143 [abstract].

116. Ito K, Ito M, Elliott WM, et al. Decreased histone deacetylase activity in chronic obstructive pulmonary disease. New Engl J Med 2005;352:1967–76.

117. Vlahos R, Bozinovski S, Jones JE, et al. Differential protease, innate immunity, and NF-kappaB induction profiles during lung inflammation induced by subchronic cigarette smoke exposure in mice. Am J Physiol Lung Cell Mol Physiol 2006;290:L931–45.

118. Berclaz PY, Zsengeller Z, Shibata Y, et al. Endocytic internalization of adenovirus, nonspecific phagocytosis, and cytoskeletal organization are coordinately regulated in alveolar macrophages by GM-CSF and PU.1. J Immunol 2002;169:6332–42.

119. Stanley E, Lieschke GJ, Grail D, et al. Granulocyte/macrophage colony-stimulating factor-deficient mice show no major perturbation of hematopoiesis but develop a characteristic pulmonary pathology. Proc Natl Acad Sci U S A 1994;91:5592–6.

120. Robb L, Drinkwater CC, Metcalf D, et al. Hematopoietic and lung abnormalities in mice with a null mutation of the common beta subunit of the receptors for granulocyte-macrophage colony-stimulating factor and interleukins 3 and 5. Proc Natl Acad Sci U S A 1995;92:9565–9.

121. Kikly K, Liu L, Na S, Sedgwick JD. The IL-23/Th(17) axis: therapeutic targets for autoimmune inflammation. Curr Opin Immunol 2006;18:670–5.

122. Weaver CT, Hatton RD, Mangan PR, Harrington LE. IL-17 family cytokines and the expanding diversity of effector T cell lineages. Annu Rev Immunol 2007;25:821–52.

123. Molet S, Hamid Q, Davoine F, et al. IL-17 is increased in asthmatic airways and induces human bronchial fibroblasts to produce cytokines. J Allergy Clin Immunol 2001;108:430–8.

124. Chen Y, Thai P, Zhao YH, Ho YS, DeSouza MM, Wu R. Stimulation of airway mucin gene expression by interleukin (IL)-17 through IL-6 paracrine/autocrine loop. J Biol Chem 2003;278:17036–43.

125. Jones CE, Chan K. Interleukin-17 stimulates the expression of interleukin-8, growth-related oncogene-alpha, and granulocyte-colony-stimulating factor by human airway epithelial cells. Am J Respir Cell Mol Biol 2002;26:748–53.

126. Vanaudenaerde BM, Wuyts WA, Dupont LJ, Van Raemdonck DE, Demedts MM, Verleden GM. Interleukin-17 stimulates release of interleukin-8 by human airway smooth muscle cells in vitro: a potential role for interleukin-17 and airway smooth muscle cells in bronchiolitis obliterans syndrome. J Heart Lung Transplant 2003;22:1280–3.

127. Park H, Li Z, Yang XO, et al. A distinct lineage of CD4 T cells regulates tissue inflammation by producing interleukin 17. Nat Immunol 2005;6:1133–41.

128. Langrish CL, McKenzie BS, Wilson NJ, de Waal Malefyt R, Kastelein RA, Cua DJ. IL-12 and IL-23: master regulators of innate and adaptive immunity. Immunol Rev 2004;202:96–105.

129. Oppmann B, Lesley R, Blom B, et al. Novel p19 protein engages IL-12p40 to form a cytokine, IL-23, with biological activities similar as well as distinct from IL-12. Immunity 2000; 13:715–25.

130. Aggarwal S, Ghilardi N, Xie MH, de Sauvage FJ, Gurney AL. Interleukin-23 promotes a distinct CD4 T cell activation state characterized by the production of interleukin-17. J Biol Chem 2003;278:1910–4.

131. Steinman L. A brief history of T(H)17, the first major revision in the T(H)1/T(H)2 hypothesis of T cell-mediated tissue damage. Nat Med 2007;13:139–45.

132. Cua DJ, Sherlock J, Chen Y, et al. Interleukin-23 rather than interleukin-12 is the critical cytokine for autoimmune inflammation of the brain. Nature 2003;421:744–8.

133. Lubberts E, Koenders MI, Oppers-Walgreen B, et al. Treatment with a neutralizing anti-murine interleukin-17 antibody after the onset of collagen-induced arthritis reduces joint inflammation, cartilage destruction, and bone erosion. Arthritis Rheum 2004;50:650–9.

134. Murphy CA, Langrish CL, Chen Y, et al. Divergent pro- and antiinflammatory roles for IL-23 and IL-12 in joint autoimmune inflammation. J Exp Med 2003;198:1951–7.

135. Taraseviciene-Stewart L, Scerbavicius R, et al. An animal model of autoimmune emphysema. Am J Respir Crit Care Med 2005;171:734–42.

136. De Boer WI. Cytokines and therapy in COPD: a promising combination? Chest 2002; 121(5 Suppl.): 209S–18S.

137. Strieter RM, Kunkel SL, Elner VM, et al. Interleukin-8. A corneal factor that induces neovascularization. Am J Pathol 1992;141:1279–84.

138. Arenberg DA, Kunkel SL, Polverini PJ, Glass M, Burdick MD, Strieter RM. Inhibition of interleukin-8 reduces tumorigenesis of human non-small cell lung cancer in SCID mice. J Clin Invest 1996;97:2792–802.

139. de Boer WI, van Schadewijk WAAM, Stolk J, et al. Pulmonary expression of IL-8 and its receptor CXCR2 in chronic obstructive pulmonary disease. Am J Respir Crit Care Med 1999; 159(Suppl. 3): A802 [abstract].

140. Thatcher TH, McHugh NA, Egan RW, et al. Role of CXCR2 in cigarette smoke-induced lung inflammation. Am J Physiol Lung Cell Mol Physiol 2005;289:L322–8.

141. Stevenson CS, Coote K, Webster R, et al. Characterization of cigarette smoke-induced inflammatory and mucus hypersecretory changes in rat lung and the role of CXCR2 ligands in mediating this effect. Am J Physiol Lung Cell Mol Physiol 2005;288:L514–22.

142. Mukaida N, Matsumoto T, Yokoi K, Harada A, Matsushima K. Inhibition of neutrophil-mediated acute inflammation injury by an antibody against interleukin-8 (IL-8). Inflamm Res 1998;47(Suppl. 3): S151–7.

143. Folkesson HG, Matthay MA, Hebert CA, Broaddus VC. Acid aspiration-induced lung injury in rabbits is mediated by interleukin-8-dependent mechanisms. J Clin Invest 1995;96:107–16.

144. Boring L, Gosling J, Chensue SW, et al. Impaired monocyte migration and reduced type 1 (Th1) cytokine responses in C-C chemokine receptor 2 knockout mice. J Clin Invest 1997;100:2552–61.

145. Kurihara T, Warr G, Loy J, Bravo R. Defects in macrophage recruitment and host defense in mice lacking the CCR2 chemokine receptor. J Exp Med 1997;186:1757–62.

146. Lu B, Rutledge BJ, Gu L, et al. Abnormalities in monocyte recruitment and cytokine expression in monocyte chemoattractant protein 1-deficient mice. J Exp Med 1998;187:601–8.

147. Mack M, Cihak J, Simonis C, et al. Expression and characterization of the chemokine receptors CCR2 and CCR5 in mice. J Immunol 2001;166:4697–704.

148. Conti P, Boucher W, Letourneau R, et al. Monocyte chemotactic protein-1 provokes mast cell aggregation and [3H]5HT release. Immunology 1995;86:434–40.

149. Taub DD, Proost P, Murphy WJ, et al. Monocyte chemotactic protein-1 (MCP-1), -2, and -3 are chemotactic for human T lymphocytes. J Clin Invest 1995;95:1370–6.

150. Schweickart VL, Epp A, Raport CJ, Gray PW. CCR11 is a functional receptor for the monocyte chemoattractant protein family of chemokines. J Biol Chem 2001;276:856.

151. de Boer WI, Sont JK, van Schadewijk A, Stolk J, van Krieken JH, Hiemstra PS. Monocyte chemoattractant protein 1, interleukin 8, and chronic airways inflammation in COPD. J Pathol 2000;190:619–26.

152. Rolfe MW, Kunkel SL, Standiford TJ, et al. Expression and regulation of human pulmonary fibroblast-derived monocyte chemotactic peptide-1. Am J Physiol 1992;263:L536–45.

153. Warhurst AC, Hopkins SJ, Warhurst G. Interferon gamma induces differential upregulation of alpha and beta chemokine secretion in colonic epithelial cell lines. Gut 1998;42:208–13.

154. Penton-Rol G, Polentarutti N, Luini W, et al. Selective inhibition of expression of the chemokine receptor CCR2 in human monocytes by IFN-gamma. J Immunol 1998;160:3869–73.

155. Gunn MD, Nelken NA, Liao X, Williams LT. Monocyte chemoattractant protein-1 is sufficient for the chemotaxis of monocytes and lymphocytes in transgenic mice but requires an additional stimulus for inflammatory activation. J Immunol 1997;158:376–83.

156. Gonzalo JA, Lloyd CM, Wen D, et al. The coordinated action of CC chemokines in the lung orchestrates allergic inflammation and airway hyperresponsiveness. J Exp Med 1998;188: 157–67.

157. Hautamaki RD, Kobayashi DK, Senior RM, Shapiro SD. Requirement for macrophage elastase for cigarette smoke-induced emphysema in mice. Science 1997;277:2002–4.

158. Weber KS, Nelson PJ, Grone HJ, Weber C. Expression of CCR2 by endothelial cells: implications for MCP-1 mediated wound injury repair and in vivo inflammatory activation of endothelium. Arterioscler Thromb Vasc Biol 1999;19:2085–93.

159. Salcedo R, Ponce ML, Young HA, et al. Human endothelial cells express CCR2 and respond to MCP-1: direct role of MCP-1 in angiogenesis and tumor progression. Blood 2000;96:34–40.

160. Furukawa Y, Matsumori A, Ohashi N, et al. Anti-monocyte chemoattractant protein-1/monocyte chemotactic and activating factor antibody inhibits neointimal hyperplasia in injured rat carotid arteries. Circ Res 1999;84:306–14.

161. Gharaee-Kermani M, Denholm EM, Phan SH. Costimulation of fibroblast collagen and transforming growth factor beta1 gene expression by monocyte chemoattractant protein-1 via specific receptors. J Biol Chem 1996;271:17779–84.

162. Jiang Y, Beller DI, Frendl G, Graves DT. Monocyte chemoattractant protein-1 regulates adhesion molecule expression and cytokine production in human monocytes. J Immunol 1992;148:2423–8.

163. Gong JH, Clark-Lewis I. Antagonists of monocyte chemoattractant protein 1 identified by modification of functionally critical NH2-terminal residues. J Exp Med 1995;181:631–40.

164. Mirzadegan T, Diehl F, Ebi B, et al. Identification of the binding site for a novel class of CCR2b chemokine receptor antagonists: binding to a common chemokine receptor motif within the helical bundle. J Biol Chem 2000;275:25562–71.

165. Rodriguez-Frade JM, Vila-Coro AJ, de Ana AM, Albar JP, Martinez AC, Mellado M. The chemokine monocyte chemoattractant protein-1 induces functional responses through dimerization of its receptor CCR2. Proc Natl Acad Sci U S A 1999;96:3628–33.

166. van der Vaart H, Koeter GH, Postma DS, Kauffman HF, ten Hacken NH. First study of infliximab treatment in patients with chronic obstructive pulmonary disease. Am J Respir Crit Care Med 2005;172:465–9.

167. Dentener MA, Creutzberg EC, Pennings HJ, Rijkers GT, Mercken E, Wouters EF. Effect of infliximab on local and systemic inflammation in chronic obstructive pulmonary disease: a pilot study. Respiration 2008;76:275–82.

168. Rennard SI, Fogarty C, Kelsen S, et al. The safety and efficacy of infliximab in moderate to severe chronic obstructive pulmonary disease. Am J Respir Crit Care Med 2007;175:926–34.

169. Bongartz T, Sutton AJ, Sweeting MJ, Buchan I, Matteson EL, Montori V. Anti-TNF antibody therapy in rheumatoid arthritis and the risk of serious infections and malignancies: systematic review and meta-analysis of rare harmful effects in randomized controlled trials. JAMA 2006;295:2275–85.

170. Mahler DA, Huang S, Tabrizi M, Bell GM. Efficacy and safety of a monoclonal antibody recognizing interleukin-8 in COPD: a pilot study. Chest 2004;126:926–34.

171. Newbold P, Bayley D, Sapey E, et al. Evidence to support a role for IL-1beta in the COPD disease process. Proc Am Thorac Soc 2005: A395.

172. Lappalainen U, Whitsett JA, Wert SE, Tichelaar JW, Bry K. Interleukin-1beta causes pulmonary inflammation, emphysema, and airway remodeling in the adult murine lung. Am J Respir Cell Mol Biol 2005;32:311–8.

173. Castro P, Legora-Machado A, Cardilo-Reis L, et al. Inhibition of interleukin-1beta reduces mouse lung inflammation induced by exposure to cigarette smoke. Eur J Pharmacol 2004;498: 279–86.

174. Churg A, Zhou S, Wang X, Wang R, Wright JL. The role of interleukin-1{beta} in murine cigarette smoke-induced emphysema and small airway remodeling. Am J Respir Cell Mol Biol 2009;40(4):482–490. Epub 2008 Oct 17.

14

'Triple therapy' in the management of COPD: inhaled steroid, long-acting anticholinergic and long-acting β₂-agonist

Ronald Dahl

Department of Respiratory Diseases, Aarhus University Hospital, Denmark

14.1 Introduction

Chronic obstructive pulmonary disease (COPD) is a multi-component lung and airways disease with inflammation playing a key role in early as well as late phases of the disorder.[1] Although inflammation and structural changes are the essential components of COPD, it is characterized in the clinical setting by crude respiratory physiology measurements of airflow obstruction, often performed as a forced expiratory manoeuvre and after inhaled bronchodilator.[2] The obstruction in COPD is progressive, especially in smokers. In ex- and non-smokers the progression may be related to the normal age-related decline in lung function. The airways obstruction in COPD has different degrees of reversibility, but by definition the forced expiratory function values cannot be normal. Pharmacological and non-pharmacological treatments for COPD aim to control symptoms, maximize pulmonary function and reduce exacerbation rates. Ultimately we want to improve survival, and we strive for therapies that regenerate the destroyed lung and bronchial tissue.

14.2 Long-acting inhaled anticholinergic (LAMA) and β₂-agonist (LABA) bronchodilators

The inhaled anticholinergic drug tiotropium (TIO) provides effective bronchodilation over 24 h, reduces symptoms and reduces exacerbation rates.[3–5] The long-acting

Advances in Combination Therapy for Asthma and COPD, First Edition. Edited by Jan Lötvall.
© 2012 John Wiley & Sons, Ltd. Published 2012 by John Wiley & Sons, Ltd.

beta-agonists (LABA) currently available provide alternative inhaled bronchodilator therapy that provides bronchodilation for 12 h, reduce symptoms and are often prescribed in a combination inhaler with corticosteroid.[6–9] This combination has demonstrated a broad range of anti-inflammatory effects that are greater than those seen with inhaled corticosteroid (ICS) monotherapy. This is likely caused by additive effects from the two drugs with different mechanisms of action; a possible explanation for this could be a molecular interaction (synergy) between the LABA and ICS. The anti-inflammatory and bronchodilator effects of the salmeterol/fluticasone combination (SFC) provide greater symptom control, pulmonary function improvement and exacerbation reduction compared with treatment with either component individually. Current COPD guidelines recommend that long-acting bronchodilators should be used in patients who are symptomatic in spite of therapy with short-acting bronchodilators.[10–14]

14.3 Treatment strategies for COPD

Many patients with severe or very severe COPD are not adequately treated with one therapeutic principle alone, even using the highest recommended dose. For this reason, national and international treatment guidelines recommend a stepwise addition of therapeutic options.[15, 16] A fixed-dosed combination of salmeterol and fluticasone propionate and of formoterol and budesonide is approved for the symptomatic treatment of patients with severe COPD and a history of repeated exacerbations who have significant symptoms despite regular bronchodilator therapy.

The risk of side effects increases with increasing doses of any drug, therefore an important rationale for combination therapy, or multi-pharmacy, is probably a more favourable therapeutic ratio (i.e. between efficacy and safety/side effects). Knowing that anticholinergic and beta-adrenergic agents achieve their bronchodilating effects by different mechanisms, the combination of these agents in particular has proven to be beneficial in the management of COPD.[17–19]

14.4 Inhaled corticosteroids and COPD

Inhaled corticosteroid therapy is recommended for patients with a forced expiratory volume in 1 second (FEV_1) of 60% of the predicted value and who are having two or more exacerbations requiring treatment with antibiotics or oral corticosteroids in a period of 12 months. However, the dose–response relationships and long-term safety of ICS in COPD are unknown, and careful consideration of whether ICS may or may not be beneficial to the individual patient is needed. It has not been evaluated whether the different COPD phenotypes, i.e. demonstrating different degrees of emphysema, numbers of eosinophils in biopsies/sputum, etc., may have differences in responsiveness to ICS.

Only four studies have investigated the effect of withdrawal of ICS in COPD.[20–23] The studies showed that patients previously treated with ICS were more likely to exacerbate upon withdrawal. The large majority of exacerbations occurred in the first 7 weeks after withdrawal. One study reported the effect of ICS withdrawal on exacerbations in COPD patients who received regular treatment with a LABA (salmeterol). There was a doubling of the incidence rate of mild exacerbations, but no influence on the occurrence of moderate-to-severe exacerbations in the year after withdrawal. All studies gave no evidence that withdrawal of ICS treatment was of significant risk to COPD patients.

14.5   Combination treatment with ICS, LAMA and LABA: 'triple therapy'

'Triple therapy' with long-acting anticholinergics, LABA and ICS is widely used in clinical practice. Each component of the 'triple therapy' has a different molecular mechanism of action, so there is a good rationale for the use of these drugs in combination to maximize clinical benefits in COPD.

Treatment with such 'triple therapy' is inevitably used in clinical practice for patients with COPD to optimize lung function, improve symptoms and reduce exacerbations. However, the evidence base for the clinical consequences and outcomes of this approach is limited.

A pilot study by Yildiz et al. 38 patients with moderate COPD showed that there was no effect on lung function when budesonide 800 μg was given on top of treatment with formoterol and ipratropium bromide for 12 weeks. But an effect on quality of life as measured by the St George's Respiratory Questionnaire was determined.[24]

Villar and Pombo[25] reported a crossover study in patients who were on continuous treatment with inhaled fluticasone dipropionate (FP) 500 μg twice daily, comparing 1 week of therapy with ongoing FP plus addition of salmeterol 50 μg twice daily and ongoing FP plus TIO 18 μg once daily versus a 'triple therapy' arm with ongoing FP plus TIO plus salmeterol. The combination inhaler SFC was not used and components were given from individual inhalers. The 'triple therapy' was found to have the greatest effect on FEV_1.

The 1-year study named the Optimal Therapy of Chronic Obstructive Pulmonary Disease To Prevent Exacerbations and Improve Quality of Life (OPTIMAL) study[26] showed that SFC 50/500 μg twice daily plus TIO 18 μg once daily was superior to TIO alone in terms of pulmonary function and symptoms, and results for TIO plus salmeterol 50 μg twice daily were similar to TIO alone. The primary endpoint of this study was exacerbations, but the number of subjects was too small to provide adequate statistical power for the observed treatment difference. The proportion of participants with moderate or severe COPD who had an exacerbation did not differ among those receiving monotherapy with TIO (62.8%), those receiving combination TIO plus salmeterol (64.8%), or those receiving all three therapies (60.0%). Mean number of exacerbations per patient year were 1.61 in the TIO group, 1.75 in the TIO and salmeterol group, and 1.37 in the TIO and SFC group. Many patients went off the trial groups treated with monotherapy and onto open-label SFC.

Cazzola et al. studied 90 patients for 3 months in a parallel group design and evaluated three treatment arms: SFC + TIO, SFC and TIO. The primary endpoint was FEV_1, which was significantly higher after 'triple therapy' compared to the single components.[27]

In a retrospective analysis the relative efficacy of tiotropium and salmeterol as a function of the concomitant use of ICS in patients with moderate COPD was evaluated by means of the combined results of two 6-month studies of TIO 18 μg once daily compared with salmeterol 50 μg twice daily.[28] The result showed that TIO and salmeterol are effective bronchodilators. However, dyspnoea, health status and frequency of exacerbations were superior with TIO compared to salmeterol, regardless of concomitant ICS use. The direct effect of ICS on COPD outcomes was not studied in this post hoc analysis, and concurrent use of ICS seemed neither to augment nor to impede the relative efficacy of the two bronchodilators.

The effects of 'triple therapy' on measurements of airflow obstruction and hyperinflation have been addressed in a recently published 2-week crossover study by Singh et al.[29] The combination of one inhaler containing salmeterol and fluticasone propionate (SFC) and another with tiotropium bromide (TIO) is frequently prescribed in clinical practice. The effects of SFC 50/500 μg twice daily in addition to TIO 18 μg once daily were compared with the individual treatments alone in 41 patients with COPD in a randomized, double-blind, double-dummy, three-way crossover study with 2-week washout periods between treatments. The primary outcome parameter was post-dose specific airway conductance (sG_{aw}) area under the curve (AUC 0–4 h) on day 14. Other efficacy measures were spirometry data including FEV_1, forced vital capacity (FVC), inspiratory capacity (IC), residual volume (RV) and total lung capacity (TLC); the Transition Dyspnoea Index (TDI) total score; mean morning peak expiratory flow (PEF); and the mean number of occasions of rescue salbutamol use in a 24 h period. The results showed that AUC 0–4 h sG_{aw} was significantly higher on day 14 after SFC+TIO compared with TIO or SFC alone (22% and 27% respectively) (both $P < 0.001$). SFC+TIO significantly improved trough FEV_1 by 212 mL compared to TIO alone ($P < 0.001$) and 110 mL compared to SFC alone ($P = 0.017$) on day 14 (Figure 14.1). Also, on day 14 IC measurement was significantly higher on triple therapy compared to treatment periods with individual components. It is important to notice that IC is a more frequently used measure of pulmonary hyperinflation that is related to the degree of breathlessness that patients suffer.[3] Subjects on 'triple therapy' had clinically relevant improvements in TDI total score of 2.2 compared with TIO alone ($P < 0.001$) but not compared with SFC, and treatment with 'triple therapy' resulted in significantly less rescue medication, amounting to 1.0 and 0.6 fewer dosages daily compared to TIO ($P < 0.001$) and SFC ($P = 0.01$), respectively. This short study concentrating on respiratory function and symptoms showed that SFC+TIO triple therapy led to greater improvements in lung function indices compared with TIO and SFC alone. The 'triple therapy' gave improved outcome in all physiologically important parameters tested, including airway conductance and lung volumes. 'Triple therapy' also led to less symptomatic use of rescue medication.

The benefits from 'triple therapy' were only evident after 14 days of treatment whereas measurements on the first day of treatment showed no differences in pulmonary function test responses. The advantages of 'triple therapy' seem to occur after repeated

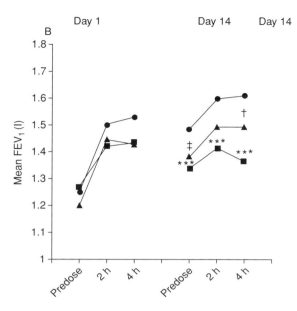

Figure 14.1 Effects in chronic obstructive pulmonary disease (COPD) of triple combination of salmeterol/fluticasone and tiotropium bromide on lung function at 2 and 4 hours after inhalation before and after 2 weeks of regular treatment.

dosing, and appear to be a time effect of cumulative dosages. More extended trials are needed to find out if these beneficial effects increase, remain constant or disappear with long-term treatment.

All these referenced studies provide strong evidence that 'triple therapy' is the best way of optimizing pulmonary function in patients with COPD of an appropriate severity.

14.6 Extracted data from TORCH and UPLIFT studies

Some information may be derived from the two recent large studies of TORCH[6] and UPLIFT[7] in relation to the value of 'triple therapy' in COPD. These studies showed a reduction in COPD exacerbations with the combination of salmeterol/fluticasone and regular tiotropium (Figure 14.2), as well as tendencies to reduced mortality (Figure 14.3).

The Towards a Revolution in COPD Health (TORCH) study was a 3-year placebo-controlled, randomized, double-blind parallel-group study to find out if a significant reduction in all-cause mortality in 6184 COPD patients could be the result of treatment with the fixed combination of fluticasone 500 μg or salmeterol 50 μg twice daily (SFC) or either component alone.[6] In addition a post hoc analysis was performed on the rate of decline in FEV_1.[8] The reduction in death from all causes among patients with COPD in the combination therapy arm did not reach the predetermined level of statistical significance. The risk of death in the salmeterol group and the fluticasone group did

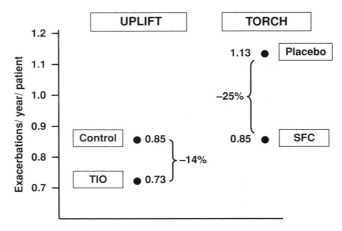

Figure 14.2 Reduction in chronic obstructive pulmonary disease (COPD) exacerbation frequency with regular treatment with tiotropium (TIO) and the combination of salmeterol and fluticasone (SFC) in two very large multicentre studies, the UPLIFT and TORCH studies, performed over several years.

not differ significantly from that in the placebo group. Of concern was the significantly increased possibility of having pneumonia in both the combination treatment and the fluticasone treatment arms.

The Understanding Potential Long-term Impacts on Function and Tiotropium (UPLIFT) trial was a 4-year randomized, double-blind, placebo-controlled, parallel-group study with inclusion of 5993 patients with moderate-to-severe COPD. Patients were randomized to receive either tiotropium or placebo in addition to their usual

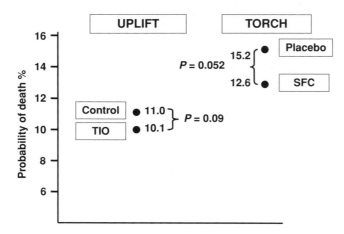

Figure 14.3 The probability of death during regular treatment with tiotropium (TIO) or the combination of salmeterol and fluticasone (SFC) after 3 years' observation in two very large multicentre studies, the UPLIFT and TORCH studies.

bronchodilator therapy. The primary outcome of the UPLIFT trial was rate of decline in FEV_1 over 4 years.

In the TORCH study, maintenance treatment with short-acting bronchodilators and short courses of oral steroids for the treatment of exacerbations was allowed. However, maintenance use of TIO was not allowed, which was also the case for LABA and ICS other than the study drugs. Patients included in any of the possible TORCH treatment arms did not have the opportunity to receive 'triple therapy' including TIO, and the placebo-treated patients were only allowed maintenance with short-acting bronchodilators. This allows an evaluation of the effect of treatment without TIO in a large cohort.

In the UPLIFT study the use of ICS, LABA and their combination was allowed and the only anticholinergic allowed was TIO. Any medication could be used for treatment of exacerbations. In this way, irrespective of whether patients were randomized to the placebo or the TIO group, the UPLIFT trial mimicked everyday COPD care except for inhaled anticholinergics.

In principle the UPLIFT trial was a placebo-controlled trial but the placebo group should rather be called a control group as 60% of patients at inclusion were being treated with ICS or LABA. During the study additional patients seem to have received therapy with ICS and LABA. This gives a unique opportunity to evaluate these two trials in the light that COPD patients in the TORCH study had LABA and/or ICS whereas most cases in the UPLIFT study in addition to ICS and/or LABA had TIO, which means that the TIO group in the UPLIFT trial broadly can be regarded as a 'triple therapy' group.

Exacerbations in the TORCH and UPLIFT studies

Exacerbations were defined differently in TORCH and UPLIFT, and the way the exacerbations are analysed may also differ. In UPLIFT, an exacerbation was defined as 'an increase or new onset of more than one of the following respiratory symptoms (cough, sputum, sputum purulence, wheezing, and dyspnoea) with a duration of three or more days requiring treatment with an antibiotic and/or systemic (oral, intramuscular or intravenous) steroid.' In TORCH, exacerbations were defined as symptomatic deterioration requiring treatment with systemic corticosteroids and/or antibiotics (moderate exacerbation) or hospitalization (severe exacerbation).

In TORCH the annual exacerbation rate was 1.13 in the placebo group, which reduced to 0.85 in the SFC group at the 3-year analysis. The exacerbation rate in the control group of UPLIFT – i.e. the group in which most cases were treated with ICS and LABA – was 0.85 in the 4-year analysis. The exacerbation rate was reduced to 0.73 in the TIO group – i.e. in the group that may be considered as receiving 'triple therapy' (Figure 14.2).

Probability of death in the TORCH and UPLIFT studies

A similar analysis may be performed regarding the probability of death in the TORCH and UPLIFT studies (Figure 14.3). In the TORCH placebo group the probability

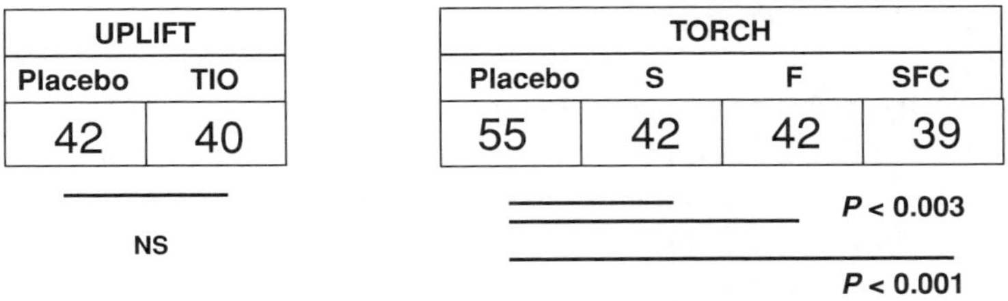

UPLIFT	
Placebo	TIO
42	40

NS

TORCH			
Placebo	S	F	SFC
55	42	42	39

$P < 0.003$

$P < 0.001$

Figure 14.4   The annual decline in postbronchodilator forced expiratory volume in 1 second (FEV_1; mL/yr) in chronic obstructive pulmonary disease (COPD) patients was significantly reduced by the combination of salmeterol/fluticasone (SFC) in the TORCH study, but not by tiotropium (TIO) in the UPLIFT study. NS, not significant.

of death after 3 years was 15.2% while in the SFC-treated group this was reduced to 12.6%.

The data for three years of treatment in UPLIFT show in the control group the mortality was 11.4% and in the TIO (here regarded as the 'triple therapy') group this is further reduced to 10.1%. This comparison of the two separate trials of TORCH and UPLIFT has no firm scientific foundation, but illustrates the possibly positive interaction of the three different pharmacological interventions.

Rate of decline in FEV$_1$ in TORCH and UPLIFT

The prospective 4-year data in UPLIFT[32] showed no difference between the TIO and the control group in the rate of decline in FEV_1. The difference in postbronchodilator FEV_1 was only 2 mL/yr, i.e. -40 ± 1 versus -42 ± 1 mL/yr, respectively ($P = 0.21$) (Figure 14.4), and for prebronchodilator FEV_1 the difference was zero, i.e. -30 ± 1 mL/yr in each group ($P = 0.950$).

The retrospective analysis of TORCH[33] found that all three active treatment groups reduced the rate of decline in postbronchodilator FEV_1 as the only spirometric parameter reported. The adjusted rate of decline was -42 ± 3 mL/yr for salmeterol (S) and fluticasone (F) alone, -39 ± 3 mL/yr for the SFC combination, and -55 ± 3 mL/yr for the placebo group (Figure 14.4). There was no significant difference between the SFC group and individual drug treatment groups. However, a significant reduction in decline was found between the single components and placebo ($P < 0.003$) and between the SFC combination and placebo ($P < 0.001$).

14.7   Conclusions

The few studies available provide an important addition to our knowledge, and prove that 'triple therapy' with SFC plus TIO is more effective than SFC or TIO alone in terms of pulmonary function. Adequately powered, long-term studies of the benefits of 'triple therapy' on exacerbation rates and other clinical endpoints are now needed to fully justify this approach in clinical practice.

The added benefit that ICS may give to patients with severe or very severe COPD who are regularly treated with LABA and TIO as two potent long-acting bronchodilators remains to be elucidated. Further, it is unknown whether the presumed benefit of ICS in terms of reduced exacerbations can be assigned to a responsive subgroup.

References

1. Hogg JC, Chu F, Utokaparch S, et al. The nature of small-airway obstruction in chronic obstructive pulmonary disease. New Engl J Med 2004;350:2645–53.
2. Global strategy for the diagnosis, management, and prevention of chronic obstructive pulmonary disease. Global Initiative for Chronic Obstructive Lung Disease, 2006.
3. Casaburi R, Mahler DA, Jones PW, et al. A long-term evaluation of once-daily inhaled tiotropium in chronic obstructive pulmonary disease. Eur Respir J 2002;19:217–24.
4. O'Donnell DE, Flüge T, Gerken F, et al. Effects of tiotropium on lung hyperinflation, dyspnoea and exercise tolerance in COPD. Eur Respir J 2004;23:832–40.
5. Maltais F, Hamilton A, Marciniuk D, et al. Improvements in symptom-limited exercise performance over 8 h with once daily tiotropium in patients with COPD. Chest 2005;128:1168–78.
6. Mahler DA, Donohue JF, Barbee RA, et al. Efficacy of salmeterol xinafoate in the treatment of COPD. Chest 1999;115:957–65.
7. Jones PW, Bosh TK. Quality of life changes in COPD patients treated with salmeterol. Am J Respir Crit Care Med 1997;155:1283–9.
8. Dahl R, Greefhorst LAPM, Nowak D, et al. Inhaled formoterol dry powder versus ipratropium bromide in chronic obstructive pulmonary disease. Am J Respir Crit Care Med 2001;164:778–84.
9. Van Noord JA, deMunck DRAJ, Bantje TA, et al. Long-term treatment of chronic obstructive pulmonary disease with salmeterol and the additive effect of ipratropium. Chest 2000;15:878–85.
10. Soriano JB, Vestbo J, Pride NB, et al. Survival in COPD patients after regular use of fluticasone propionate and salmeterol in general practice. Eur Respir J 2002;20:819–25.
11. Man SF, McAlister FA, Anthonisen NR, Sin DD. Contemporary management of chronic obstructive pulmonary disease: clinical applications. JAMA 2003;290:2313–6.
12. Mahler DA, Wire P, Horstman D, et al. Effectiveness of fluticasone propionate and salmeterol combination delivered via the Diskus device in the treatment of chronic obstructive pulmonary disease. Am J Respir Crit Care Med 2002;166:1084–91.
13. Calverley PMA, Pauwels R, Vestbo J, et al. Combined salmeterol and fluticasone in the treatment of chronic obstructive pulmonary disease: a randomised controlled trial. Lancet 2003;361:449–56.
14. Hanania NA, Darken P, Horstman D, et al. The efficacy and safety of fluticasone propionate (250µg)/salmeterol (50µg) combined in the Diskus inhaler for the treatment of COPD. Chest 2003;124:834–43.
15. Rabe KF, Hurd S, Anzueto A, et al. Global strategy for the diagnosis, management and prevention of chronic obstructive pulmonary disease: GOLD executive summary. Am J Respir Crit Care Med 2007;176:532–55.
16. Celli BR, MacNee W, Agusti A, et al. Standards for the diagnosis and treatment of patients with COPD: a summary of the ATS/ERS position paper. Eur Respir J 2004;23:932–46.
17. Van Noord JA, deMunck DRAJ, Bantje TA, et al. Long-term treatment of chronic obstructive pulmonary disease with salmeterol and the additive effect of ipratropium. Chest 2000;15:878–85.

18. Van Noord JA, Aumann J, Janssens E, et al. Comparison of tiotropium once daily, formoterol twice daily and both combined once daily in patients with COPD. Eur Respir J 2005;26:214–22.

19. Di Marco F, Verga M, Santus P, et al. Effect of formoterol, tiotropium, and their combination in patients with acute exacerbation of chronic obstructive pulmonary disease: A pilot study. Respir Med 2006;100:1925–32.

20. Jarad NA, Wedzicha JA, Burge PS, Calverley PM. An observational study of inhaled corticosteroid withdrawal in stable chronic obstructive pulmonary disease. ISOLDE study group. Respir Med 1999;93:161–6.

21. O'Brien A, Russo-Magno P, Karki A, et al. Effects of withdrawal of inhaled steroids in men with severe irreversible airflow obstruction. Am J Respir Crit Care Med 2001;164:365–71.

22. Wouters EF, Postma DS, Fokkens B, et al. Withdrawal of fluticasone propionate from combined salmeterol/fluticasone treatment in patients with COPD causes immediate and sustained disease deterioration: a randomised controlled trial. Thorax 2005;60:480–7.

23. van der Valk P, Monninkhof E, van der Palen J, et al. Effect of discontinuation of inhaled corticosteroids in patients with chronic obstructive pulmonary disease: the COPE study. Am J Respir Crit Care Med 2002;166:1358–63.

24. Yildiz, F, Basyigit I, Yildirim E, Boyaci H, Ilgazli A. Does addition of inhaled steroid to combined bronchodilator therapy affect health status in patients with COPD? Respirology 2004;9:352–5.

25. Villar AB, Pombo CV. Bronchodilator efficacy of combined salmeterol and tiotropium in patients with chronic obstructive pulmonary disease. Arch Broncopneumol 2005;41:130–4.

26. Aaron SD, Vandemheen KL, Fergusson D, et al. Tiotropium in combination with placebo, salmeterol, or fluticasone–salmeterol for treatment of chronic obstructive pulmonary disease: a randomized trial. Ann Intern Med 2007;146:545–55.

27. Cazzola M, Ando F, Santus P, et al. A pilot study to assess the effects of combining fluticasone propionate/salmeterol and tiotropium on the airflow obstruction of patients with severe-to-very severe COPD. Pulm Pharmacol Ther 2007;20:556–61.

28. Hodder R, Kesten S, Menjoge S, et al. Outcomes in COPD patients receiving tiotropium or salmeterol plus treatment with inhaled corticosteroids. Int J Chron Obstruct Pulm Dis 2007;2:157–67.

29. Singh D, Brooks J, Hagan G, Cahn A, O'Connor BJ. Superiority of "triple" therapy with salmeterol/fluticasone propionate and tiotropium bromide versus individual components in moderate to severe COPD. Thorax 2008;63:592–8.

30. O'Donnell DE, Webb, KA. Exertional breathlessness in patients with chronic airflow limitation: the role of lung hyperinflation. Am Rev Respir Dis 1993;148:1351–7.

31. Calverley PM, Anderson JA, Celli B, et al. Salmeterol and fluticasone propionate and survival in chronic obstructive pulmonary disease. New Engl J Med 2007;356:775–89.

32. Tashkin DP, Celli B, Senn S, et al. A 4-year trial of tiotropium in chronic obstructive pulmonary disease. New Engl J Med 2008;359:1543–54.

33. Celli BR, Thomas NE, Anderson JA, et al. Effect of pharmacotherapy on rate of decline of lung function in chronic obstructive pulmonary disease: results from the TORCH study. Am J Respir Crit Care Med 2008;178:332–8.

Index
